MR. I. J. SWANN, F.R.C.S.D.F.M.
Consultant in Administrative Charge
Department of Accident and Emergency Medicine
Glasgow Royal Infirmary
84, Castle Street
Glasgow, G4 0SF

MINOR TRAUMATIC BRAIN INJURY HANDBOOK

Diagnosis and Treatment

MINOR TRAUMATIC BRAIN INJURY HANDBOOK

Diagnosis and Treatment

GARY W. JAY, M.D., D.A.A.P.M

NATIONAL MEDICAL DIRECTOR

PHYMED PARTNERS, INC.

CRC Press

Boca Raton   London   New York   Washington, D.C.

Library of Congress Cataloging-in-Publication Data

Jay, Gary W.
    Minor traumatic brain injury handbook : diagnosis and treatment / Gary W. Jay.
        p.   cm.
    Includes bibliographical references and index.
    ISBN 0-8493-1955-2 (alk. paper)
    1. Brain damage. I. Title.
    RC387.5 .J39 2000
    617.4′81044—dc21

                                                                        00-037818
                                                                        CIP

This book contains information obtained from authentic and highly regarded sources. Reprinted material is quoted with permission, and sources are indicated. A wide variety of references are listed. Reasonable efforts have been made to publish reliable data and information, but the author and the publisher cannot assume responsibility for the validity of all materials or for the consequences of their use.

© 2000 by CRC Press LLC

No claim to original U.S. Government works
International Standard Book Number 0-8493-1955-2
Library of Congress Card Number 00-037818
Printed in the United States of America 1 2 3 4 5 6 7 8 9 0
Printed on acid-free paper

Dedication

This book is dedicated to many people, especially the patients who have survived and even prospered after an MTBI, as well as to the physicians, other clinicians, and the attorneys who fought for them.

As always, this book could not have been written without the loving support of my wife Suzanne and my daughter Samantha, who has begun to write her own books.

Finally, this book is also dedicated to Alvin Arakaki, who learned early and taught the right thing to do. He is missed.

Authors

Gary W. Jay, MD, FAAPM, DAAPM
National Medical Director
PhyMed Partners
Longwood, FL

Denise E. Baugh, MS, PT
Denver, CO

Richard H. Cox, PhD, MD, ABRP, ABPP
President and Clinical Professor
Forest Institute of Professional Psychology
Springfield, MO

Richard S. Goka, MD
Fresno, CA

Edward J. Jacobson, PhD, DABFE, DABFM
Northglenn, CO

Pamela A. Law, CBIS/CI-CE, CCC-SLP
Pamela Law and Associates
Westminster, CO

Karen E. Lee, PsyD
Clinical Professor, Director of Neuropsychological Services
Forest Institute of Professional Psychology
Springfield, MO

Thomas Politzer, OD
Denver, CO

Stacy Rogers, OT
Vail, CO

Michael J. Sawaya
Sawaya and Rose
Denver, CO

Contents

Foreword

Did you know that there is no such thing as mild (acquired) traumatic brain injury (MATBI)? For two of the largest automobile liability insurance companies, this is their reality.

Don't you love it?

And if you don't believe them, there are a host of clinicians, many of the neuropsychological persuasion as well as neurologists and other physicians who are, apparently, charter members of the "If I Don't Want to Believe It, It Ain't True School of Medicine."

So, is MATBI (in this book, synonymous with MTBI) a form of mass hallucination? Is it a form of mass hysteria?

Neither explanation can answer the question: Why do patients from all over the country who experience similar types of trauma have such similar if not identical complaints? Do they all read the same Cliff Notes®? Are they all determined to "rip off the insurance companies?"

Of course not! The facts of the matter are simple: MATBI does exist. It is real. It can devastate a patient and his or her family. It is not a wastebasket diagnosis that is used by unprofessional clinicians when they don't know what is going on. It is not a different way of saying, "depressed."

Over the last eight years, since the advent of more mangled — uh — managed care, I have had to hire a full time person just to get approvals for treatment from the automobile medical liability companies. I have watched my patients undergo Independent Medical Examinations (IMEs), one after the other, demanded by the insurance companies for the sole purpose of stating that there is absolutely nothing wrong with a patient. This, while the patients lose their jobs, their families, even undergo bankruptcy, all because the insurance company or their trusty henchman, the third-party administrators, refuse to accept or acknowledge the diagnosis.

I have undergone deposition after deposition at the request of the insurance company, typically, where their pet attorney does his or her best to try to disprove what I have stated and written about a patient's medical problems and diagnosis.

My patients have never lost a case, with the exception of a 72-year-old gentleman, who for other reasons did his own case in, on his own.

For the most part, the purpose of this book is to present the facts in a coherent manner which is relatively easy for physicians to read and understand and to help them sharpen their diagnostic skills regarding MTBI; to give the attorneys who care about their clients another source of medical information they can use to help them; and to be useful to all of the above when some microcephalic minion of an insurance company states that there is no such thing as a mild traumatic brain injury.

That being said, I want to explain this textbook. It has two parts. Part One is a medical overview of most of the important aspects of MTBI. I wrote it in the same style I used in the *Headache Handbook*, as I have received many wonderfully complimentary comments about that book. The second half of this text is written by a number of different professionals, and details the clinical aspects of diagnosis and treatment by specific specialty. I was even lucky enough to find an attorney, who I respect greatly, to write a chapter on the legal aspects of MTBI.

I have included patient case studies in Part One, along with the now infamous "Ah-Has" from the headache book, which are now the *Bottom Line*, important points that really need to be considered.

In my clinical experience, patients with MTBI are remarkably underserved, underdiagnosed, and generally, misunderstood. Because of the seriousness of the consequences of those two "uns" and one "mis," I hope that the reader will take the time to learn the facts and use them to help the patients who experience the trauma of a minor acquired traumatic brain injury.

Because of the breadth of the topic, I have included information about, but not dwelt on, the moderate to severe traumatic brain injury patients. This book is for the clinicians and others who deal or need to deal with the patients with minor or minor to moderate traumatic brain injury.

I have tried to maintain the "just like I lecture" style, but I have greatly supplemented that with very pertinent information from hundreds of authors.

Other clinicians have been good enough to read though this manuscript in draft form. Both were unsure about including my comments on the insurance problems faced by the MTBI patient. After several discussions, they agreed that this information, like the clinical information, is fact, and should therefore be fair game for a textbook.

Facts are facts, whether you like them or not.

To all of you clinicians and readers who help to care for these patients, as well as for all of you patients who may access this book, "God Bless You." This one's for you!

I hope you will find this text useful.

Part One

1 What is Mild Traumatic Brain Injury?

The problem of mild acquired traumatic brain injury is an old one. It was described in the 1860s by Erichson and Trimble[1,2] and called the "postconcussion syndrome," as well as the "posttraumatic syndrome." Dr. Page, in the mid 1880s, began a good bit of controversy by expressing doubts that the closed "spinal concussions" seen in the railway accidents described by Erichson were real.[3] He went so far as to indicate that patients suffering from closed brain or spinal nondefinable injury were malingerers.

The workers' compensation laws were introduced in the late 1880s and made much more worker friendly in 1906. This had a significant effect on the growing debate, as more complaints of similar work-related injuries were made.

The medical investigations into the pathophysiology of closed head trauma and closed head acceleration/deceleration injuries began in the 1940s.[4] Over the following two decades several medical papers notably concluded that minor closed head injury and/or simple concussion could cause significant neuronal loss and profound clinical changes.[5,6] While the pathophysiological mechanisms were not known, MTBI was seen as a real clinical entity.

A major problem was noted. It appeared that minimal or minor closed head trauma frequently induced emotional or "neurotic" changes in patients. The early difficulties delineating cerebral function and/or dysfunction which had resulting characterological changes were problematic.[7-11] As the neurological examination was frequently found to be essentially normal, such posttraumatic sequelae were felt to be fallacious and the patient a slacker.

These problems were exacerbated by the members of the medical-legal field, with attorneys in workers' compensation and personal injury law trying to prove or disprove real clinical dysfunction, while physician experts had very little in the way of objective clinical or radiological evidence to make their point.

Starting in the 1960s, more research began to support Erichson's original contentions that minor head trauma could induce severe disturbances of cerebral function.[12-14] Evidence of true dysfunction was identified by more sophisticated neurological and vestibular testing.[14] Clinicians only infrequently used neuropsychological testing early on, but it added more data showing cognitive dysfunction after minor head or soft tissue trauma, including the medical problem legally known as "whiplash", or cervical extension/flexion or acceleration/deceleration injury.

The so-called posttraumatic syndrome, which was called the postconcussion syndrome if there was an attendant loss of consciousness, was found to produce, in some patients, a host of varied symptoms with or without accompanying objective clinical neurological findings. These symptoms were found to vary, in many cases secondary to, it was initially felt, the age and emotional or psychological predispositions of those injured.

Mild (acquired) traumatic brain injury (MATBI or MTBI — used interchangeably in this book) is the clinical entity in which the brain has sustained a pathological injury. The pathology can be secondary to a direct contusion, or neurochemical, axonal, or circulatory injury.

The nosology of the term "minor TBI" must be called into question. It is noted that MATBI may induce neuronal dysfunction which may produce persistent symptoms, indicating that such "mild" injuries to the brain may produce effects which are not "minor" at all, and which may last for indeterminate periods of time.[15]

At this time there is, thankfully, a consensus definition of mild traumatic brain injury which has been published by the members of the Mild Traumatic Brain Injury committee of the Brain Injury Interdisciplinary Special Interest Group (BISIG) of the American Congress of Rehabilitation Medicine.[16] This definition states:

A patient with mild traumatic brain injury is a person who has had a traumatically induced physiological disruption of brain function, as manifested by at least one of the following:

1.   Any period of loss of consciousness
2.   Any loss of memory of events immediately before or after the accident
3.   Any alteration in mental state at the time of the accident (e.g., feeling dazed, disoriented, or confused)
4.   Focal neurological deficit(s) that may or may not be transient

The severity of injury does not exceed:

1.   Loss of consciousness of approximately 30 minutes or less
2.   After 30 minutes, an initial Glasgow coma scale (gcs) of 13 to 15 is found
3.   Posttraumatic amnesia is not greater than 24 hours.

It is extremely important to note that the definition includes patients with direct head trauma *as well as* those who suffer an acceleration/deceleration injury ("whiplash") without specific direct head trauma. Loss of consciousness *is not a clinical requisite for a classification of MATBI*, in spite of the pronouncements of multiple pseudoexperts, including those who do know better, those who should know better, and those who get paid to skirt the truth. (I am trying to be nice here!) These are the good folk who should know the difference between "lies, damn lies, and statistics."

The members of the BISIG note that the symptoms of MATBI may last for varying lengths of time and can consist of persistent physical, emotional, cognitive, and behavioral symptoms that may produce a *functional* disability.

Zasler stated, "Clinicians should remember that gross absence of proof is not necessarily proof of absence. In unsophisticated hands there may be no evidence whatsoever that someone has had a significant injury, whereas in different hands and to other eyes, the patient may indeed have objective examination findings clinically as well as neurodiagnostically."[17]

To that, I add, "It depends on who is looking, and *why*: if they are patient-oriented, or working for an insurance company or defense attorney, their findings may be very different from those of someone who cares for the truth and medical accuracy as it pertains to a specific patient."

MATBI is a contentious issue in very litigious times. The diagnosis, and especially the treatment, of MTBI can be rather expensive, and in the managed care environment, no one wants to be responsible for fulfilling an insurance contract. It may injure the insurance companies' bottom line. It would also cause a loss of income for attorneys who work for insurance companies, who get paid to "prove" that no one ever suffers an MATBI.

Now, if a person is injured and his brain is literally oozing out of his ear, it is extremely difficult to declare that such a patient does not have a brain injury. Fortunately or unfortunately, the patient who suffers an MATBI may look normal. That makes it easier to sell the lie to a jury.

The purpose of the rest of this book is to make the pathophysiology, diagnosis, and treatment issues of an MATBI perfectly clear. To anyone and everyone.

Personally, I am tired of seeing patients who have suffered an MATBI be made worse by the deadly combination of iatrogenic and nomogenic factors. This will be dealt with later in this text.

For now, we'll move on to the epidemiology of the problem. If there is no such thing, how come it is found in multiple societies by multiple people who can't even read about, never mind practice, the symptoms of the disorder that isn't there?

2 Epidemiology and Causation

One of the major problems clinicians face when attempting to obtain any idea of the true epidemiological aspects of MATBI is that the literature is rife with studies which utilized different criteria for the diagnosis of this entity.

INCIDENCE

Studies performed during the 1980s and early 1990s that attempted to quantify the incidence of MATBI were methodologically different and may not necessarily be considered equivalent. Inclusion criteria were different in most of these studies. A large number relied on subjective patient information, with both urban and rural patients being given the same written or verbal questionnaires.[18-27] The incidence of MATBI ranged from 152 to 367 per 100,000 people. Again, significant differences were found in the methodologies of these studies.

Krause,[28] in 1993, felt that the general incidence was 200/100,000 population. More recently, Krause again stated that there were approximately 2,000,000 brain injuries occurring each year, an incidence of 175–200 per 100,000 population, with an associated 56,000 deaths per year.[29] For now, these figures appear to be the most commonly cited.

In these figures, from the way Kraus evaluated the numbers, there may be a significant number of individuals who experience an MATBI and who do not go to an emergency room or immediately to their primary care provider, an MD, or a chiropractor. The actual number of these patients has not been established.

Another problem is the clinical acumen of primary care physicians, as well as specialists, who may not make the diagnosis when a patient presents to them. Some counties that have regional centers appear to do better at diagnosis, as will be discussed below.

Stewart and his associates[30] tried to determine the frequency of cognitive deficits in emergency room patients with MATBI, and to identify the factors in the initial history and physical examination that would be predictive of cognitive deficits. Seventy patients were admitted into their study, all having a history of blunt trauma or deceleration injury to the head, and a Glasgow coma scale (See Chapter 9) of 14–15. Only 36 completed the follow-up, and 42% of those patients completing the study had either mild or moderate cognitive deficits one week post injury. The authors concluded that history and initial physical examination were poor predictors of these deficits. They also reported that the patients who completed the study were more commonly employed and less likely to have used alcohol or "sensorium-altering" drugs. Of interest was that the finding of abnormal cerebellar function noted in the initial evaluation was associated with cognitive deficits at one week. Only 4 of 15 patients with initial cognitive deficits had abnormal cerebellar examinations at follow-up.

Another study found the importance of immediate expert care for traumatic brain injury. Gabella et al.[31] compared urban to rural traumatic brain injuries in Colorado for 1991 and 1992. Annual, average traumatic brain injury varied from 97.8 per 100,000 population for residents of the most urban group, to 172.1 per 100,000 population for the residents of rural, remote counties. Mortality rates ranged from 18.1 per 100,000 in the urban setting to 33.8 per 100,000 people in the remote rural populations.

Another report from the same year, 1997, indicated that the data from Colorado, Missouri, Oklahoma, and Utah, when evaluated from 1990–1993, included a decreased annual rate of TBI, and that the rates of TBI were highest in association with motor vehicle accidents and falls.[32] In 1992 a report in the *Oklahoma State Medical Association Journal* stated that 4000 people were disabled or killed after head injury each year in Oklahoma.[33]

The Virginia Brain Injury Registry analyzed statistics for 1988–1993. They found age-adjusted incidence rates of TBI were greatest for children under 6 years of age at 237/100,000, and least for persons aged 40–69 years of age, at 56/100,000. They noted that TBI occurred more frequently in males (1.4:1), and mortality rates were also higher in males as compared to females (1.6:1).[34]

Surveillance of TBI cases requiring hospitalization or that were fatalities in Utah during 1990-1992 found an annual incidence rate of 108.8 per 100,000 population. This rate was significantly lower than previous identified rates of TBI.[35] The Alaskan Trauma Registry looked at hospital trauma admissions in 1991–1992 and found an incidence rate of 129.5 per 100,000 population.[36]

Note that the differences between the incidence rates appear to depend on a number of factors, including hospitalization and mortality. Very little comment is made regarding mild traumatic or mild to moderate traumatic brain injury, as the ability to diagnose this problem is dependent on follow up not typically performed by a hospital emergency room.

The epidemiology of TBI has been looked at in various countries, but specific incidence data has not always been given.[37-42]

A national survey conducted by Statistics Canada in 1986–1987 found the overall household prevalence rate of TBI was 62.3/100,000 adults, with a male predominance. They found that the TBI rates were highest in the 45–64 age group, which was three times greater than the 15–24 age group.[43] They also determined that 84% of adults with TBI have co-occurring disabilities, particularly limited mobility and agility. Again, no specific information regarding MTBI was garnered.

Two Australian studies looked at the incidence of TBI in north versus south Australia. The incidence of hospital-treated TBI in the North Coast region found an annual incidence of approximately 100/100,000 population. They noted that most of the injuries were mild (62.2%).[44] South Australia had a much higher incidence of TBI, 322/100,000 population, which exceeded studies with comparable methodologies in areas of the United States and Europe. Young males had the highest incidence of TBI, typically secondary to a motor vehicle accident. Hospitals in the area surveyed accepted more than 4000 new cases of TBI each year. At discharge, over 1000 of these cases had some degree of residual impairment and required postinjury services.[45]

A New Zealand study attempted to identify the incidence of MTBI.[46] This study defined MTBI by the acute management needed, including care out of the hospital or hospital admission of not more than 48 hours, including the presence of posttraumatic amnesia. The incidence seen at the four Auckland hospitals was 437/100,000 population for ages 15 and over, and 252/100,000 population for ages under 15. The major causes were motor vehicle accidents and falls. Persistent symptoms occurred in 5% of patients 15 years or older.

The epidemiology of TBI in Johannesburg, South Africa, was evaluated.[47] The overall incidence was 316/100,000. The incidence in whites was 109/100,000 overall, with a male-female ratio of 40.1. The data for blacks showed an incidence of 355/100,000 population, with a male-female ratio of 4.4:1. There was an incidence in black males aged 25–44 of 763/100,000 population. Whites had a 419/100,000 incidence in the same age group. The overall incidence of fatal TBI was 80/100,000. The nature of the injuries showed interpersonal violence accounting for 51% of nonfatal TBI among blacks, and only 10% among whites. Motor vehicle accidents caused 27% of black nonfatal TBI and 63% for whites. In spite of the large incidence, no data on the diagnosis of MTBI was given.

In northern Sweden a retrospective study found the incidence of TBI to be 24.9/10,000 population for the age range of 16–60. It was found that many of the patients with an early diagnosis of brain concussion, who were hospitalized for one day, experienced losses in preinjury functions and abilities.[48]

Northern Norway's incidence of TBI was found to be 229/100,000 population during 1993, with a male preponderance of 1.7:1. In this retrospective population-based survey, the most common causes were found to be falls in 62%, motor vehicle accidents in 21%, and assaults in 7%.[49]

A study from Taiwan found 58,563 TBI cases over a six-year period (July 1, 1988 – June 30, 1994). The major etiology of trauma was traffic accidents (69.4%), followed by falls and assaults. Motorcyclists accounted for the majority of TBI cases among traffic accidents. Using the Glasgow coma scale, 79.5% of cases were considered mild, 8.9% moderate, and 11.6% severe. Outcomes were determined by the Glasgow Outcome Scale (GOS), and good recovery was found in 87.2% of cases.[50] Note that the percentage of "good outcomes" was higher than the number of "mild" TBI patients. Using the GOS, a "good outcome" may be associated with moderate disability.

BOTTOM LINE

The epidemiological studies rarely looked at MTBI. Those that did specifically, and those that did not (the vast majority), had different diagnostic criteria and methodologies. The outcome determinations were different.

It appears that the lack of specific studies belies the true incidence of MTBI. Part of this is most probably specific diagnostic criteria. A good bit of it is the lack of emergency room follow-up. That is, ER folks don't know, usually, what happened to a patient after discharge from the ER. This is not a criticism. Follow-up is not their job.

On the other hand, many patients may not immediately go for follow-up with their primary care physicians. If they do, and I've seen this far too often, their symptoms are discounted and the diagnosis of MATBI is usually not made, or the patient is bluntly told that they should be all better in three to six months, that any problems that persist are either illusionary or secondary-gain related.

Then there is the issue of patients who experience head trauma, with alterations in mental state at the time of the accident, possibly with a short period of loss of consciousness or minimal memory loss, who do not seek medical attention. This may be secondary to lack of insurance, or lack of close medical facilities for rural patients. It may also be secondary to the immediate feeling that, "I'm all right." These patients then experience the full brunt of medical and legal antagonism if indeed they are not "all right" and see a physician weeks or months later after being unable to deal with any persistent symptoms.

So, it appears that the real incidence of MATBI may not as yet be known.

Two recent studies give one pause. A look at the incidence of TBI in a New Zealand prison population found that 86.4% of 118 respondents had sustained a TBI, with 56.7% reporting more than one. All reported problems with general memory and socialization.[51]

An attempt to evaluate the prevalence of TBI in a psychiatric population was done.[52] It was found that a greater percentage of psychiatric patients reported TBI than control groups of medical patients and students. The TBI was typically considered mild, according to the Traumatic Brain Injury Questionnaire used to assess TBI. The authors note that the role of TBI in the emergence, expression, and treatment outcome of psychiatric patients needs to be further examined.

Yes, it does.

CAUSE OF INJURY

As noted in the brief review above, motor vehicle accidents (MVAs) are the most common cause of TBI, followed by falls, violence, and recreation.[18,21,23,25,53] MVAs appear to account for approximately 50% of the TBIs.

It has always been fascinating for me to observe the sophistic machinations of the (typically) insurance defense industries which utilize nonmedical criteria to state that a patient could not have been injured in a low velocity (or a high velocity) motor vehicle accident. They claim that it just isn't possible. While I don't feel that this textbook is the place to evaluate the physics and biomechanics that these people cite, it is very much worth mentioning.

The things which are important in the evaluation of an MVA include: the physical attributes of the driver and passengers (size, age, strength, immediate knowledge that the accident will occur, use of alcohol or drugs, physiologic impairment, and experience), vehicle design, and environmental factors. At the time of the actual accident or crash, important factors include physical attributes of the occupants of the vehicle, use of restraint systems, and safety modifications to the vehicle.

At the time of the accident, did the patients have the time to brace themselves, or were they taken totally by surprise and unprepared? Was the patient's head turned at the time of the vehicle crash? What were the physical characteristics of the patient?

Clinically, I see fewer physical problems in patients who were prepared and had braced themselves immediately prior to the crash. Fewer of these patients appear to develop significant cognitive deficits, particularly if their heads are braced sufficiently to prevent an acceleration/deceleration injury (whiplash), but, the physics must be considered.

When a two-ton vehicle strikes another massive piece of metal, the force of the impact is imparted "down-line," to the part of the vehicle (or its occupant(s)) which is least connected to the frame. That is typically the occupant(s). The least massive part of the occupant is the neck, which is connected to the body at one end and to the head at the other. The head is heavier than the neck, so the physical force of the crash is most commonly directed to the most moveable part — the head. A forward then backward (acceleration/deceleration) movement occurs, many times more than once, and is frequently associated with the back of the head striking the headrest or, in a small truck, the rear window. If the head is well-braced, the forces from the crash may still effect the lesser-braced entity — the brain, which floats in fluid and cannot be tethered down. The brain itself can undergo the brunt of the physical forces by being forced forward and backward onto the bony cage (skull) that encases it. If the head itself is not braced and undergoes the resultant acceleration/deceleration, these movements may amplify the injurious effects on the soft, essentially gelatinous brain tissue.

If the occupant's head is rotated at the time of the crash, these rotational forces, which accompany the forward/backward acceleration/deceleration forces on the brain, make the patient far more likely to sustain a cerebral injury.

There are many variables, starting with the ability of the patient to brace prior to the impact forces. The size of the automobile's occupant is important. A low velocity impact would possibly have much less physical damage associated with it if the driver was the phenomenal Denver Broncos quarterback John Elway, as compared to someone who is not in good physical condition strengthwise, does not have an 18-inch neck, is less than 5 foot 6 inches tall, is female, and so on.

I've never heard these types of facts dealt with by the so-called defense experts whose stories depend on who is paying their bills. This is disgraceful, nonmedical, and sophistic, but the courts of law tolerate it, much to the detriment of truly injured patients.

Gennarelli et al.[54] noted that pedestrians who are struck by motor vehicles are most likely to sustain head injuries. In motor vehicle versus bicycle accidents, between 1984-1988, there were an estimated 2,985 TBI deaths and 905,752 bicycle-associated head injuries.[55,56] Motorcycle riders (or donor-cycle riders, if you prefer) have a 5- to 6-time higher risk of TBI than people in other fatal MVAs.[57] Between 1979–1986 there were 15,194 motorcycle deaths associated with head injury in the United States.[57] In 43% of motorcycle fatalities, the drivers did not use helmets.[58]

And still, people fight for their right to forego wearing helmets when they ride motorcycles or bicycles. We pay for their freedom to donate their lives and their organs.

The second leading cause of TBI is falls, which account for 20%–30% of injuries. The majority of falls involve in children under 5 years of age and people over 75 years of age.[18,21,23,28,59]

Recreational injuries, particularly sports-related injuries, are routinely underestimated.[60] TBI may occur in 5% of football injuries.[61] Football also has the greatest percentage of concussive injuries of all contact sports.[62]

Boxing is the only sport whose sole purpose is to render an opponent unconscious. The "punch-drunk" syndrome was first identified in 1928. Subsequent studies have identified pathognomonic, neuroanatomical changes associated with this syndrome, including fenestrated *cavum septi pellucidi* and neurofibrillary tangles without senile plaques.[63,64] Neurocognitive changes are also seen.

Another major factor in the pathogenesis of TBI is alcohol and drug abuse. Alcohol use is a predisposing factor in 35%–72% of all TBIs, particularly in relationship to MVAs, assaults, falls, firearm accidents, and other causes.[65-66] While illegal drugs were found in significant numbers of tested patients in an urban trauma center, the role of prescription drugs is less well defined.[67]

BOTTOM LINE

The majority of causes of TBI are controllable or, at the very least, amenable to change. New technology in motor vehicles is attempting to decrease the overall morbidity and mortality of MVAs. Injuries secondary to bicycle and motorcycle accidents can be lessened by the use of appropriate protective equipment, such as motorcycle helmets. The use of alcohol and drugs is a very difficult societal problem, but laws are striving to make the use of alcohol or drugs while driving more serious offenses.

It is obvious that we can work to decrease the incidence of TBI, but it will be slow going, to say the least.

Next, we go into a gray area to some. The postconcussion syndrome has been thought to be another term for TBI. But, is it?

3 The Post-Concussion Syndrome

The post-concussion syndrome (PCS) appears to include multiple signs and symptoms consisting of neuropathological, neurophysiological, and neuropsychological, as well as physical and psychological or emotional aspects, secondary to a mild traumatic brain injury.[68]

The most common medical problems found in the patient with PCS (and MTBI) include:

- Posttraumatic headache
- Posttraumatic musculoskeletal pain syndromes
- Vestibular disturbance
- Visual disturbance
- Fatigue
- Posttraumatic seizure disorder

The most common cognitive, emotional, and behavioral deficits include:

- Memory impairment
- Depression
- Irritability
- Anxiety
- Loss of self-esteem
- Job loss/disruption
- Denial
- Difficulties with social interactions and family relationships

* Lack of initiative
* Work finding problems
* Decreased ability to concentrate
* Poor impulse control
* Slowed behavioral processing
* Behavioral/personality changes
* Perseveration

The PCS can be both chronic and disabling, or short-lived and benign. A possible explanation for this may be the interaction between organic and psychological factors.[69] It is very difficult to differentiate between the effects of primary neurological, neurophysiological, and neuropathological injury and secondary psychosocial factors. It is felt by some that the typical PCS symptoms, including headache, dizziness, and irritability, result from emotional stress associated with diminished cognitive performance secondary to MATBI.[70]

The influence of accident mechanisms associated with more severe symptoms was studied and it was found that patients with more severe deficits had, at the time of a motor vehicle accident: been an unprepared occupant; been in a rear-end collision, with or without subsequent frontal impact; and had a rotated or inclined head position at the moment of impact.[71]

The "postconcussional disorder" (PCD) has been recently accepted and is found in an appendix of the DSM-IV. A major criterion is loss of consciousness. It is felt that it would be better to utilize the BISIG definition (see chapter 2).[72]

Many researchers have looked for a primary psychological/emotional etiology for the PCS.[73]

Gasquoine[74] felt that symptom persistence was associated with increased emotional distress. He notes that this fact is also true in patients with severe head injury as well as back injury, and relates more to the patient's interpretation of the effect of the trauma than to objective "indicators of brain injury severity."

Landy[75] looked at the more objective symptoms of headache and cervical pain and found that 70% of patients "get better" within a few weeks post MVA, while about 30% continued to complain of headaches and/or cervical pain. He felt that prolonged management and slow court settlement lead to extensive introspection by the patient and, thus, prolongation of symptoms. His results also repeat the long held knowledge that patients with more severe head or neck injuries had a lesser incidence of chronic post-traumatic headaches or cervical symptoms.

Barrett et al.[76] compared two groups of PCS patients, one of which was hospitalized for observation following a brief loss of consciousness, while the others went to the emergency department, and then home. It was found during follow up at two and twelve weeks that the type and frequency of complaints were similar in both groups. However, at twelve weeks, the number of complaints/symptoms were significantly less in the group of hospitalized patients.

Several groups noted that the PCS was more frequently found after blunt head trauma and other trauma than would have been predicted.[77,78]

Using a questionnaire, Bohnen et al.[79] evaluated the longevity of long-term PCS complaints. Their results indicated that in a percentage of patients, MTBI might not ever resolve.

In an attempt to evaluate the importance of psychological factors in the outcome of whiplash injuries, Mayou and Bryant[80] utilized interviews at 3 and 12 months postinjury. The majority of the patients in their study continued to complain of persistent cervical symptoms, while a "sizeable minority" reported specific posttraumatic psychological symptoms such as intrusive memories as well as phobic travel anxiety, which was felt to be "similar to those described by patients suffering multiple injuries". They concluded that travel, social and psychological morbidity was more prevalent than previously recognized. They did not deal with the issue of the recognized posttraumatic stress disorder (PTSD).

Cicerone and Kalmar[81] urged clinicians to use a great deal of caution before attributing PCS symptoms or neuropsychological deficits to a preexisting affective disorder. Leininger et al.[82] looked into the idea that MTBI patients do not develop persistent neuropsychological deficits. They found that patients with the PCS/MTBI had measurable neuropsychological deficits, and the severity of those deficits was independent of gross neurological status immediately post injury.

Looking at symptomatic patients two years post whiplash injury, Di Stefano and Radanov[83] evaluated complaints of memory and attentional difficulties with neuropsychological testing. They found that memory problems were minimal, while problems in selective aspects of attentional functioning after whiplash were present. These could explain the patients' cognitive complaints, and could induce adaptational problems in daily life.

An interesting study was performed by Parker and Rosenblum,[84] who looked at intelligence and personality difficulties after whiplash or MTBI in adults, an average of 20 months post MVA. They found a mean loss of 14 points of Full Scale IQ from the estimated preinjury baseline (using WAIS-R) with no evidence of recovery. They also found a number of personality dysfunctions including organic or cerebral personality disorder. Thirty of 33 patients had psychiatric diagnoses including post-traumatic stress disorder, psychodynamic reactions to impairment, and persistent altered consciousness. They concluded that cognitive loss was induced by the interaction of brain injury with distractions including pain and emotional distress. The report also repeated the fact that the presence of MTBI after MVAs was probably consistently underestimated.

While the PCS has been thought of as a reflection of the psychological response to injury, there is considerable evidence suggesting that the PCS is primarily a physiological disturbance.[77] Reaction time testing, for example, has been used to support a structural, organic etiology for the PCS.[85]

It has been found likely that cervical injury contributes to the symptomatology post PCS/MTBI, and vice-versa.[86] Testing has shown that cervical injuries secondary to whiplash can induce a distortion of the posture control system as a result of disorganized cervical proprioceptive activity.[87] Others note that restricted cervical movements and changes in the quality of proprioceptive information from the cervical spine region affect voluntary eye movements. Acceleration/deceleration (flexion/extension) injury to the neck secondary to whiplash may result in a dysfunction of the proprioceptive system. Oculomotor dysfunction after cervical trauma may therefore be related to disturbances in cervical afferent input.[88] Patients who have sustained head or cervical trauma appear to exhibit an increased reliance on accurate visual input, and are unable to utilize vestibular orienting information to resolve conflicting information from the visual and somatosensory systems.[89]

Soustiel et al.[90] evaluated 40 patients post mild head trauma using brainstem trigeminal and brainstem auditory-evoked potentials (BTEP, BAEP) and middle-latency auditory-evoked potentials (MLAEP) within 48 hours of injury and again at 3 months. They defined PCS as the presence of at least four of the following: failure to resume previous professional activity, memory deficits, headache, dizziness and vertigo, behavioral and emotional disturbances, and other neurological symptoms. Initially, all three evoked potentials were abnormal, showing prolonged latencies indicative of disseminated axonal damage. Only the MLEAPs correlated to outcome at three months, particularly in its psychocognitive aspects, suggesting that organic diencephalic-paraventricular primary damage may account for the presence of the PCS.

PET, SPECT, and MRI studies have been done to attempt to correlate cerebral dysfunction to PCS symptoms. (See Chapter 4 for further information on this technology.) PET looks at glucose metabolism (in these studies), while single photon emission computed tomography (SPECT) looks at cerebral perfusion.

Six patients with PCS and 12 normal controls were tested. The patient group had significant hypometabolism and hypoperfusion in the bilateral parieto-occipital regions, as compared to the controls. In some patients there was also hypometabolism found in other regions. It was hypothesized that parieto-occipital hypometabolism can be caused by activation of nociceptive afferent nerves from the upper cervical spine.[91]

Another study examined 13 patients with a late whiplash syndrome, using PET and SPECT. The authors did not find hypometabolism in the parietotemporo-occipital regions. They did find hypometabolism in the frontopolar and lateral temporal cortex, and in the putamen. They did not recommend that PET or SPECT be used as diagnostic tools for routine examination of patients with a late whiplash syndrome.[92]

SPECT was compared to MRI/CAT scans in 43 patients. The SPECT was found to be abnormal in 53% of patients, MRI was abnormal in 9%, and CAT scan was abnormal in 4.6% of patients post MTBI/PCS. The SPECT scan appeared to be more sensitive to post MTBI changes, especially in patients with persistent PCS (see below), than MRI or CAT scan. No statistical relationships were found between the SPECT scan results and age, previous psychiatric history, history of substance abuse, history of multiple MTBI, or concurrent neuropsychological symptoms.[93]

BOTTOM LINE

"The truth is out there," but we don't seem to have determined the best method of identifying it. The tests noted above were given to patients with PCS, by author statement. The relationship between PCS and MTBI is discussed below, as well as in the next chapter.

Nosologically, it is difficult to determine exactly what constitutes PCS. Evans[94] states that PCS refers to the large number of signs and symptoms found alone or in combination following MATBI, including headache, memory problems, dizziness, fatigue, irritability, anxiety, insomnia, and sensitivity to light and sound. He further indicates that studies have substantiated the existence of PCS, that it is common, with resolution in three to six months, but with persistent symptoms and cognitive deficits persisting for months or years.

Headache, dizziness, and memory deficits are the most common combination of PCS symptoms.[95] There is no specific symptom complex found in the majority of patients with acute or chronic PCS.[96] The multiplicity of signs and symptoms of PCS have been well documented.[69,95,97-105]

One group has suggested that PCS should include all of the consequences of head injury, regardless of its severity and the nature of the injury.[106]

Berrol[107] states that the term mild traumatic brain injury (MTBI) is preferable, as it identifies the etiology of the injury, its degree, and the pathological substrate much better than other past terms: minor head injury, traumatic head syndrome, postconcussive syndrome, posttraumatic syndrome, postbrain-injury syndrome, and traumatic cephalgia.

The term postconcussive syndrome (PCS) continues to be frequently used in the literature. The important nosological question is whether PCS is secondary to the MTBI, or are the cognitive/neurological deficits found after MTBI separate entities.

The term PCS would then encompass the nonneurological, neurocognitive, and neurophysiological deficits, leaving the term PCS to be used specifically for the other organ (noncerebral) systems that display posttraumatic signs and symptoms.

BOTTOM LINE

Teleologically, it appears to make more sense to separate the etiologies of the problems encountered post MATBI. A patient with physical findings such as posttraumatic headache may indeed, post trauma, have a postconcussive syndrome. Patients with neurocognitive deficits and other neurological difficulties have direct evidence of a (mild) traumatic brain injury. The author feels it more appropriate to differentiate the two disorders. This would mean that a patient may indeed have both an MTBI and a PCS. Both entities must be treated, and, as will be discussed later, the PCS should be treated first.

Soon after injury, patients have complaints referable to several different organ systems. Alexander[108] identifies this as the PCS. He notes that the MTBI, which can lead to brain injury, can also cause injury to the head, neck (whiplash and soft tissue damage), the vestibular system, and psychological functioning. The initial complaints of deficits in cognition and sleep disorder are, he feels, secondary to neuronal injury, while the headache may be secondary to cervical injury, neuronal injury, or a combination; cervical pain secondary to soft tissue problems; dizziness secondary to peripheral vestibular dysfunction or cervical injury; and the anxiety, moodiness, and irritability secondary to neurological injury, pain, and/or psychological factors.

BOTTOM LINE

The term PCS should not include central nervous system deficits. Vestibular dysfunction secondary to brainstem injury should be included in the MTBI while peripheral dysfunction should be a part of the PCS.

To the extent plasticity allows, neuronal recovery is certainly taking place at one month after injury.[109-113] Neurological recovery is thought to be "substantial," by some, at three months.[114] At this point, post injury, 30% to 50% of patients have continued complaints.[115] Over the next 6 to 12 months (longer than a year post injury) most patients will show continued improvement and "recovery."[116]

It has been found that even "well recovered" patients are still susceptible to periodic impairments secondary to physiological or psychological stress,[117,118] which indicates that recovery is most likely the wrong term. That these patients have "compensated" for their injury may be more correct. To say that patients may have a permanent sense of decreased mental or cognitive efficiency[119] would also be a function of incorrect terminology, i.e., recovered versus compensated.

PERSISTENCE OF SYMPTOMS

At one year, 85%–90% of patients are felt to be "recovered" but are still symptomatic,[106,120] leaving 10%–15% of patients who are not only "not recovered," but are also "not compensated" and still very symptomatic. The literature is replete with studies showing persistence of symptoms after the magic, if not mythic, 3-month period. This literature indicates that the symptoms and deficits following MTBI and PCS may last for six to twelve months or even longer.[82,94,107,119,121-125]

Problem

Much of the literature equates MTBI and PCS, essentially using the terminology interchangeably. Therefore, breaking the literature reviews and thoughts into PCS and MTBI chapters by the author does not delineate both syndromes as "Bottom Lined" above. The majority of the literature includes cognitive and other neurological deficits in PCS.

A survey of rehabilitation specialists who followed patients with MTBI for 6 to 18 months found that 21% of the patients experienced symptoms of PCS 2 to 6 months after their initial injury, and that 20% of these patients had the "post-MTBI syndrome."[126] In another survey of 51 patients, where 23 responded, 25% of the respondents reported continued sequelae from their injuries. The patients with sequelae after one year were found to have reported more symptoms one week after injury.[127]

Cicerone[128] indicated that there was considerable evidence to show that PCS symptoms persisted in a significant proportion of patients after MTBI, and such symptoms were particularly prevalent in patients who indicated that they needed clinical attention.

Symptoms with organic etiologies, it has been noted, can mimic functional disorders.[129] Alves[130] indicated that as recovery occurred, persistent symptoms could be secondary to an interaction between organic and psychosocial factors. These persistent symptoms are more than would be expected from the initial organic damage alone. Alves further stated that a significant percentage of patients would exhibit persistent problems with symptoms 12 months post injury. He felt that recovery from MTBI should also be considered in the social context in which it occurred. By recognizing the complexity of the recovery process, we should extend the concept of morbidity to include the specific socioeconomic and emotional sequelae that the patient experienced.

Mateer[131] found that patients post MTBI were more acutely aware of their cognitive deficits and difficulties with functional abilities. These patients would go to a physician and would have a negative neurological examination. They would be told that there is no organic reason for their problems, that they should wait longer for recovery, learn to live with their problems, or seek psychiatric help.

These iatrogenically-induced problems (cause and effect) most likely lengthen the patients' symptomatic period as they begin to feel an ever increasing loss of control, fear of the unknown, and concern that they must be "going crazy."

BOTTOM LINE

It doesn't matter what the medical problem is, particularly when, like most patients with MTBI, they look "normal." Physicians with little or no background in the diagnosis of MTBI or PCS, or bought and paid for consultants, do a great disservice to MTBI patients. Constant repetition by physicians of the mantra, "There is nothing wrong with you. You look fine. There's no problem here," will demonstrably disrupt a patient's sense of self, their life, and their feelings that there are indeed people (specifically doctors and insurance companies) out to get them. This induces iatrogenic exacerbation of their symptoms as they strive, consciously or unconsciously, to prove to *someone* that they do have a problem. Then, to add insult to injury, this iatrogenically induced problem is used against them both by other physicians and the legal "warriors" who are bound and determined to prove that there is nothing wrong with them, thus saving their insurance company client's money.

PERSISTENT POSTCONCUSSIVE SYNDROME

Alexander[108,132] has written extensively about the "persistent post concussive syndrome" (PPCS). These patients, after one year, continue to have symptoms commonly seen in acute PCS, such as headache, sleep disorder, balance problems, dizziness, sensory hyperesthesias, and cognitive symptoms including deficits in attention, memory, and executive functioning. They are also frequently noted to have prominent emotional symptoms including irritability, depression, nervousness, discouragement, and anger.

Alexander[108] identifies some "predictors" of the development of PPCS, including the female sex, litigation, low socioeconomic status, prior MTBI, headache, and serious associated systemic injury. While these factors may be implicated, he states that none accounts for more than a small percentage of cases of PPCS.

Other authors identify pain severity post injury as a predictor of the development of the PPCS post MTBI.[133,134] Additional data suggests a greater frequency of anxiety and depression months after initial injury.[135]

Dizziness is a frequent symptom of the PCS. It is noted that peripheral vestibular injury with dizziness also has a close relationship with psychiatric disorders, particularly with affective disease and anxiety. Unfortunately, the significant aspects of dizziness secondary to myofascial problems are often ignored. Zasler[136] discusses cervicogenic dizziness. Dizziness secondary to myofascial trigger points in the sternocleidomastoid muscles, which is also frequently overlooked. In contradistinction, Alexander[108] does not appear to anticipate the psychological aspects secondary to this problem, making it seem more of a primary psychological problem than being secondary to a true organic problem.

Chronic pain and headache are fairly universal accompaniments of the PPCS. It is also known that patients who experience chronic headache not associated with a PCS have many of the same complaints, including fatigue, sleep disorder, depression, and occasionally, dizziness, as well as difficulties with concentration and memory. Psychological factors may aggravate these headaches.

It is also recognized that anxiety may decrease concentration and complex mental processes.[68,137] Depression can cause decreased cognitive functioning, particularly in concentration, memory, and executive functions.[128,138,139] The latter problem has also been called "depressive pseudodementia."[140]

Therefore, one cannot consider that if everyone with a PCS/MTBI has impaired concentration, then everyone with impaired concentration after PCS/MTBI has a neurological etiology. The problem is that patients with PCS/MTBI associated with pain and affective difficulties may have impaired concentration for multiple reasons, including post MTBI neuropathological changes.

Alexander[108] asks the question, "When does the physiogenesis of a clinical problem become psychogenesis?" This may be difficult to determine and may have an iatrogenic component. Alexander does indicate that while the major issue is physiogenesis transforming to psychogenesis, physiogenesis can be very underestimated. He also indicates that there is no single psychological factor, physiological factor, or demographic factor leading to the PPCS.

STILL MORE

Fenton[141] attempted to reappraise the PCS. He reviewed data from two UK prospective studies of the initial aspects and course of postconcussive symptomatology using parallel psychosocial, neuropsychiatric, quantitative EEG (electroencephalogram, or QEEG), and brainstem-evoked potentials. Abnormal, prolonged brainstem-evoked potentials were seen in between 27% and 46% of patients. Prolonged symptomatology was noted in 13% of patients and was associated with a high percentage of brainstem dysfunction. The degree of QEEG recovery related to the intensity of early symptom reaction to trauma. Fenton felt that levels of perceived stress at the time of the injury or afterwards were not related to symptom formation, but chronic social difficulties were seen in 21% of patients who initially showed improvement but later, between 6 weeks and 6 months post trauma, experienced an exacerbation of symptomatology.

Taylor et al.[142] compared 15 whiplash patients to 10 patients with moderate to severe brain injury, and 24 chronic pain patients. They were assessed 4 years after initial injury via neuropsychiatric testing. It was concluded that the theory of neuronal degeneration in the etiology of whiplash-related cognitive complaints was not supported, nor was the specificity of neuropsychological tests in detecting the subtle effects of brain trauma.

Not to be outdone, Greiffenstein et al.[143] compared the motor skills "which are sensitive to central lesions, but…. also affected by peripheral injury and motivation" in a group of "proven brain injury" patients versus "healthy postconcussion patients." They concluded, "Motor skill deficiencies in postconcussion syndrome (PCS) are probably functional in nature."

I don't get it, either.

BOTTOM LINE

I think Bob Dylan said something like, "I don't know what it is, but there's something out there, Mr. Jones."

The PCS as well as the PPCS are not symptoms or syndromes looking for patients. As I indicated above, I believe that the PCS is different from an MTBI. Still, patients from around the country, around the globe, complain of the same symptoms after an acceleration/deceleration injury. There are tests and many studies that show the presence of abnormalities. Again, we don't yet seem to know the best tests, the best window to perform them, or the best way to interpret them.

As clinicians, we also know that we have to listen to our patients. If something they say doesn't make sense, make like Sherlock Holmes (who was modeled after Dr. Bell, a neurologist) and investigate, actively, what the patient is telling you. It's your job.

To be antagonistic to a diagnosis, to not accept the presence of a diagnosis because of preconceived notions or thoughts of patient malingering — right off the bat, or because your opinion depends on who pays you — puts us back into the era of the Inquisition. That's not our job.

4 Pathophysiology

The primary mechanisms of traumatic brain injury (TBI) may include focal injury, as well as diffuse axonal shearing and neurochemical damage. Before we deal with these issues, let's take a brief tour of the normal physiology.

NORMAL COGNITIVE FUNCTIONING: THE VERY BASICS

The frontal and temporal lobes deal with complex, high-level behaviors including complex thought, memory, and language. The parietal and occipital lobes subserve sensation, vision, and perceptual information processing. All aspects of cerebral function are influenced by the others.

Normal frontal lobe activity includes executive functioning, or "Master Control." This includes integration of information from all other parts of the brain, including problem solving, planning, and emotional control.

After injury, abnormal frontal lobe activity includes: behavioral problems, inappropriate behaviors, poor problem solving, memory deficits, difficulties with routine activities, and poor insight into the presence of existing deficits.

The temporal lobes include the hippocampus regions, which are immensely important to memory. They also deal with speaking and understanding language, and correlation of sensory input including smell, taste, and hearing.

After injury to the temporal lobes, patients will develop memory problems, affective problems, and sensory and language problems. Also associated with temporal lobe injury is a higher incidence of seizure disorder.

The parietal lobes normally work to process various types of sensory information, including touch and position sense. After injury, patients will demonstrate problems with reading and writing, as well as spatial disorientation.

The occipital lobes normally enable effective processing and interpretation of visual information. When injured, they can induce difficulties in perception and interpretation of objects, words, and people.

When injured, the cerebellum can induce difficulties with coordinated movement of the extremities and the trunk, as well as difficulties with several other forms of information processing.

PRIMARY NEUROPATHOLOGY

Focal lesions are large enough to be visualized by the naked eye. They include cortical contusions, subdural hematomas, epidural hematomas, and intracerebral

0-8493-1955-2/00/$0.00+$.50
© 2000 by CRC Press LLC

hematomas. Subarachnoid hemorrhages are more diffuse, but stem from a focal area of bleeding.

Focal lesions induce neurological problems secondary to local brain damage and by causing intracranial mass lesions which may lead to brain shifting, herniation, and possible brainstem compression and death.

Diffuse injury is associated with more global or widespread neurological dysfunction not associated with macroscopically visible cerebral lesions. Such difficulties may follow mechanical injury such as the acceleration/deceleration injury, also known as cervical flexion/extension injuries or, by our legal brethren, "whiplash."

FOCAL LESIONS

CEREBRAL CONTUSION

- Focal areas of brain injury with areas of hemorrhage, infarction, necrosis, and edema; gray and white matter involvement.
- At coup and/or at contre coup sites (the area "under" the part of the head that is struck is coup, and the area of the brain exactly opposite the initial blow which strikes the hard surface of the skull is contre coup).
- Can be secondary to an acceleration/deceleration injury.
- May be secondary to impact on the irregular bony floor of the skull (especially in the frontal and middle fossa); may be secondary to coup or contre coup forces.
- Frontal and temporal regions are contused more frequently than the parietal region, more so than the occipital lobes.
- Most often multiple.
- More severe with associated skull fracture.

INTRACEREBRAL HEMATOMA

- Well-defined hemorrhagic regions within the cerebral parenchyma.
- Incidence found to range from .6% to 4%–23%.
- Most common mechanism is moving head striking a fixed object.
- 80%–90% are located in the white matter of the frontal or temporal lobes.

One study of 852 patients found 218 with intracerebral lesions only. Neurological deterioration after admission was seen in 71% of these patients. Patients with intracerebral hematoma seemed to improve after evacuation of the lesion, particularly if it was larger than 50 ml.[144]

Another study[145] found 22 patients of 1500 with posttraumatic intracerebral hematomas in the posterior cranial fossa. The most common etiology was motor vehicle accidents. Ninety percent of these patients had a history of direct trauma to the occipital region. Also, 90% of the patients with a Glasgow Coma Scale (GCS) between 13 and 15 had a good recovery. Statistical analysis found that patients with a GCS of below 9 had poor outcomes.

ACUTE SUBDURAL HEMATOMA

- Primary etiologies: motor vehicle accidents and falls.
- Occurrence is 1% of all brain injury and 5% of serious injury.
- Other studies show an incidence from 5% to 13%.
- Most commonly found after brain contusion leads to torn vessels via stretching or tearing.
- May fool clinicians who see a patient with a GCS of 15 and are neurologically intact; the subdural may occur within 24 hours of injury.

A retrospective study of 113 patients found that age and associated intracranial lesions were related to outcome, 91% of these patients had an initial GCS score of 9–15 and achieved functional recovery. [146]

Another retrospective study[147] assessed the specific variables with regard to morbidity and mortality: mechanisms of injury, age, neurological presentation, time delay from injury to intervention, and CAT scan findings on admission. The GCS and CAT scan findings were most important prognostically. The rapidity of hematoma development was not taken into account. It was concluded that the extent of primary brain injury underlying the subdural hematoma was the most important factor affecting outcome.

In a study evaluating criteria for conservative treatment of supratentorial acute posttraumatic subdural hematomas, it was found that patients with a midline shift of less than 10 mm on a CAT scan and with an initial GCS of 15 could be treated conservatively under close observation. Surgical intervention was utilized for those patients with deteriorating neurological conditions. It was felt that a midline shift of more than 5 mm in patients with a GCS of less than 15 predicted an exhaustion of cerebral compensatory mechanisms within 3 days of injury. The authors advised repeat CAT scan studies be done before discharge, along with close follow-up for the first month post injury.[148]

It was noted that traumatic interhemispheric subdural hematomas typically presented acutely or subacutely with contralateral monoparesis of a lower extremity, or hemiparesis or in bilateral hematomas, even with paraparesis. They typically needed early surgical evacuation. In the author's series of five cases, none followed the "classical" clinical pattern, and three recovered without surgery.[149]

Lee, et al.[150] found that in 436 patients, the mean interval from injury to diagnosis of acute posttraumatic subdural hematoma was 0.4 days; for subdural hygroma it was 13.4 days; and for chronic subdural hematomas, 51.6 days.

Another study showed that the mean volume of blood in extradural and subdural hematomas was essentially not space-consuming within the first hour after injury, but increased rapidly in the second and later hours post injury.[151]

Posterior fossa subdural hematomas are rare. One group reported on three cases. They noted that of the (inclusive) 16 reported cases, 60% had a sudden clinical worsening within 24 hours of injury. Seven cases had an occipital fracture.[152]

BOTTOM LINE

Patients who present to the emergency room with a GCS score of 15 should not be trundled out of the ER as soon as possible. A number of these patients, who may have an initially normal cerebral CAT scan, may develop an acute subdural hematoma within the first 24 hours post injury.

EXTRADURAL HEMATOMA

- Low incidence.
- Typically secondary to motor vehicle accidents and falls.
- Secondary to direct trauma to the skull and underlying meningeal vessels, not "brain injury" and not acceleration/deceleration injuries.

Riesgo et al.[153] described three cases of delayed extradural hematoma after mild head injury (GCS 12–15) and without associated intracranial or traumatic systemic lesions. Diagnosis was made by sequential CAT scans after neurological impairment was noted.

SUBARACHNOID HEMORRHAGE

- May be spontaneous, secondary to aneurysm, or posttraumatic in origin.
- Typically followed by vasospasm, which can cause secondary ischemic damage.
- May be secondary to the increase in conduction of calcium across the cell membrane.

Shigemori et al.[154] looked at the clinical significance of posttraumatic subarachnoid hemorrhage (TSAH) in 20 head-injured patients. Nine were classified as mild and 11 were classified as severe by their initial GCS scores. They concluded that a TSAH in the Sylvian fissure was suggestive of focal brain contusion around the fissures. Massive TSAH in the basal subarachnoid cisterns was not necessarily associated with severe parenchymal injury of the brainstem.

Another study found that the outcome of patients with TSAH was significantly worse when used as a prognostic factor, when compared to those patients whose initial CAT scan did not show subarachnoid blood, but who subsequently developed an SAH.[155]

In a prospective study of 130 patients with closed head trauma who exhibited subarachnoid blood on admission CAT scans, ten developed delayed ischemic symptoms between days 4 and 16 post injury. Three of these patients had minimal blood on initial evaluation, while seven had massive quantities of blood on CAT scan. Severe vasospasm was demonstrated on angiography performed after ischemic symptoms were identified. The authors concluded that massive TSAH is a predictable indicator of delayed ischemic symptoms.[156]

Gaetani et al.[157] also noted that TSAH is a negative prognostic factor. The degree of TSAH was related to clinical conditions at admission, while the presence of subarachnoid blood clots in both the basal cisterns and over the cerebral convexity were indicative of poor outcomes.

Terson's syndrome consists of retinal or vitreous hemorrhage in association with subarachnoid hemorrhage. Medele et al.[158] noted that Terson's syndrome may be related to an acute elevation in ICP, independent of its etiology, and may occur with similar incidence in patients with severe brain injury and those with an SAH. They also felt that recognition and treatment of this entity was important to avoid secondary damage to the eye and visual impairment.

CLINICALLY SPEAKING

Mlay[159] noted both delayed epidural and subdural hematomas in seven patients. Clinical signs of neurological deterioration necessitated reinvestigation.

Meyer et al.[160] investigated traumatic brainstem hemorrhage (TBH). They found that the most common site of TBH is the anterior rostral midbrain, secondary to sudden craniocaudal displacement of the brain upon impact. The authors also noted the high percentage of survival after a TBH in this region.

Kurth et al.[161] evaluated the effect on neuropsychological outcome of the number of acute hemorrhages, lesion volume, and lesion location after a TBI. They could find no specific relationship.

The concept of "inner cerebral trauma" (ICT) has been defined as a characteristic topographic pattern of deep brain lesions secondary to physical forces occurring within the cranial cavity in an acceleration/deceleration type injury, inducing closed head injury or TBI. These lesions are typically located in the "centro-axial" regions of the brain. Birbamer et al.[162] found that the extent of ICT is very often underestimated by CAT scan. MRI scans correlated well with the neuropathological studies, which showed a multifocal pathogenesis of severe TBI.

As noted above, brainstem lesions are thought to be comparatively rare, yet the literature is growing. Ezzat et al.[163] found that a pontomedullary rent or tear is a primary brainstem injury which can occur in high-speed injuries. In their group of 13 patients, 7 had associated basal skull fractures, while 3 had fractures of the cervical spine. They note that a partial rent is compatible with survival. It was also noted that many authors feel that these tears are mostly induced by traumatic craniocervical hyperextension; others feel the injuries can be a form of diffuse axonal injury caused by the angular acceleration of the head.

Traumatic lesions of the brainstem can be considered primary, those induced at the moment of trauma/impact, or secondary, those lesions associated with a supratentorial mass lesion.

In a Japanese study of 239 patients with significant brain injury who had severe disturbances of consciousness when first seen, CAT scans done on admission revealed 21 patients (8.8%) to have had a primary brain stem lesion. The injuries were primarily secondary to motor vehicle accidents. Sixteen of the 21 patients were found to have brain stem lesions along with other cerebral pathology, including cerebral contusion of the white and gray matter, callosal injury, intraventricular hemorrhage, and subarachnoid hemorrhage, which are considered to be caused by diffuse shearing injury. The primary brainstem lesions in their study were found on the dorsal side of the midbrain, which would differentiate them from secondary brainstem lesions. These lesions were felt to be secondary to shearing injury in and around the brainstem, close to the tentorial edge, or to an injury of the lower brainstem caused by hyperextension of the cervical vertebrae. They again noted that the prognosis of the patient with a primary brainstem lesion is usually poor, but exceptions can be found in patients with a single brainstem lesion. [164]

Goscinski et al.[165] described nine cases of posttraumatic primary brainstem hematoma. All of the patients presented with ocular and vegetative symptomatology. Hyperextension during injury was the primary mechanism of pathology. After conservative treatment, half of the patients had good outcomes.

Inner cerebral trauma (ICT) has also involved the corpus callosum, the neuronal "bridge" between cerebral hemispheres. An extensive neuropathological study by Zarkovi et al.[166] found that the lesions in the corpus callosum were related to the pattern of ICT, with a correlation between the shape and distribution of periaxial lesions of the ICT and the direction of the linear translation of acceleration forces. It was felt that the axonal lesions were more focal or diffuse.

A complete corpus callosal disconnection syndrome after closed head injury has been described. Zarkovi et al. also felt that posttraumatic callosal disconnection may be frequently overlooked.[167]

Another study found abnormal MRI signals in small percentages of patients with mild, moderate, and severe brain injuries (2%, 10%, and 38%, respectively). The findings appeared to mirror those of paracontusional edema in the subcortical white matter. The authors suggested that some of the lesions in the corpus callosum post closed head injury were reversible and resembled edema which may have been secondary to a relatively mild shear strain force to the corpus callosum.[168]

Primus et al.[169] looked at the possibility of a "subcortical" syndrome which differentially affected memory in TBI subjects. Using neuropsychological testing protocols, they were unable to find any unique patterns of subcortical pathology secondary to corpus callosum involvement.

Porencephaly, or the development of a porencephalic cyst, can be secondary to traumatic brain injury. A porencephalic cyst is a cavity within the cerebral hemisphere filled with cerebral spinal fluid that communicates directly with the ventricular system. It is frequently associated with opthalmic and neurological signs such as visual field deficits, optic nerve hypoplasia, nystagmus, strabismus, hemi-inattention, seizures, mental deficits, and abnormal pupillary responses. Yang et al.[170] report two patients who developed porencephalic cysts from traumatic head injury. They note that the visual field defects resulting from a porencephalic cyst can imitate those visual findings from a stroke or brain tumor, making appropriate differential diagnosis imperative.

The author has, several times, seen patients injured by electrical shock or lightning strike. The typical nonclinical problems were of a legal nature: could a person develop a TBI post electrical injury? Clinically, the answer appears to be yes. One of the few groups to do neuropsychological evaluations of patients status-post lightning strike, van Zomeren et al.[171] found that lightning strikes can induce mild or subtle cognitive impairments. They speculate that most of the difficulties in such patients stem from "vegetative dysregulation," a disorder that has often been noted in the literature to be secondary to the effects of electrical injury on the central nervous system. They conclude that such dysregulation may cause both fatigue and mild cognitive impairments. They don't go into the behavioral sequelae of electrical injury, which, clinically, can include frontal lobe behavioral problems such as increased irritability as well as increased aggression.

Another important clinical point was made by Aoki et al.[172] who noted that a symptomatic subacute subdural hematoma can present with focal neurological deficits. This point must be kept in mind when performing nonsurgical management of an acute subdural hematoma. In their study, a patient had a traumatically-induced acute SDH that was managed nonsurgically because he complained only of mild headache, which resolved within a week. Twelve days later, the patient developed amnestic aphasia, a craniotomy was performed, and he needed several months of speech therapy to return to his baseline status.

Work continues to try to better determine the relationship between cognition, generally and specifically, and specific neurological deficits.

Memory, concentration, and problem-solving deficits are noted after mild and moderate TBI. These functions are at least partially mediated by forebrain cholinergic and catecholaminergic systems.

Using fluid percussion head injury techniques in the rat, Schmidt and Grady[173] found no visible effects of head injury on forebrain dopamine or noradrenergic systems. They did find a significant loss of ventrobasal forebrain cholinergic neurons after brief concussive injury in rats. This can produce significant disturbances in cognitive tasks linked to the neocortical and hippocampal cholinergic systems. Remember that this was done in rats, and its specific correlations in humans, other than the above, is not demonstrated.

Rogers et al.[174] compared 12 patients with focal frontal cortex damage to 12 patients with mild, medicated, early Parkinson's disease in a series of number- and letter-naming tasks. They found that both left and right frontal cortical areas are involved in the organization of cognitive and motor processes in situations dealing with novel task demands. It appeared to them that only the left frontal cortex is involved in the dynamic reconfiguring between already established tasks, and that it is also the site of an executive mechanism responsible for the modulation of exogenous task activity. They also noted that dopaminergic transmission via the nigrostriatal pathway may be associated with sustaining various cognitive and motor processes over prolonged periods, including the operation of executive control mechanisms which enable reconfiguring between different tasks.

Executive functions, which will be dealt with in greater detail in following chapters, refer to a patient's ability to plan, initiate, follow through, and monitor the success of activities.

Coolidge and Griego,[175] using a self-rating scale to test the executive functions of the frontal lobes, compared 17 head-injured patients and a matched control group. They found that the head-injured patients scored significantly higher on the overall measures of executive dysfunction and higher on the decision-making subscale of the 200-item Coolidge Axis II inventory.

Minderhoud et al.[176] also reviewed the fronto-temporal component in both mild and moderate TBI.

Verbal fluency is a part of frontal lobe activity, as well as other areas of the brain. Field potentials from intracranial electrodes in humans were used to evaluate language-related processing. A large negative field potential was found with a peak latency near 400 msec, which was found in the anterior medial temporal lobe and associated with anomalous sentence-ending words. This field potential at 400 msec shares a number of characteristics with the N400 potential typically recorded from scalp electrodes and associated with semantic processing.[177]

Stuss et al.[178] evaluated patients with focal brain injures compared to normal controls on tasks of letter-based and category-based list generation. They found that damage to the right dorsolateral cortical or connecting striatal regions, the right posterior area, or the medial inferior frontal lobe of either hemisphere did not significantly affect letter-based fluency performance. Superior medial frontal damage, right or left, resulted in moderate impairment, while patients with left dorsolateral and/or striatal lesions were most impaired. Left parietal damage led to performance that was essentially equivalent to the superior medial and left dorsolateral patient groups. The same lesion sites produced impairments in category-based fluency, but so did lesions of the right dorsolateral and inferior medial regions. Different cognitive processes related to different brain regions appeared to underlie performance on verbal fluency testing.

In general, three principal syndromes have been associated with regions of the frontal lobes. These include the disinhibited syndrome associated with a lesion to the orbital area, the apathetic syndrome associated with damage to the frontal convexity, and the akinetic syndrome associated with lesions to the medial structures.

Crowe[179] found that injuries to all three areas produced, in his experimental group, lower overall levels of responding than did normals when looking at verbal fluency.

Smith et al.[180] found that patients with unilateral frontal or temporal lobe injuries were more susceptible to interference with spatial memory than controls.

The dorsolateral prefrontal cortex is known to be involved with working memory. Experimental work finds that this area also plays a role in the retrieval of visuospatial information used for guiding a response program.[181] Other research has shown that patients with prefrontal lesions suffer from deficits in both divided and focused attention, which corresponded to behavioral changes.[182]

An excellent study by Bechara et al.[183] also looked at the prefrontal cortex. Prior work has shown that lesions in this area will induce severe difficulties in real-life decision-making, even in the presence of normal intellect. These patients may recognize the consequences of their actions, but fail to act in their own best interests, therefore appearing oblivious to the future. This group's work showed, by measuring skin conductance responses (SCRs), there was an absence of anticipatory SCRs in patients with prefrontal damage, which is correlated with their insensitivity to future outcomes.

Another group found that patients with anterior frontal lobe lesions have an exaggerated willingness to adopt bizarre hypotheses, again showing a failure to anticipate future consequences or effects from decision making.[184]

Patients with unilateral lesions of the medial frontal region which involved the supplementary motor area were found to have a dual motor function, rather than a single function, when reaction time was tested.[185]

Several times over the last decade I have been asked to comment on the loss of fluid intelligence in a TBI patient, usually by an attorney implying how ridiculous the entire idea of loss of intelligence after a supposed TBI can be. In some patients general intelligence may be preserved after TBI in spite of significant deficits in memory and/or executive functioning. Duncan et al.[186] found that patients with superior IQs on the Wechsler Adult Intelligence Scale can show impairments of 20 to 60 points on conventionally-measured fluid intelligence or novel problem solving. They found that general intelligence may be a reflection of frontal lobe functioning.

It doesn't take much to see how complex frontal lobe functioning is in terms of the number of aspects of cognition and behavior it involves. And we haven't really scratched the surface.

Unilateral injury to the posterior parietal or frontal lobe affects patterns of oculomotor scanning. The posterior parietal lesion affected the visuospatial guidance of visual scanning, while the frontal damage impaired the planning involved in such visual scanning. It appears that the posterior parietal and frontal brain structures have reciprocal connections and act together as part of a distributed neural network subserving visually-guided oculomotor scanning; the spatio-temporal organization of a scanpath depends on both stuctures.[187]

The left parietal cortex, especially the supramarginal gyrus, is associated with motor attention. Lesions there were associated with ideomotor apraxia and problems performing sequences of movements. It is felt that left hemisphere and apraxic impairment in movement sequencing is secondary to difficulty in shifting the focus of motor attention from one movement in a sequence to the next.[188]

Trauma to the left hemispheric temporal and parietal lobes induced disturbances in both verbal and nonverbal short-term memory.[189]

The possibility of "whiplash" producing an amnestic syndrome secondary to bilateral paramedian thalamic infarctions has been noted.[190] Even a decrease of thalamic volume was found to be associated with an increase in sensory-perceptual errors, showing that diencephalic injuries can affect specific types of cognitive functioning.[191]

BOTTOM LINE

The main purpose of this little trip into clinical correlations is to show the reader a little bit of the immense complexity of the problem, the surface of which, as noted, was barely scratched. It is very important to show that when dealing with the brain, things may not always be as they seem. This must never be forgotten by the clinicians who diagnose and treat mild and moderate (even severe) TBI.

OTHER PRIMARY AND SECONDARY LESIONS

Other neurological problems may follow focal lesions, including:

HYPOXIC/ISCHEMIC DAMAGE

- Secondary to decreased blood flow from a mass effect, increased ICP (intra-cranial pressure), and edema.
- Also secondary to brainstem dysfunction of respiratory system.
- May be secondary to aspiration and airway obstruction.
- Hypothalamic injury can cause "neurogenic" pulmonary edema.

CEREBRAL EDEMA

There are five types of cerebral edema, three of which may be associated with TBI.

- Vasogenic: a plasma filtrate secondary to increased capillary permeability; found extracellularly in white matter; the blood-brain barrier (BBB) is disrupted; may be secondary to TBI.
- Hydrocephalic: Secondary to increased ventricular pressure effecting the cerebral spinal fluid (CSF); in extracellular white matter; the BBB is intact.
- Cytotoxic: Plasma ultrafiltrate (electrolytes) secondary to disturbed intra-cellular metabolism; in white and/or gray matter, intracellular BBB is intact.
- Ischemic: Some characteristics of cytotoxic edema; secondary to diminished oxygenation; found in white and gray matter; variable intactness of BBB.
- Osmotic: From water intoxication.

Other posttraumatic difficulties include:

BRAIN SWELLING

- Not the same as edema.
- Secondary, at least in part, to increased intravascular blood within the brain.
- Secondary to any type of head injury.
- Magnitude of brain swelling does not correlate to severity of brain injury.

INCREASED INTRACRANIAL PRESSURE (ICP)

- Trauma may disturb normal homeostatic mechanisms controlling ICP (< 15 mm Hg) and induce continued increases in ICP and eventual herniation and neurological death.
- Can be secondary to mass lesion with volume/pressure interactions disturbing steady state.
- Major clinical significance of ICP and its intracranial dynamics is its usefulness in recognizing impending cerebral herniation.

VENTRICULAR ENLARGEMENT (HYDROCEPHALUS)

- Non-acute.
- Found in 72% of a series of young adults and adolescents with moderate or severe TBI.
- In another study, 30.5%; with 90% of the patients developing ventricular enlargement within three months of the injury.
- Most common cause: *ex vacuo* hydrocephalus, with loss of brain tissue due to injury.

There is a great deal of contention between the facts and relationships between posttraumatic blood flow, intracranial hypertension, metabolic stability, and postinjury outcome. Most of the work has been done in the more severely injured patients, but the information remains important in our discussions of mild and moderate TBI.

The various aspects of hyperemia (cerebral blood flow (CBF) greater than 55ml/100 g/minute), intracranial hypertension (ICP) (greater than 20 mm Hg), and particularly their relationship(s) have been explored.

The literature suggests that global posttraumatic hyperemia is an acute, malignant phenomenon associated with increased ICP, profound unconsciousness, and poor outcome. Sakas et al.[192] found that posttraumatic hyperemia may occur across a wide spectrum of brain injury severity, and may be associated with favorable patient outcomes.

One study showed that the majority of patients with hyperemia-associated ICP had severe initial insults with gross impairment of metabolic vasoreactivity and pressure autoregulation. In some patients, it was noted that hyperemia was coupled to a hypermetabolic state, and other patients had hyperemia without ICP. In the latter group, it was felt that an increased CBF was a manifestation of appropriate coupling to increased metabolic demand, which was consistent with a favorable outcome. It was felt that there were multiple etiologies of both increased CBF and ICP after head injury.[193]

In contradistinction, another study found that phasic elevation of CBF immediately after TBI was a necessary condition for achieving functional recovery, as the rise in CBF resulted from increased metabolic demands in the presence of intact vasoreactivity. It was felt that in a minority of patients the constellation of hyperemia, severe ICP, and poor outcome were indicative of badly impaired vasoreactivity with an uncoupling of the congruent mechanisms of blood flow and metabolism.[194] This suggests an associated period of cerebral/neuronal vulnerability.

Another study looked specifically at the blood flow velocity of the middle cerebral artery (MCA) using transcranial Doppler ultrasonography. Patients with mild, moderate, and severe injury were evaluated. The initial mean velocity was significantly lower in severe injury than in minor and moderate injury. The MCA velocity remained low in the severely injured patients but returned to normal in the minor and moderately injured patients. It was felt that a significant increase in MCA velocity was associated with good recovery or moderate disability, while patients with MCA velocities of less than 28 cm/s did not show these outcomes.[195]

Looking at a smaller group of patients, another group found that patients without surgical lesions had low CBF in the first hours post injury, and this was followed by a hyperemic state that typically peaked in 24 hours.[196]

Associated with the phenomena of vasoregulation is the role of ischemia. A group looked at the question of cerebral ischemia being an early finding after injury, and that CBF measurements have not been performed early enough to register these changes. They felt the above statement was true, and that early ischemia after TBI was an important factor in determining neurological outcome. Of great interest was the interpretation of their data to indicate that early hyperventilation or lowering blood pressure to prevent cerebral edema may be harmful,[197] which would make teleological sense.

Cerebral vasospasm would have a significant effect on the brain. Collecting transcranial Doppler data with CBF data from 85 patients, Lee et al.[198] calculated a "spasm index." This consisted of the velocity of blood flow in the middle cerebral artery (MCA) and the basilar artery (BA). The spasm index was the V/(MCA) or V/(BA) divided by the hemispheric or global CBF. They found that hemodynamically significant spasm was a significant predictor of poor outcome, independent of the GCS score. They concluded that cerebral vasospasm was a pathophysiologically important posttraumatic secondary insult, and was best diagnosed by the combined measures of transcranial Doppler and CBF measurement. Another report indicated cerebral vasospasm was an important secondary posttraumatic insult post TBI and could, in some cases, be treated with intravenous calcium channel-blockers.[199]

Somatosensory evoked potentials (SSEPs) were utilized to evaluate outcome after severe head injury. It was noted that increased oxygen utilization and lowered CBF in patients showing deteriorating SSEPs implied that early ischemia was responsible for associated SSEP deterioration, and not failure of O_2 extraction or utilization.[200]

Another group found that even in the presence of adequate cerebral perfusion, limited improvement in elevated cerebral arteriovenous oxygen post-treatment (either mannitol administration or craniotomy) would predict delayed cerebral infarction and poor outcome post TBI.[201]

Techniques for monitoring and measuring hemodynamic responses in patients post TBI include transcranial Doppler monitoring, as well as 123I-iodoamphetamine single-photon emission CT (IMP SPECT).[202,203] No matter what the instrumentation, hemodynamic measurements are imperative in patients post severe TBI.

McLaughlin and Marion[204] looked at the CBF and vasoresponsivity around cerebral contusions. They concluded that the CBF within intracerebral contusions is very variable and often above 18 ml/100 g/min, the assumed threshold for irreversible ischemia. Intracontusional CBF is significantly decreased when compared to surrounding brain parenchyma; CO_2 vasoresponsivity was found to be intact. Vasoresponsivity in the contusion and the surrounding tissue may be three times normal, which suggests hypersensitivity to hyperventilation therapy. The relative hypoperfusion within and around cerebral contusions makes these areas very vulnerable to secondary injury from hypotension or overly aggressive hyperventilation.

In a study of cerebral autoregulation after minor TBI, Junger et al.[205] looked at 29 patients with GCS scores of 13–15 within 48 hours of injury via transcranial

Doppler and blood pressure. It was found that a significant number of patients with minor TBI may have impaired cerebral autoregulation and an increased risk of secondary ischemic neuronal damage. Strebel et al.[206] also found that a mild TBI can result in the loss of cerebral autoregulation.

For many years, cerebral edema and vascular engorgement have been terms used interchangeably to describe brain swelling associated with severe TBI. It appears that brain edema, and not blood volume, is the major contributor to brain swelling.[207] Diffuse brain swelling after TBI has also been found to be relatively benign in children as compared to adults, unless there is a severe primary injury or secondary hypotensive episode.[208,209]

The importance of cerebral temperature alterations and the existence of a possible defect in the central thermoregulatory system post TBI have also been discussed.[210-213]

DIFFUSE INJURY

There are four categories of diffuse injury:

MILD CONCUSSION

- There is no loss of consciousness, but transient neurological disturbance may be seen.
- The patient may be confused, disoriented, and may or may not have amnesia.
- Posttraumatic headache is frequently seen.

"CLASSICAL" CEREBRAL CONCUSSION

- The patient may show temporary, reversible neurological deficits secondary to trauma, associated with a brief loss of consciousness (less than 1 hour) with some degree of posttraumatic amnesia.
- A mild or moderate degree of microscopic neuronal abnormalities can be found.
- There may be an associated focal brain injury (contusion).
- Posttraumatic headache, tinnitus, subtle changes in memory, or psychological functioning may be seen.

DIFFUSE INJURY

- Prolonged loss of consciousness (greater than 24 hours) with residual neurological, psychological, or personality deficits frequently seen.
- There are no sympathetic nervous system changes.
- No decerebrate posturing.
- There may be acute cerebral swelling.

- Widespread neuropsychological dysfunction(cortical and diencephalic) is frequently seen.
- The degree of recovery depends on the amount and location of anatomic damage.

DIFFUSE WHITE MATTER (AXONAL) SHEARING

- The injury is associated with anatomical disruption of white matter in both hemispheres and may extend into the diencephalic and brainstem regions.
- Prolonged loss of consciousness.
- Abnormal brainstem signs such as posturing.
- Autonomic nervous system dysfunction, including increased blood pressure, temperature and hyperhydrosis.
- Recovery is related to the amount of anatomical damage — 50–70% die.
- Principal findings on microscopic examination.
- CAT scan may show small hemorrhages in the corpus collosum and periventricular regions.

VERY IMPORTANT CAVEATS

- Physiological and (neuro) psychological dysfunction may occur in the absence of anatomical (macroscopic) lesions.
- Functional disruption, which precedes anatomical disruption, is always the greater.
- Clinically, patients with mild concussion syndromes and "classical" cerebral concussion may have physiological dysfunction as well as microscopic anatomical disruptions that may be in contradistinction to the apparent severity of the injury.
- TBI deficits are additive.

The neuropathology of TBI is, as most aspects of the disorder, replete with knowns, unknowns, and variables. Research has established many of the basic facts noted above, but the exact how, when, why, and where are still subject to debate.

Clinical practice indicates that a CAT scan should be performed on patients post TBI. However, as noted above, the timing of the test is important. It is important to repeat a CAT scan on a patient who begins to decompensate neurologically. As previously mentioned, an acute subdural hematoma or subarachnoid hemorrhage may occur in patients with normal GCS scores (GCS = 15), typically within 24 hours. Other authors feel that when the first CAT scan is performed within 3 hours of injury, another should be done within 12 hours.[214]

Quantitative MRI analyses have shown significant differences in TBI patients — unimodal gray-white matter histograms — as compared to normals, who demonstrate bimodal gray matter-white matter histograms.[215] The MRI is also better than the CAT scan at determining other postinjury pathology, including diffuse axonal injury (DAI) and glial scarring. The MRI scan is also useful in morphometric analysis of the brain showing diffuse neuronal degeneration after TBI with more severe injury. This may include larger ventricle-to-brain ratios and temporal horn volumes, which may relate to neuropsychological outcome.[216]

A host of structural changes occur after TBI. In looking at the evolution of a contusion, it is found that initial BBB disruptions from trauma will induce extracellular edema. Microscopic analysis will reveal multiple vacuoles in the edematous region, which, over time, may induce small cysts in the white matter. Short-term cerebral edema may clear, with the neuropil being returned to normal. Long-standing edema typically induces reactive gliosis, which may remain indefinitely. Neurons may swell and/or shrink, which is associated with eosinophilia and nuclear pyknosis. These changes, at the periphery of a contusion, may last for six months or longer. Nuclear pyknosis may remain in the tissue and become mineralized (ferruginated neurons), which remain for years. After trauma, axons may become swollen and ballooned in and around the contusion, but also at great distances from it (DAI). The axonal ballooning may be seen between 24 and 48 hours post trauma and can remain for many years, with selective axonal calcifications seen in humans as well as in animals that have undergone experimental trauma. Astroglia begin to proliferate after 7 to 10 days post injury. They continue to increase in number and with fibrillary appearances finally resulting in a glial scar over ensuing months and years. It has been noted that the reactive gliosis may result in the restoration of the blood brain barrier in the damaged area.[217]

Timing, being everything, has been investigated by numerous researchers. Many utilize paraffin sections with hematoxylin and eosin stains, as well as special staining preparations. Many patients who survive severe brain injury for less than one hour are found to have eosinophylic neurons, particularly in the areas of contusion, the hippocampus, and the arterial boundary zones of the cerebral cortex. Neuronal incrustation is seen beginning after 3 hours and up to 48 hours in a contusion. Axonal swelling and white matter spheroids are seen in the regions of laceration and hemorrhage within one hour, and continue to be noted through all time periods. Glial swelling is also noted. Polymorphonuclear leukocytes (granulocytes) are seen early after injury and persist, increasing in number over time. In one study, axonal swelling, eosinophilia of neurons, and neuronal incrustation were noted at earlier time periods than previously reported.[218]

DIFFUSE AXONAL INJURY

Diffuse axonal injury is one of the most prevalent and well-acknowledged primary and secondary post injury pathophysiological phenomena. The brain tissue, or parenchyma, can be severely injured secondary to axonal shearing forces during acceleration/deceleration and rotational injures in a closed head injury. The most common locations of DAI include cerebral hemispheric gray/white matter interfaces and subcortical white matter, the body and the splenium of the corpus collosum, the basal ganglia, dorsolateral aspects of the brainstem, and the cerebellum. MRI technology is continually evolving. Nonhemorrhagic lesions can be seen via MRI using fluid attenuated inversion recovery (FLAIR) techniques, proton-density, and T2 weighted images. Old hemorrhagic lesions are best seen with the use of gradient echo sequences.[219]

A good tool utilized in the investigation of DAI is beta-amyloid precursor protein (beta-APP). In one series, DAI was seen in 65% to 100% of all cases of closed head injury, fatal cerebral ischemia/hypoxia, and brain death with a survival time of greater than 3 hours. Cases with a posttraumatic interval of less than 180 minutes did not express beta-APP.[220] The extent and severity of DAI cannot be predicted from biomechanical data alone, such as the height of a fall; total axonal injury in a given patient is a variable mixture of nonfocal axonal injury (DAI) and focal axonal injury from secondary mechanisms. Beta-APP immunostaining is not able to distinguish between primary and secondary axonal injury.[221] Still another study found beta-APP immunostaining demonstrations of positive axonal swelling 1.75 hours post injury in both mild and severe TBI groups, and demonstrated a spectrum of axonal injury in TBI. The study found that axons were more vulnerable than blood vessels, and those axons in the corpus callosum and fornices were the most vulnerable of all.[222]

Findings from another study express that neurofilamentous disruption is a pivotal event in axonal injury. The authors studied the progression of TBI- induced axonal change at the ultrastructural level using two antibodies (NR4, used to target light neurofilament subunits; and SMI32, used to target the heavy neurofilament subunit). Changes were noted at six hours post injury, which entailed focally enlarged, immunoreactive axons with axolemmal infolding or disordered neurofilaments. By 12 hours, some axons showed continued neurofilamentous misalignment, pronounced immunoreactivity, vacuolization and, on occasion, disconnection. Between 30 and 60 hours, further accumulations of neurofilaments and organelles induced further expansion of the axis cylinder and disconnected reactive swellings were recognized. During later times, focally enlarged disconnected axons were observed in relation to axons showing less advanced reactive changes.[223]

Currently, limited sampling methods are used for screening brain tissue for DAI using antibodies to beta-APP and microglial-associated antigen CD68 (PG-MI) and for GFAP. It is noted that a restricted number of blocks from injured or vulnerable areas is typically not sufficient to make the diagnosis. Also, with limited sampling, beta-APP and PG-MI immunochemistry can involve interpretive problems.[224]

Another study of brain tissue from contused areas found that fluid accumulations were seen around microvessels. Endothelial cells showed marked intracellular edema. Pinocytotic activity was increased, and swelling of astrocytic perivascular processes and increased macrophages with very large lysosomes were seen. It was concluded that endothelial cell edema may be a central fact in the pathophysiology of posttraumatic edema.[225]

Other studies used both light and electron microscopy to look at morphological changes of cerebral tissue post TBI. Vasogenic brain edema was correlated with clear and dense astrocytes, bi- and multinucleated astrocytes, and hypertrophic astrocytes; swollen clear and dense perineuronal astrocytes were seen compressing and indenting degenerated pyramidal and nonpyramidal nerve cells. Glycogen was depleted in many astrocytes, astrocytic ensheathment of synaptic contacts was lost, the perivascular astrocyte end-feet appeared dissociated from the capillary basement membrane, and the interastrocytary gap junctions were disrupted. The posttraumatic neurological deficits and neurobehavioral disorders of the patient studied were correlated to astrocyte ultrastructural changes and the disruption of the BBB.[226] In addition, phagocytosis of degenerated myelinated axons and synaptic endings by neuroglial cells was seen, along with nonnervous system-invading cells.[227] Reactive oligodendrocytes were found to induce myelinolysis. Vasogenic and cytotoxic edema from BBB dysfunction and the subsequent neuronal and neuroglial cell reactive and degenerative processes were also thought to be the morphological substrate which mediated TBI neurobehavioral disorders.[228] In another study, phagocytosis of isolated presynaptic endings or of entire synaptic contacts by astrocytes, microglial cells, and non-nervous-system-invading cells (monocytes and macrophages) was seen. Also noted were osmiophylic bodies, necrotic membranes, lipid inclusions, and glycogen granules in synaptic terminals. Synaptic disassembly was also seen.[229]

Axonal injury, including DAI, was noted by several authors in the brains of patients who were victims of blunt head trauma/assault.[230-232]

Other studies reinforce the fact that neuronal loss after head injury is secondary to both primary and secondary mechanisms. One study also found that microglial activation was a delayed result of TBI.[233] Another study, which evaluated Purkinje cell vulnerability to mild TBI, found that there was a close anatomical association between activated microglial cells and Purkinje cells, which suggests that Purkinje cell injury is the cause of microglial cell activation.[234]

Povlishock's work comes to some of the same conclusions, but he arrives there by a different road. He feels that the TBI itself does not cause axonal disruption. Rather, it is focal, subtle axonal changes that occur over time that lead to impaired axoplasmic transport, continued axonal swelling, and, finally, disconnection. He attributes the trauma to altering the axolemmal permeability, direct cytoskeletal damage, or disruption or more overt metabolic and functional disturbances. Trauma may induce axonal change, but also Wallerian degeneration and, finally, deafferentation. He feels that traumatically induced DIA will lead to diffuse deafferentation. He also notes that posttraumatically, the cerebral parenchyma is involved with increased neuronal sensitivity to secondary ischemia. Furthermore, he feels that this increased sensitivity is secondary to the neurotransmitter storm that follows a TBI, which can induce sublethal neuro-excitation. Most importantly, he indicates that the damage noted does not take place immediately post trauma, but over days, or even weeks.[235,236]

NEUROCHEMICAL ASPECTS OF TRAUMATIC BRAIN INJURY

Now we get into some heavy-duty neurophysiology/neuropharmacology. Those of you who feel lost should do some reading in basic neuropharmacology.

Abnormal agonist-receptor interactions related to excitotoxic processes may contribute to the pathophysiology of TBI. Activation of the muscarinic cholinergic or N-methyl-D-aspartate (NMDA) glutamate receptors appear to contribute to TBI pathophysiology.

TBI-induced membrane depolarization induces a massive release of excitatory neurotransmitters, particularly acetylcholine (ACH) and glutamate. The posttraumatic overproduction/release of these chemicals may induce abnormal activation of receptors that can produce changes in intracellular signal transduction pathways and, thereby, induce short-term, long-lasting, or irreversible changes in cell function. Such deficits can occur with sublethal cell disruption or cell death.

Experimental TBI is known to produce widespread neuronal depolarization, which is demonstrated by large increases in extracellular potassium (K+) resulting from neuronal discharges and not neurotransmitter release.

Increased neurotransmitter release is recruited to increase depolarization as injury severity increases. The release of these excitatory amino acids (EAAs) significantly contributes to the high levels of K+ release following TBI.

After moderate and, most probably, mild TBI, tissue deformation may open ion channels resulting in an influx of K+ large enough to induce abnormal levels of excitatory neurotransmitter release and, therefore, further depolarization.

Mild to moderate TBI induces increases in glutamate and ACH. Increased ACH release and increased cholinergic neuronal activity in some regions of the brain (such as the hippocampus) may persist for hours or longer after injury.

Posttraumatic changes in the BBB may also contribute to posttraumatic receptor dysfunction by allowing the abnormal passage of bloodborne excitatory exogenous neurotransmitters and neuromodulators into the brain. These additional excitatory neurochemicals may act synergistically with endogenously increased excitatory neurotransmitters (ENTs).

Moderate experimental TBI without contusion in the rat leads to acute BBB dysfunction in the hippocampus and the cortex that may last more than 12 hours.

Other research suggests that dysfunction of the BBB secondary to TBI may allow blood plasma constituents such as ACH (at levels seven times greater than in the CSF) to gain access to the brain and influence injury processes.

Moderate TBI can induce significant reductions in muscarinic cholinergic receptor binding. Decreased binding by glutaminergic receptors, specifically the NMDA receptors, also occurs following moderate TBI.

The predominant changes seen only in the NMDA receptors suggest that the ENT agonist-receptor interaction secondary to moderate TBI occurs predominately at this receptor subtype. This is supported by the protection given by administration of NMDA antagonists.

Pharmacological antagonism of muscarinic cholinergic receptors or pharmacological depletion of ACH can provide protection from TBI pathophysiology. Pre- or posttreatment with scopolamine significantly reduces functional motor deficits associated with fluid percussion TBI in the rat. Dicyclomine, a selective M1 muscarinic antagonist, provides protection similar in nature to scopolamine. (See Chapter 10.)

The reduced duration of posttraumatic unconsciousness may be produced by pre-treatment with the (anticholinergic) scopolamine, and is probably secondary to the inhibition of a muscarinic brainstem system which, when activated, produces reflex inhibition associated with profound behavioral suppression or loss of consciousness. The mechanisms mediating posttraumatic loss of consciousness are probably different from those mediating more enduring behavioral deficits.

Reduced motor and memory deficits can be seen with pharmacological antagonism of NMDA receptors using Phencyclidine (PCP), MK-801, Dextrorphan, and others. This appears to be secondary to their ability to restore MG++ (magnesium) levels post injury.

Receptor activation by ENTs may contribute to cellular metabolic alterations after TBI. Further results indicate that EAA neurotransmitters may be involved in injury-induced disruption of ionic homeostasis and ion-induced cytotoxic cerebral edema.

In rats, the probable therapeutic window for NMDA and muscarinic antagonists post TBI may be less than or up to 30 minutes. The window for humans is unknown.

Currently, the clinical usefulness of NMDA and muscarinic cholinergic antagonists is problematic. Cytotoxicity with MK-801 is greater than PCP, which is greater than Ketamine (an NMDA antagonist). Scopolamine may protect against the neurotoxic side-effects of MK-801, which have adverse effects on neural functioning and behavior. More than one type of receptor antagonist may be needed.

We need to know more about the neurochemical intracellular cascade coupled to pathological receptor activation, and thereby attack the problem during the initial EAA neurotransmitter agonist surge, and then modulate intracellular effects after the initial surge period.

Hypothermia may be used in association with pharmacological interventions aimed at attenuating the initial excitotoxic response, and also by enhancing inhibitory processes.

TBI produces widespread neuronal excitation causing prolonged, usually sublethal, pathological changes in neuronal activity which disrupt many functions, including memory. Inhibitory neurotransmitters such as GABA (gamma-aminobutyric acid) and the opiods may also be released with TBI to try to decrease the excitatory state.

Oxygen free radicals (OFRs) may also be important mediators of TBI and cerebral edema. Sources for oxygen free radicals include catecholamines, amine oxidases, and peroxidases, among others. Pharmacological agents being considered to decrease OFR damage include Vitamin E, DMSO, and lipid peroxidation inhibitors (Lazaroids).

Some conclusions can be drawn:

- Excitotoxic phenomena may render neurons dysfunctional, but not necessarily kill them.
- TBI results in widespread depolarization and nonspecific release of many excitatory and inhibitory neurotransmitters.
- Significant changes in the BBB are found.
- The resultant sublethal toxicity appears to be mediated via increases in intracellular calcium levels.
- There are three subtypes of glutamate receptors: NMDA, Quisqualate, and Kainate.
- The NMDA receptors may protect against TBI secondary to trauma and cerebral ischemia.
- Cholinergic systems have roles in mediation of TBI and neuronal recovery, including behavioral suppression. Long-term motor deficits may be decreased by the ACH medications blocking release of excitotoxins.

- Catecholamines (especially norepinephrine) appear to help in TBI recovery.
- Alpha noradrenergic agonists and probably dopaminergic agonists accelerated motor recovery after experimental injury to the sensorimotor cortex. Their antagonists retarded recovery.
- Early post-injury use of benzodiazipines may slow neural recovery and possible restoration of neural recovery.
- Most likely, "therapeutic cocktails" of more than one agent will probably be necessary for appropriate treatment of TBI.

Now, let's look at some of the more pertinent information dealing with the effects of TBI on the neuropharmacological environment of the brain.

BIOGENIC AMINES AND THE ENDOGENOUS OPIATE SYSTEM

Acute traumatic injury of any type will engender the production of beta-endorphin (BE) as well as other endogenous opiates. One group looked at BE levels in the blood after trauma and found, to little surprise, that there was no correlation between serum BE and pain severity.[237] When looking at cerebral spinal fluid (CSF) BE levels, it was discovered that significant changes in CSF BE levels are found in patients with the full range of TBI, mild to severe. Interestingly, the patients with mild TBI had significantly higher levels of BE than those with severe head trauma. The BE levels did not correlate with early prognosis.[238]

Another group of patients had lumbar punctures done on days 1, 4, and 7, post head injury, and the levels of leucine, or leu-enkephalin (LENK), and methianine, or met-enkephalin (MENK), were determined in the CSF. It was found that MENK levels were constantly elevated, while LENK levels decreased in patients with GCS scores of 8 or less, and might provide a poor prognostic factor. It was indicated that LENK and MENK appeared to be linked to different pathophysiological functions.[239]

While endogenous opiates are found in the human gut, BE is produced in the hypothalamus. It is broken down to the smaller forms of endogenous opiates, LENK and MENK. It would therefore be more likely to be found in the CSF, along with enkephalins and dynorphins, which together help mediate the central perception of pain.

Primary metabolites of norepinephrine (methoxyhydroxyphenylglycol- MHPG), serotonin (5-hydroxyindole-acetic acid- 5HIAA), and dopamine (homovanillic acid- HVA) were assayed in CSF taken from comatose patients after severe head injury. Samples were taken within days of the injury, and again after clinical improvement (13/20 patients) or deterioration (7/20 patients) was seen. Clinical improvement was associated with significant decreases in HVA and 5HIAA. The levels of all three metabolites remained high in patients who deteriorated. These results appeared to indicate that increased turnover of CNS neurotransmitters in severe head injury normalized during recovery.[240]

In another study, CSF levels of serotonin (5-HT), substance P (SP), and lipid peroxidation (LPx) products were measured in patients with TBI and compared to controls. The levels of SP and 5-HT in patients with head trauma were lower than those found in controls. The CSF LPx products were significantly increased in the TBI patients. There was no correlation between the CSF levels and the GCS at admission.[241]

The loss or decrement of cholinergic neurotransmission has been implicated in both cognitive dysfunction and memory impairment after TBI. One group looked at presynaptic markers related to cholinergic neurotransmission via choline acetyltransferase activity, as well as high-affinity nicotinic receptor binding sites in the inferior temporal gyrus, cingulate gyrus, and superior parietal cortex in postmortem brains. They found that the correlation of choline acetyltransferase activity with synaptophysin immunoreactivity revealed a deficit of cholinergic presynaptic terminals in the postmortem human brain after TBI.[242]

An inverse relationship between plasma norepinephrine and thyroid hormones is found in patients with hyper- or hypothyroidism, or severe stress. Head-injured patients were found to have low thyroxine (T4), low triiodothyronine (T3), and high reverse T3. When phenytoin was used for seizure control, T3 and T4 were lowered, but thyroid-stimulating hormone was increased. In these patients there was no correlation between NE and T3.[243]

A great deal of evidence indicates that dopamine neurotransmission dysfunction after mild to moderate TBI is involved in the induction of posttraumatic memory deficits. Using anesthetized animals that were given mild traumatic brain injuries, it was found that mice were impaired in task performance. They had prolonged latencies for finding and drinking in a retention test and retest. If these animals were injected with haloperidol 15 minutes post trauma, they had a shortened latency in both of the tests, which appeared to show that the use of dopamine receptor antagonists was beneficial for recovery of posttraumatic memory dysfunction. Looking closer at the receptor sites, a D1 receptor antagonist, SCH-23390, was used, as was sulpiride, a D2 receptor antagonist, in the same experimental protocol. The use of sulpiride, but not SCH-23390, improved the deficits in task performance, indicating that the D2 receptors were the major sites of action. A positive interaction was noted when both D1 and D2 receptor antagonists were given together at individually subtherapeutic levels, indicating that interaction between the two receptors was involved. The dopaminergic mechanisms appear to contribute to memory dysfunction after TBI.[244]

NEUROPHARMACOLOGICAL DATA — CLINICAL FACTS

I've already mentioned the excitotoxic theory of cell damage and death. Research has focused on this aspect of TBI because of the possibility of providing a pharmacological response to decrease the excitotoxic injury.

Glutamate is one of the prime "suspects" in excitotoxic injury. We know it is a part of the post-TBI neuropharmacological cascade that produces injury. Glutamate release, which forms a significant part of the net release of cerebral amino acids, appears to be impaired in patients with head injury, with or without other associated injuries. When the brain is injured, other aspects of normal neuroendocrine function are disrupted. For example, hepatic glucose production and hypoglutaminemia are more pronounced in injured patients with associated TBI.[245]

Profound hypoglutaminemia is frequently seen in TBI patients and may be caused by the diminished release of glutamine from the brain to the systemic circulation. At the same time, glutamine in the brain is producing neuronal injury and death secondary to overproduction. When looking at the relationship in plasma of glutamine, and the product of its precursor, glutamate, the ratio of these chemicals is reduced in the plasma post TBI. It may be secondary to defective amidation of glutamine, as GABA is only minimally effected. Nutritional support should increase the release of glutamine from the brain.[246]

Anaerobic glycolysis with increased lactate production and release of excitatory amino acids into the extracellular space is seen in both primary TBI and secondary ischemic/hypoxic injury. Induction of a thiopental coma (barbiturate coma) will decrease ICP. This is also associated, in one study, by a 37% reduction of lactate, 59% reduction of glutamate, and 66% decrease in aspartate in the cerebral extracellular spaces.[247]

Again, in spite of the excitotoxicity of glutamate as a putative mechanism of secondary damage, no dose-response relationship has been found in relation to CSF glutamate concentrations and severity of injury, degree of electrophysiological deterioration, or prediction of clinical outcome in severely brain-injured patients.[248] We are left with the important question of whether this is also true in mild and moderate TBI.

Another important question is the timing of the neuro-metabolic cascade(s) and their duration. When looking at the CSF of comatose patients, high levels of the excitatory amino acid glutamate are found. Possibly more importantly, these severely brain injured patients are exposed to high concentrations of this excitotoxic amino acid for days following initial injury.[249] Treatment with an appropriate antagonist may be very beneficial.

Another excitotoxin, quinolinic acid, is a tryptophan- derived, N-methyl-D-aspartate (NMDA) agonist produced by macrophages and microglia. A large increase in the CSF concentration of quinolinic acid is found after TBI.[250] Again, it is possibly another place to intervene, or interfere, with the damage via the use of an appropriate antagonist.

The principal glucose transporter at the BBB is the Glut1 isoform, and the transporter density is thought to be an index of the cerebral metabolic rate. Using quantitative electron microscopic analysis, a Glut1 density is observed in capillaries from acutely injured brains. This appears to be seen concomitantly with BBB dysfunction.[251] In other analyses via positron emission tomography (PET) and L-[11c]methylmethionine (11c-MET) for assessment of amino acid accumulation, it is noted that focal increases of 11c-MET were mild. They could be seen in a core area of ischemia, indicating BBB breakdown, with a poor prognosis for the tissue. Focal increases are also seen during or after ischemic compromise in areas of focal cerebral infarction, possibly representing changes in amino acid transport or changes of protein synthesis in brain tissue that will recover.[252]

The determination of prognosis soon after initial TBI is a major goal. One approach is to evaluate the role of the sympatho-adrenal system (SAS) and hypo-thalamo-pituitary-adrenocortical system (HPAS) after TBI via the relationships of plasma epinephrine (E), norepinephrine (NE), adrenocorticotropic hormone (ACTH), and cortisol levels, along with clinical condition. The degree of activation of these systems appears to depend on the severity of TBI. An inverse correlation between the levels of E, NE, and the GCS was found, indicative of the severity of injury. ACTH and cortisol levels were also related to clinical condition. Catecholamines and ACTH levels were low in severely brain-injured patients who also had significant findings on CAT scan in the mesencephalic-diencephalic area.[253] It is helpful to remember that ACTH and beta-endorphin are found in the same hypothalamic neurons.

Neuroendrocrine function studies performed on patients an average of 6.3 years after trauma, specifically the combined pituitary anterior lobe test, showed dysfunction in the somatotropic, adrenocorticotropic axis, as well as a decrement in FSH secretion. There were no specific hypothalamic injuries noted on neuroradiological testing.[254]

The use of alcohol is one of the possible instigators of TBI. After TBI, alcohol decreases sympatho-adrenal activation post TBI. It changes the rise in catecholamine levels post TBI in a dose-dependent manner, and changes the relationship between neurological dysfunction and sympathetic nervous system activation.[255] In patients with acute brain injury who did not lose consciousness in a motor vehicle accident, alcohol intoxication induced a significant elevation in serum ionized calcium and magnesium. The Ica2+/Img2+ ratio is a sign of increased vascular tone and reactivity, and it was significantly increased in intoxicated patients.[256] This group of patients, alcohol abusers post TBI who are at risk for the Wernicke-Korsakoff syndrome, may also have a thiamine deficiency, which would necessitate thiamine prophylaxis.[257]

As with many things, glucose metabolism in patients post TBI has its good and bad aspects. Remember that glucose metabolism is one of the most important sources of energy for the brain. When metabolized, glucose will increase lactic acid. The administration of glucose during the early recovery period after severe head injury is a major cause of suppressed ketogenesis, and can increase production of lactic acid by the injured brain by decreasing the availability of nonglycolytic energy substrates.[258]

The PET scan, using [18F]-2-deoxyglucose, can evaluate the state of glucose metabolism in the different areas of the brain. Looking at mild traumatic brain injury patients, and comparing glucose metabolism, neuropsychological testing, and continuing behavioral dysfunction, retrospectively, several interesting observations were made. Abnormal cerebral metabolic rates of glucose (rLCMs) were found, most prominently in the midtemporal, anterior cingulate, precuneus, anterior temporal, frontal white matter, and corpus callosum regions of the brain. The abnormal rLCMs were significantly correlated with overall clinical complaints, particularly with problems with attention and concentration, and with overall neuropsychological test abnormalities. It appears that even mild TBI patients may express continuing brain behavioral deficits. Using the PET scan can help elucidate dysfunctional brain regions in patients with neurobehavioral problems, and specific cerebral areas may correlate with deficits in daily neurobehavioral functioning as well as neuropsychological test results.[259]

There are a lot of pieces to the neuropharmacological puzzle. The more we recognize them, the more we can hope to put all of the pieces together in a coherent way.

When the cell surface molecule Fas is triggered by its agonist Fas ligand, the result is apoptosis of the cells and tissue destruction. Levels of Fas ligand in the CSF of patients with severe brain injury are very high. This chemical is not found in the CSF of controls, including injured patients without brain injury. The Fas-Fas ligand system may be very important in inducing local tissue destruction and edema in the brain after a severe brain injury.[260]

Protein S-100 is a calcium binding protein that is synthesized in astroglial cells throughout the central nervous system. Serum levels of this protein were evaluated in two groups of patients after mild traumatic brain injury. While no overall cognitive dysfunction was found on neuropsychological testing, there were specific dysfunctions in reaction time, attention, and speed of information processing. The Protein S-100, when present in serum, may be indicative of diffuse brain damage. It may also be prognostic for long-lasting neurocognitive deficits after minor TBI.[261,262]

After TBI, cerebral tissue acidosis appears to play a role in the traumatic neurochemical cascade. Mild brain tissue acidosis can recover within hours of experimental injury. However, hypoxia combined with trauma produces relative ischemia that exacerbates the acidosis, from which recovery may not be possible.[263]

Plasma and CSF nitrite and nitrate concentrations are indicators of nitric oxide production. Increases in CSF nitrites and nitrates peak within a day or two after a severe TBI, with the highest concentrations correlating with nonsurvivors, linking CSF nitric oxide with injury severity and death.[264]

Earlier we talked about glucose as an energy source for the brain. Another major source of metabolic energy is adenosine triphosphate, or ATP. After it is used, it becomes ADP, and then AMP as the bonds with the phosphate atoms are broken. In comatose patients, cerebral blood flow (CBF) and oxidative metabolism become uncoupled. Adenosine can produce cerebral vasodilatation and decrease neuronal activity, and may mediate this uncoupling. This association between increased CSF adenosine and reduced global cerebral extraction of oxygen is indicative of a regulatory role for adenosine in the balance between CBF and oxidative and nonoxidative metabolism after severe TBI in humans. It is possible that hyperglycolysis or occult ischemic foci are sources of ATP breakdown and adenosine formation. It also appears that adenosine is playing a neuroprotective role.[265,266]

Thrombin, the proteolytic enzyme for the blood coagulation cascade, affects multiple cell types, including neurons and astrocytes; in these cells it prevents process outgrowth, and can induce significant morphological degeneration and cell death. Thrombin is synthesized in the central nervous system along with prothrombin, its precursor. It appears that prothrombin may gain access to the CSF via an intact or compromised BBB, in amounts increasing with age. CSF levels of prothrombin are reduced in TBI patients.[267] Erythropoietin (EPO) has been found to be produced in the brain of humans. EPO concentrations in CSF appear to correlate with the degree of BBB dysfunction. EPO may function as a protective factor against hypoxia-induced neuronal damage.[268]

There appear to be an ever-increasing number of CSF markers regarding the extent of brain injury. These include neuron-specific enolase (NSE), creatine kinase (CK), creatine kinase BB isoenzyme (CK-BB), lactate dehydrogenase (LDH), gamma-glutamyltransferase, aldolase, and leucine aminopeptidase (LAP). In CSF there is a significant correlation between the severity of brain trauma and levels of CK, CK-BB, LDH, LAP, and aldolase. Significant plasma and CSF levels of NSE have also been found in patients with major brain injury and appear to be reliable indicators of the degree of brain damage; they may also provide an early prognostic indicator.[269-271]

We talked about the beta-amyloid precursor protein above. It appears that beta-APP is a marker for diffuse axonal injury. Beta-APP may also be found in non-traumatically injured brains, including those with Alzheimer's disease and Down's syndrome. Only specific forms of beta-APP were found in the latter two disorders.[272-276]

The immune system can be our friend. It can also be responsible for some of the most horrible disorders known to man, including AIDS, multiple sclerosis, and systemic lupus erethematosis. The significance of the immune system changes post TBI are emerging, and may present us with one of our best opportunities to obtain treatment, or at least some ability to ameliorate the destructive secondary TBI processes.

The intracellular adhesion molecule-1 (ICAM-1) is expressed by endothelial cells and is very important for the promotion of adhesion and transmigration of circulating leukocytes across the BBB. After these immunocompetent cells migrate into the central nervous system, they release mediators that stimulate glial and endothelial cells to express ICAM-1 and release cytokines, which may also induce cerebral damage. After this activation, proteolytic activity cleaves the membrane-anchored ICAM-1, resulting in measurable levels of soluble ICAM-1, which is found in high levels in the CSF of patients with significant cerebral damage and a dysfunctional BBB. Serum sICAM-1 is found to correlate to neurological outcome and the GCS score, suggesting that the inflammatory response of the CNS to TBI may be detrimental to the patient. This indicates another possible avenue of therapy.[277, 278]

Cerebral lesions may affect nonspecific immune responses. That neutrophil activation exacerbates brain injury is known. It may be possible to find a medication therapy that can induce a transient suppression of neutrophil function and decrease associated secondary damage. Complement proteins associated with immunological events have been found in the CSF of patients with severe traumatic brain injury, secondary to BBB dysfunction. They may also contribute to secondary cerebral damage.[279-281]

Tumor necrosis factor from traumatized cerebral parenchyma is found in high concentrations in the CSF of patients with severe brain injury. This may implicate the cytokines in cellular metabolic derangement post TBI.[282] Yes, the cytokine story is incomplete, but very important.

Cytokine receptors and receptor antagonists (RAs) have been identified in TBI patients. After TBI, as part of the immunological cascade, a sequential release of soluble cytokine receptors and RAs may exist. After subarachnoid hemorrhage, for example, an inflammatory reaction may lead to ischemic brain damage. Experimentally, ischemia is known to be connected with the alarm-reaction cytokines interleukin-1 receptor antagonist (IL-1Ra), and tumor necrosis factor-alpha (TNF-alpha). Both of these cytokines are known to induce fever, malaise, leukocytosis, and nitric oxide synthesis, as well as mediate ischemic and traumatic brain injury. High CSF levels of these cytokines correlate with brain damage.[284] Other studies indicate that severe head injury can cause cellular immune function suppression, with a resulting high rate of infection.[285-286]

Cytokines also play a role in nerve regeneration by modulating the synthesis of neurotrophic factors. Interleukin-6 (IL-6) promotes nerve growth factor (NGF) after brain injury. There is a concordance between the two, as the NGF is not found if the IL-6 levels are not high or not present.[287] IL-6 is found in markedly high concentrations after acute TBI, apparently produced by the intracranial cells.[288] IL-6 is also a mediator of the pathophysiological acute-phase response (initial proteins including C-reactive protein, alpha 1-antitrypsin, and fibrinogen). The high correlation between CSF and serum IL-6 is most probably secondary to a severe dysfunction of the BBB. The increase of IL-6 levels in CSF and serum is followed by a profound acute-phase immunological response.[289]

Elevations in CSF interleukin-8 and interleukin-12 both appear in the CSF in association with TBI. They are both made via intracerebral cytokine synthesis, and both appear important in the pathophysiology of TBI.[290-291] Impaired immunity is seen with lower levels of interleukin-12.[292]

BOTTOM LINE

Understanding the basic neuropharmacological data is needed to help the clinician in the development of an appropriate determination of the problem, as well as to help with possible treatment paradigms.

This information will, I believe, one day help in the development of new treatments, which is a Good Thing.

5 Clinical Aspects of MTBI

NOMENCLATURE

In spite of the BISIG definition of mild traumatic brain injury quoted in Chapter 1, questions still arise regarding the diagnosis/definitions of MTBI and the PCS. It has been stated that "minor" or "mild" traumatic brain injury is typically not, clinically, mild at all, as it may induce significant sequelae. Any injury to the most complex system in the human organism, the brain, is rarely if ever truly mild.

The terminology, or nomenclature — mild or minor — by themselves may indicate to those who are not cognizant of the reality that the problem is relatively innocuous, unimportant, or insignificant. A minor laceration is certainly not a cause for alarm, and sutures may not even be necessary. Mild or minor abnormalities found in blood workups may mean nothing and may even be functions of laboratory or test errors.

When a patient is determined to have a "minor" or "mild" traumatic brain injury, the terminology alone may convey the wrong message to clinical and nonclinical people (insurance folk, for example) who are not experienced in dealing with brain injury.

The classification comes originally from the GCS scoring: minor or mild is 13–15; moderate, 8 to 12; and severe, 3 to 7. *These terms relate to the level of coma, and **not** necessarily the severity of the sequelae.*

It becomes easy, unfortunately, to see that the current terminology may possibly hinder treatment.

THE CLINICAL PICTURE

Remember the statistics: an estimated 400,000–500,000 patients are hospitalized in the United States for head trauma each year. Between 60 to 82% of all admissions to the hospital are for head trauma.[94,114,293] These numbers do not include those patients who visit an emergency room secondary to trauma, and who have suffered an injury to their brain which is not visible or even noticed in the typical ER frenzy to help a patient with multiple trauma. The number of patients who experience a minor concussion and/or head trauma who never even make it into an emergency room is felt to be significantly higher, possibly as high as 2,000,000 patients per year.[294] Economically, costs are felt to exceed $3.9 billion per year.[295] This figure does not take into account the non-economic costs of vocational, familial, and social morbidity.

These facts account for the term frequently used for patients with MTBI: members of the "silent epidemic."[296]

CLINICAL EVALUATION

After an injury, with direct or indirect trauma from accidental injury such as a slip and fall or an acceleration/deceleration injury, a patient's choices bifurcate. Many decide to go to the emergency room, particularly those who experienced a loss of consciousness. Many do not.

The problems encountered by those patients who do not go to an emergency room magnify, particularly if they do not see their primary care physicians within a day or so after injury. When these patients finally seek medical attention it is because they have had problems — with memory, balance, or emotional lability — but otherwise do not show physical evidence of an acute injury. These are the unfortunates who are told that their problems are referable to psychiatric etiologies. They begin their health care odyssey and their problems accumulate almost logarithmically. Finding someone who even believes that they have the problems they describe can be difficult. Many need to find an attorney to help them receive any help at all. And that only works if their insurance company recognizes the medical entity of MTBI.

The patient who goes to the emergency room is evaluated for what can be seen, and the signs and symptoms noted by the patient. A simple mental status examination is typically done, which may or may not be abnormal, and, because of the nature of emergency room medicine, is typically not as thorough as it will be when the patient sees a neurologist or rehabilitation specialist. Appropriate examination may or may not show clinical abnormalities. If it does, the patient may be kept overnight or on a 23-hour hold for observation.

Most patients are sent home with a sheet of appropriate precautions: they should be awakened frequently, if they have problems with waking up, vomiting, diplopia, etc., they should immediately go back to the emergency room. A cerebral CAT scan may be done, particularly if a skull fracture is suspected.

The patient may be given pain medications for musculoskeletal pain or for more severe problems such as a concurrently broken bone. The patient is told to see their primary care physician if they have further problems. This may or may not occur within several days or so. If their symptoms persist, and the PCP is unsure why, the patient may be sent for a neurological evaluation.

In patients with a suspected MTBI, neurological history is best performed with the patient and any significant others who can verbalize what, if any, difficulties they have witnessed. This may be particularly important in patients who exhibit varying degrees of denial, as well as patients who are emotionally labile and unable to adequately describe the problems they are having.

Prior to doing any form of mental status examination, some rapport must be established. You should know something about the patient's job, what they do, and what the job entails. You do not want to embarrass the patient, but you must be able to determine levels of function. These, in turn, must be evaluated in relationship to the patient's level of education.

When I was in medical school and residency, one of the professors used to regularly astound me when he would speak to patients. If the patient bound books for a living, this man could ask pertinent questions which revealed that he also knew at least enough about book binding to question the patient specifically about how he or she functioned in his or her job. This neurologist, Dr. Benjamin Boshes, taught me and the other students and residents that knowing what you could about all aspects of patients' lives was extremely important in helping to determine true function. Being well-read and knowing disparate information on topics as diverse as working in a slaughterhouse, binding books, working on the railroad, and so on, really is important in helping to determine function.

The actual neurological examination must be done in a manner such that you can inspect as well as touch a patient. In the initial examination, in patients with complaints of pain, you want to determine if there are any musculoskeletal problems. You must look at the patient's back and shoulders and determine if there is a difference in the levels of the acromioclavicular joints. You must palpate and determine if there are trigger points indicative of a myofascial pain syndrome.

Balance must be tested. Aside from gait and station, heel-toe, and tandem gait, hopping on one leg is good. If the patient complains of dizziness, you must try to determine if there is a musculoskeletal aspect to the complaint. Palpate for trigger points in the sternocleidomastoid muscles. If you find any, warn the patient that you may cause some discomfort, then press on the trigger points. In many cases the patient will report immediate exacerbation of their feelings of dizziness, even vertigo. In many cases, a full evaluation of dizziness must be done.

Cranial nerve examination should concentrate on the areas most likely to be injured. All 12 should be checked, of course. But remembering that the sixth cranial nerve is the longest and, therefore, most likely to be injured from trauma should make the eye examination for movement very thorough. The senses of smell and taste are "connected." (Remember the last time you had an upper respiratory infection?) So, checking for ageusea should go along with testing for anosmia. Loss of the sense of smell may occur after an acceleration/deceleration injury, as the brain is thrust forward and backward, and the cribiform plate can sever the sensory fibers of the second cranial nerve.

Check cerebellar function carefully. Disdiadokokinesis is only one aspect. Rapid alternating movements are most often just a bit off — typically on one side more than the other.

Reflex examination must go beyond the typical deep tendon reflexes. Physicians who know what to look for and, even more importantly, how to look for them, will check carefully for abnormal frontal lobe reflexes, such as the palmomental reflexes, as well as suck and snout and jaw jerk.

If the patient has a history of altered sensorium or loss of consciousness, or proclaims cognitive problems with memory, concentration, multitasking, information processing, or behavioral changes, including emotional lability, or increased irritability, or demonstrates to the examining physician problems with pragmatics, the patient should be sent for further workup to determine the presence or absence of the cognitive/emotional sequelae of an MTBI. This further evaluation is typically performed weeks or even months after the initial insult.

On the other hand, this may or may not be a bad thing. As we discussed in the last chapter, the pathophysiological changes that occur after an MTBI may last for days or weeks. The resultant deficits may therefore not become manifest for more weeks or months. This leads to an important consideration: what if the patient complains of cognitive or emotional problems within days or several weeks of the initial insult? First of all, is the patient experiencing all of the problems that are going to arise from the injury, or only those that have been detected at that time? Secondly, you can see a good reason for considering serial neurological examinations.

MYTH-TAKE #1

Somehow it has become an "urban medical legend" that all patients with an MTBI will miraculously be healed within three months. This may be true for a simple majority of patients who are not experiencing a significant MTBI. However, anywhere from 5% to 20% of these patients do not get "all better" in three months, or even twelve months.

As the clinician takes his or her history of cognitive problems, the clinician may also find frequent complaints of posttraumatic myofascial or soft tissue pain problems, including posttraumatic headache, cervical pain, low back pain, and sleep disorder.

If the patient who complains of pain is seen soon after the injury, physical therapy may be all that is needed to stop these problems before the onset of chronicity, with its attendant affective and neurochemical alterations. The use of narcotic analgesics should be strongly discouraged, as they may further enhance cognitive difficulties. If after 6 to 12 weeks there is no significant diminution of the pain and/or headache, along with depression, consideration of a specialty pain program should be given, as long as the pain practitioner understands the effects of TBI on pain.

There is an interesting dichotomy in the majority of patients with pain and MTBI. Patients in an interdisciplinary pain program are typically taught to rate their pain, on a momentary basis, on a zero (no pain) to 10 or 100 scale. When they begin treatment, the numbers are typically high and correspond with physical findings of muscle spasm, trigger points, and loss of specific function such as decreased range of motion or weakness. As treatment progresses, typically during four to six weeks, the patient's pain complaints may not change; that is, their identification of their pain level (such as 7 over 10) may not change or may change only minimally, while functional evaluation will reveal a return to a normal range of motion, for example, or absent palpable muscle spasm or trigger points.

It is extremely important to realize that this dichotomy is NOT a manifestation of malingering, but appears to be more of a learned or even perseverative response. On observation, pain behaviors are diminished and the patients' affect is improved, but they may still claim to endure what appears to be an artificially high pain level. Evaluation must be *functional* in nature, not subjective. Even more important, in the presence of severe pain, a neuropsychological evaluation or cognitive evaluation will not be accurate and should not be performed. This means, MTBI patients with pain should have their pain ameliorated and their depression lifted as much as possible prior to any cognitive evaluation and/or treatment.

NEUROLOGICAL TESTING

There are various types of tests that should be done for specific indications. You should not "shotgun" tests; have a reason for doing them.

CAT SCAN

- Superior to MRI for the diagnosis of subarachnoid hemorrhage and fractures
- Relatively insensitive to many lesions after trauma
- Best at identification of:
  - * Hematoma
  - * Ventricular enlargement
  - * Atrophy
  Note that except for various types of hematoma, the CAT scan is useful for evaluating chronic anatomical changes
- Useful in screening patients with GCS scores of 13 to 15, brief loss of consciousness, posttraumatic amnesia
- Major question is timing: Remember that patients may appear stable for hours after an injury, have a negative cat scan, and then neurologically decompensate secondary to a bleed-hematoma, subarachoid hemorrhage, etc. In select patients, serial cat scans are necessary.

CAT scans are very useful to rule out acute intracranial pathology, particularly skull fractures and hemorrhage. The vast majority of research indicates that patients with negative neurological examinations and GCS scores of 15 along with negative CAT scans can be sent home for observation by family or friends. The patients with skull fractures and no neurological signs may be sent home, if necessary. It has also been noted that initially negative CAT scans may become positive within 12–24 hours, secondary to hemorrhage associated with the patient's clinical deterioration.[297-304]

From the beginning of its use, the CAT scan was found to be extremely useful, particularly by reducing the number of burr-holes placed without worsening long-term results.[305]

CAT scan technology has also markedly improved. A number of studies have been done to determine the diagnostic course of the traumatizing force in acceleration/deceleration injury. Lesions deep in the brain in the areas of "inner cerebral trauma" appeared to indicate the presence of possible lesions in other locations within the known pattern of ICT (see Chapter 4). Minimal traumatic brain lesions are frequently seen in ICT or in all cases where the acceleration of traumatizing forces has an antero-posterior or postero-anterior direction, including coup and contre-coup lesions. Deep cerebral lesions were typically not seen with latero-lateral acceleration forces.[306, 307] When acceleration forces have acted along the long axis of the head (centroaxial), multiple lesions have been found in the majority of cases. These lesions were most frequently found in the frontal and temporal lobes. It has been noted that CAT scan may be useful for reconstruction of the site of impact and the course of the force of injury, which may have both prognostic and forensic implications.[308]

An interesting study gives us fairly intuitive information. Patients with normal CAT scans were more likely to have mild neurological dysfunction or none at all. A positive relationship between lesion size and both plasma epinephrine and norepinephrine was found.[309]

Sixty-seven (9.4%) of 712 patients who experienced amnesia or loss of consciousness and had perfect GCS scores (15) had acute traumatic lesions found on CAT scan. Two required neurosurgical intervention, and one patient died. To say it another way, intracranial lesions cannot be totally excluded clinically in patients with mild TBI who have histories of amnesia or a short period of loss of consciousness, even when the GCS is 15.[310]

The advent of the CAT scan has also all but eliminated the need for skull films to be performed in the emergency room. As previously indicated, some patients are being sent home for observation even with skull fractures.[311,312]

MRI SCAN

- More sensitive to nonhemorrhagic lesions
- Has greater efficacy in detecting diffuse axonal or shearing injury, as well as cortical contusions
- Questionable correlation between lesions found on MRI and neuropsychological testing

Cerebral MRI consistently finds more intracranial lesions than CAT scans.[313,314] Discrete areas of cerebral edema missed by the CAT scan are typically seen on MRI, along with white matter lesions which are not picked up by the CAT scan.[315,316,317] There is also the possibility that the MRI can better identify lesions which may be compatible with neuropsychological findings than CAT scan.[318,319]

In patients with MTBI, MRI can demonstrate diffuse axonal injury in those with normal CAT scan findings. Could these lesions be the primary pathophysiological substrate for the postconcussion syndrome?[320]

MRI can also be used for cerebral volumetric studies. In this way, the more predictable atrophic changes, which are time dependent, can be quantified using MRI volumetric determinations. These in turn may give some indication of functional cognitive changes.[321]

We've mentioned disruption of the BBB post TBI. MRI scanning enhanced with Gadolinium has not detected increased cerebrovascular permeability within 96 hours post injury.[322] Other studies, as previously discussed, do document BBB disruption.

Thatcher and his group[323] evaluated the biophysical linkage between MRI and EEG amplitude after a closed head injury. Their findings were consistent with clinical EEG studies showing white matter lesions are associated with increased delta wave amplitude, and gray matter lesions are related to decreased EEG alpha and beta wave amplitude. Both findings correlated with diminished cognitive abilities in 19 TBI patients. It was felt that these results correlated with a biophysical linkage between the state of cerebral protein-lipid structures (as noted via lengthened gray matter T2 weighted relation time on MRI) and the scalp-recorded EEG.

A man developed mild cerebral dysfunction after being struck by lightning. MRI showed multiple foci of hyperintensity on long TR images found throughout the supratentorial white matter.[324]

BOTTOM LINE

For initial evaluation, CAT scan is most appropriate. It may need to be repeated within a 12- to 24-hour period in specific patients. The MRI is most appropriate for later evaluation, particularly for white matter lesions indicative of axonal damage.

PET SCAN

- The method of choice for measurement of regional cerebral blood flow (rCBF)
- In general, PET abnormalities more closely corresponded to site and extent of cerebral dysfunction noted on neurological and neuropsychological examinations: late CAT scan is typically consistent with earlier PET findings
- PET has demonstrated that the frontal and temporal lobes were most vulnerable to TBI in spite of absence of focal lesions on CAT scan or MRI
- Can show problems with cerebral metabolism beyond visualized structural abnormalities
- Can show neurotransmitter function in local or regional areas

The PET scan is an extremely facile test, the total limits of which have not yet been found. Currently, it is mostly used for research, as the cost factors remain high. Its research potential is enormous.

In one study, a half-dozen bank officials were shown a video of a jointly experienced armed bank robbery, as well as a control video. Using the PET scan, it was found that traumatic stimulation increased rCBF bilaterally in the primary and secondary visual cortex, the posterior gyrus cinguli, and the left orbitofrontal cortex, as compared to the control simulation. Decreased rCBF was noted in Broca's area, the left angular guyrus, and the left operculum as well as the secondary somatosensory cortex. This demonstrated that the visual reexperience of a robbery is associated with altered activity in the paralimbic and cortical brain regions that involve cognition and affect.[325]

After an acceleration/deceleration injury in a motor vehicle accident, with cervical and back pain immediately reported, a child experienced neurobehavioral symptoms over the next two years, including "staring spells." The child's symptoms continued and, after four years, a more extensive workup was done. The child had a negative standard EEG, but two positive ambulatory EEG's with epileptiform activity. A PET scan showed marked hypometabolism in both temporal lobes, which was consistent with neuropsychological test results that showed verbal and visual memory deficits with a high average intellegence.[326]

Cerebral hyperglycosis is the pathophysiological response to injury-induced ionic and neurochemical cascades. PET scan has demonstrated that hyperglycosis occurs both regionally and globally after a severe head injury in humans.[327]

Part of the interest in this test is what more it can show in patients with an MTBI, both prognostically as well as clinically, particularly in patients with a normal neurological examination and normal GCS immediately post injury. We shall have to wait and see.

SPECT SCAN

- For regional CBF mapping, typically using 99mtc hexamethyl propylene amine oxime (HMPAO)
- Measures relative perfusion, not absolute, which may be a "limitation"
- Is a functional technique and may therefore show abnormalities with a closer relationship to neuropsychological deficits than structural methods (CAT scan, MRI)
- May demonstrate functional residuals of structural lesions
- SPECT/PET may document rCBF and regional metabolism, as well as distribution of specific neurotransmitters and receptors

The SPECT scan appears to be useful in determining cerebral dysfunction in the morphologically normal brain and showing objective evidence which appears to account for the clinical presentation of patients with chronic symptoms post TBI. These areas of damage also appear to give objective evidence from impaired neuropsychological testing results. While the SPECT scan looks at rCBF it picks up more lesions than the CAT scan, detecting abnormalities in patients with a history of MTBI.[328-332] It may also predict late deterioration in patients with a history of or who appear to have an impending intracerebral hematoma.[333]

Functional assessment of MTBI has been attempted using SPECT and neuropsychological testing. Statistical analysis in one study found that neuropsychological testing performance predicted SPECT findings, but SPECT findings did not always correlate with test performance.[334] On the other hand, in severe TBI patients, SPECT findings correlated well between frontal lobe blood flow indices and disinhibited behavior. The severity of disinhibition was increased with lower frontal lobe blood flow rates. A weaker correlation was found between flow indices of the left cerebral hemisphere and social isolation. Low CBF rates of the right brain appeared to be related to aggressive behavior.[335]

In 41 MATBI patients without loss of consciousness and normal CAT scan, 28 had abnormal SPECT scans with focal areas of hypoperfusion seen in a larger group of 228 mild and moderate TBI patients, with abnormalities found in the basal ganglia and thalami (55.2%), frontal lobes (23.8%), temporal lobes (13%), parietal lobes (3.7%), and insular and occipital lobes (4.6%).[336]

Prognostic aspects of SPECT appear to be intriguing. In one study, CBF in the initial 48 hours post injury varied greatly and was not correlated with severity and prognosis.[337] In another study, SPECT appeared to be a promising method for a more sensitive evaluation of axial cerebral lesions in patients with mild to moderate TBI.[338]

A normal initial SPECT scan done within 4 weeks of trauma may be a reliable test to exclude significant clinical sequelae of MTBI, while at 12 months post injury a positive SPECT is also a reliable indicator of a decreased functional clinical outcome. This is also true for patients with prolonged postconcussive syndrome sequelae.[339-340]

Evoked Potentials

- Probably not sensitive enough to document physiological problems, even in patients with active symptoms
- Question of timing — multimodal evoked potentials (MED), brainstem auditory evoked responses (BAER), visual evoked responses (VER), and somatosensory evoked responses (SSEP) typically not done early enough

In general, long latency cortical auditory evoked responses (CAERs) are better able to reflect the extent and degree of cerebral dysfunction than the short latency auditory nerve and brainstem-evoked responses (BAERs). [241] Intermediate (0–60 ms) and long latency (0–500 ms) somatosensory-evoked patients (SEPs) were correlated with TBI patients. Long latency SEPs correlated well when clinical disability was measured by the disability rating scale; the intermediate latency SEPs did not. The long latency SEP patterns seemed to better reflect the extent and severity of brain dysfunction and clinical condition than did the intermediate SEPs for severe TBI patients.[342] The BAER may provide some indirect evidence for the biophysical changes as well as biochemical changes (serum creatine kinase) after the occurrence of posttraumatic cerebral edema. The SEP may also help determine the severity of the edema.[343]

Event-related P300 potentials reflect cognitive functions such as stimulus discrimination (N250), processing time (P300 latencies), and attention capabilities (P300 amplitudes). In noninjured patients, women showed a greater and perhaps earlier P300 latency increase during aging than males, indicating a rather mild cognitive decline that does not increase before old age.[344] In patients with frontal lobe injuries/lesions, there is a significant reduction in P300 amplitude at the anterior, but not the posterior aspects of the electrode montage. This would indicate that the P300 wave potential is dependent upon the prefrontal cortical regions. Other diatheses, such as schizophrenia with a presumed prefrontal dysfunction, show similar amplitude reductions.[345]

Abnormal visual P300 latencies are found in patients with mild cognitive complaints without neurological findings.[346] The cognitive auditory-evoked potential (latency and amplitude of the P300) both has and has not been found to be effective in the MTBI population as a parameter or marker for cerebral dysfunction.[347-351]

Multimodal-evoked potentials (MEPs) including brainstem auditory, visual, and somatosensory-evoked potentials have been reported to be helpful in predicting outcome in severe closed head injury. BAERs have been demonstrated to be abnormal in 10%-40% of MTBI patients. While patients may have had symptoms consistent with MTBI when MEPs were done, the MEPs were not sensitive to quantifying the associated physiological changes associated with deficits in memory, lethargy, and labile emotionality after MTBI.[352]

A group of 40 MTBI patients were evaluated serially with brainstem trigeminal and auditory-evoked potentials (BTEP and BAEP), as well as middle-latency auditory evoked-potentials (MLAEP). All three evoked responses showed markedly increased latencies at the initial evaluation, indicative of disseminated axonal damage. Only the MLAEPs appeared to correlate to outcome at three months, particularly in its psychocognitive aspects, suggesting that organic diencephalic-paraventricular primary damage may account for these symptoms.[353]

In another study, 26 MTBI patients were evaluated via BAERs, reaction-time testing, and EEG. Posttraumatic symptoms persisted in half of the patients at six weeks and six months at follow-up. There were decrements in BAER conduction time in about half of the group, which remained static at the six-month time period. The findings were felt to indicate three patterns of recovery: half recovering within six weeks; a minority having persistent brainstem dysfunction over six months; and less than a third of the patients showing symptom exacerbation with no evidence of brainstem dysfunction, possibly secondary to psychological and/or social factors.[354]

Alcohol usage post TBI shows, via event-related potentials, that there is a measurable impact on electrophysiological correlates of cognition.[355]

Visual-evoked potentials (VEPs) (P100) were evaluated in a group of ten TBI patients and compared with ten normal controls. The amplitude of the VEP is a function of cortical binocular integration, which is influenced by dysfunction of the ambient visual process in the posttrauma vision syndrome (PTVS). The latter is characterized by difficulties with binocular function, possibly secondary to dysfunction of the ambient visual process, which is part of the sensory-motor feedback loop rather than a specific oculomotor disturbance.[356]

ELECTROENCEPHALOGRAPHY (EEG)

- EEG is useful in diagnosis of posttraumatic seizure disorder in many, but not all, cases.
- EEG may determine patterns of generalized (diffuse) cerebral dysfunction.
- NOT an indicator of function.
- BEAM (Brain Electrical Activity Mapping) Scan is not felt to do more than average brain wave activity, and is not felt to be appropriate by diverse organizations.
- High-resolution EEG (124-channel) with computer enhancement is superior to routine EEG (which has 19-21 channels per montage).
- Newer techniques to spatially sharpen EEG with MRI (124 channels with specific anatomical localization).

QUANTITATIVE DIGITALIZED EEG (QEEG)

- Gives information related to functional changes related to mild axonal injury.
- Assays neurophysiological deficits quantitatively. Can identify mild injury to white matter, which reduces the efficacy of communication between

different parts of the cortex; the quality of neurotransmission is diminished when axons are injured.

- Can measure time delay between two regions of the cerebral cortex and the time needed to transmit information from one region to another.
- Looks at coherence, which reflects the integrity of neuronal connections between regions of the cortex.
- Evaluates phase, the measure of lead or lag of shared rhythms between regions, which yields information on differentiation of function.
- An objective measure of cerebral cortex function.

Several bad things have happened to this particular technology. The first is that the name QEEG is thought by some to be synonymous with the BEAM scan, which shows averages and does not digitalize information and present it in a different form.

In a courtroom several years ago, an attorney was playing "Perry Mason." He was making a great deal of standing at his table, mugging at the jury, and asking me questions such as, "Isn't it true, doctor, that the American Neurological Association does not approve of the QEEG?"

"Not to my knowledge," I answered,

"Isn't it true, doctor," he continued, "that the QEEG has been declared to be a bad test?"

"Not to my knowledge," I repeated.

Now the windup was done; he threw me the pitch. He picked up a copy of an article and held it high in the air, brandishing it toward me like a sword. He stalked up to me and thrust the article in my face so I could see it and the highlighted title. "Not to your knowledge? Does that mean that you don't know anything about this article from the green neurology journal which specifically states that the QEEG is not felt to be an appropriate test?"

I shrugged, took the offered article, looked at the journal article, and said to the jury, "Sir, if you read the entire title of the article, it specifically states that the QEEG the Neurological Association is speaking about in this article is the BEAM scan. It says so right here in the title, and that is not what I am referring to."

So the guy was an ass and didn't do his homework. He also couldn't read real well. But, the confusion between the names of the two entirely different tests made it possible for the insurance industry to refuse to pay for the test, despite being given articles that plainly explained the difference between the two procedures or tests.

As medical director of brain injury services in a well-known rehabilitation hospital, I initially had no problem having the test approved by the insurance companies and then paid for. It was very much less expensive than a neuropsychological evaluation and therefore, I felt, it made a good screening tool. One insurance adjuster had the intestinal fortitude to tell me the fact that it was a good screening tool made the insurance company less than happy to see it used.

What killed the test's use in the state of Colorado was one physician who trumpeted the fact that he could fix MTBI using neuro-biofeedback. He produced QEEG results of before and after his treatment that showed that the abnormal time delays, phase, and coherence were "fixed" after his treatment. I once asked him how he thought that neuro-biofeedback repaired axonal shearing. Needless to say, I received a less than satisfactory answer. Basically, this bit of charlatanism killed the usefulness of the test by physicians who wanted to use it appropriately.

It should also be known that the QEEG worked in this manner: an EEG was done with the electrodes hooked to an electrical instrument that digitalized the brain waves. This information was saved on a disk, which was sent to a place in California where the data was downloaded into a mainframe computer, and hundreds or thousands of algorithms were run on the data. The outcome was read by a specialist and the results sent back to the folk who performed the test. The Colorado doctor, it appears, may possibly have rewritten the results he received to fit his needs. I really couldn't argue with the insurance companies who refused to reimburse on that basis. In fact, I tried to explain this fallacious use to them, but it killed the use of a test that appeared to be very useful for the MTBI population.

Thatcher et al.[357] did the initial and follow-up work to develop the QEEG, or EEG for discriminant analysis for MTBI. This work cross-validated the discriminant function with 96.2% accuracy. A second, independent cross-validation yielded classification accuracy between 77.8% and 92.8%. The discriminating power spectra analysis was able to determine three classes of neurophysiological variables that were attributed to MTBI. These included increased coherence and decreased phase in frontal and frontal-temporal regions, decreased power differences between anterior and posterior cortical areas, and decreased alpha power in the posterior cortical regions. This tool proved, clinically, to be a cost-effective method to initially rule out, or in, the presence of an MTBI.

The general, typical EEG does not appear to be of significant import in the diagnosis of MTBI. Linear skull fractures did not add any abnormality to EEGs of patients with mild concussions.[358] The slow wave changes found on EEG are good for correlating the level of coma. Computerized analysis of this same data appeared to give better information.[359] Finally, the typical sleep EEG, when compared to the EEG polygraph (EEGP), showed that the EEGP/EEG were better predictors of outcome than the GCS.[360]

FUNCTIONAL MRI/PET SCANNING AND NEUROCOGNITIVE FUNCTIONS

Personally, I find it fascinating to see what modern functional testing procedures show us, and then compare that information to what I was taught years ago about how the brain was thought to function. These pieces of data are useful in making clinical judgments regarding TBI.

PET scan evaluations found that both the striatum and the cerebellum are involved in the implicit acquisition (learning) of a visuomotor skill. The ventrolateral prefrontal cortex also works in the development of the declarative aspect of such a task.[361] Remember when the cerebellum was just for smooth, coordinated movements?

The cerebellum, as noted, is associated with higher-order behaviors. SPECT studies have demonstrated that cerebral diaschisis can occur after cerebellar lesions, and this can, in turn, cause a basis for potential neuropsychological derangement after cerebellar insults. More specifically, cerebellar stroke has resulted in impairment of motor control and a mild naming deficit, without dysfunction in declarative memory, language, visuospatial, or executive functions.[362] Using functional MRI, some more circuitry regarding the cerebellum was determined. Increased activation of the bilateral regions of the superior cerebellar hemispheres and parts of the posterior vermis was seen during both high and low working-memory tasks. It was felt that articulatory control systems of working memory were from the frontal lobes, and other activity was derived from the phonological store in the temporal and parietal regions. From these regions, it appears, the cerebellum could compute any discrepancy between real and intended phonological rehearsal and use this information to update a feedforward command to the frontal lobes, which would facilitate the phonological loop.[363]

Speech apraxia is the impaired ability of patients with brain injury to coordinate speech movements, but their ability to perceive speech sounds, including their own errors, is unaffected. All patients with a specific deficit in articulatory planning (N = 25) had lesions that included a discrete region of the left precentral gyrus of the insula, which is a cortical area beneath the frontal and temporal regions. This area appears to be specialized for the motor planning of speech.[364]

Overall test performance of 15 TBI patients who had "recurrent perseveration" found that memory dysfunction and impaired attention were most likely responsible for perseverative errors. CAT scan in the three most perseverated patients showed left temporal lobe damage.[365]

Aspects of pleasant and unpleasant emotions were evaluated with PET scan. Both forms of emotions were distinguished from neutral emotional conditions by a significantly increased CBF in the region of the medial prefrontal cortex (Brodman's area 9), the thalamus, hypothalamus, and midbrain. Unpleasant emotion was different from neutral or pleasant emotion by activation of the bilateral occipito-temporal cortex and cerebellum, as well as the left parahippocampal gyrus, hippocampus, and amygdala. Pleasant emotions were distinguished from neutral, but not unpleasant, emotions by activation of the head of the left caudate nucleus.[366]

Functional MRI (FMRI) scans were used to evaluate hyposmia. Quantitative CNS changes in olfactory functioning were found in the areas previously associated with CNS processing of olfactory stimuli in normal subjects, but in patients there was much less activation, especially in the inferior frontal and cingulate gyral regions of the frontal cortex, and in regions of the medial and posterior temporal cortex.[367]

Still another study found that FMRI confirmed the predicted rCBF changes in premotor and prefrontal areas associated with performing arbitrary mapping tasks. It also suggested that a broad frontoparietal network may show decreased synaptic activity as arbitrary rules become more familiar, or "learned."[368]

INTRACRANIAL PRESSURE MONITORING (ICP)

- "Diagnostic" only for monitoring increasing ICP, indicative of increasing fluid/pressure dynamics from intracranial mass lesions, etc. in patients with moderate to severe brain injury.

NEUROSURGICAL RISK

An important variable in the initial evaluation of patients with MTBI who are seen in the emergency room is the possibility of neurosurgical intervention, which may occur in 1% to 5% of patients who are alert on initial evaluation in the emergency room with GCS scores of 13–15.[369]

Skull fracture increases the incidence of an intracranial complication that may increase the need for neurosurgical intervention by a factor of 20.[370]

One study of 610 patients with GCS scores of 13 to 15 showed 3% of patients needed neurosurgical intervention.[371] Another study identified 183 patients, accumulated over a ten-year period, with initial GCS scores of 13–15 and who required neurosurgical intervention. It was concluded that an acute intracerebral hematoma can never be totally discounted in patients with acute MTBI, even when there are no signs of neurological abnormality on initial evaluation.[372] This reinforces the clinical finding of a "lucid interval" seen in patients who are neurologically intact on initial evaluation but then deteriorate.[373] It was noted that small numbers of patients may clinically deteriorate 12 to 48 hours after their initial assessment secondary to delayed traumatic intracerebral hemorrhage. This is most frequently seen in association with coup and contrecoup lesions of the parieto-occipital cortex that may secondarily effect the fronto-temporal lobes.[374]

The obvious conclusion has been noted several times above. A normal initial neurological examination may not mean a patient is "okay" in 3%–5% of patients with GCS scores of 15.

MORE GENERAL INFORMATION REGARDING MTBI

It has been stated that TBI is one of the leading causes of death and disability in the United States for patients under 50 years of age.[375] The results of an MTBI as well as a moderate or severe TBI will change the way a patient behaves and perceives him or herself, as well as cause familial and social problems. A total change in personality may cause patients' friends and family to have difficulty understanding and coping with the patients.[376, 377]

The MTBI is the most common form of "traumatic encephalopathy." As we have noted, there are anatomical factors secondary to the mode of injury (acceleration/deceleration injuries, blunt trauma, contusions, etc.) as well as neurochemical changes which contribute to the posttraumatic sequelae. Symptomatology may include physical, affective/behavioral, and cognitive problems with significant attentional and information processing impairments in the absence of apparent neurological problems on examination. While many symptoms will abate within the first few months, a sizable subgroup of patients remain symptomatic for a year or more.[378] These folk are not "neurotic" until possibly later, after the symptoms have existed over time. Then, other affective changes occur, including depression and anxiety, as well as feelings of helplessness and hopelessness, if they are not adequately diagnosed and taught about their medical problems.

The consequences of TBI are increased in patients under two years of age, as well as those who are older.[379] As we have discussed, functional brain imaging testing may find evidence for cerebral dysfunction not seen on structural brain imaging tests, CAT scan, and MRI.

As human beings are anything but static in nature, what occurs may be exacerbated or ignored by perception, as well as by preinjury vulnerabilities or recent, concurrent, or postinjury events. Nothing appears to happen in a vacuum. Some pseudo-experts will (and have) state absurdities. One of my patients, who was injured at the age of 38, had a past history of one, and only one, episode 20 years earlier of shoplifting a music CD. This was the reason for the diagnosis of preexisting psychopathology, with no diagnosis of MTBI in spite of both neurological findings and cognitive difficulties. I was disgusted, the patient abreacted and dealt rather poorly with what was essentially an accusation.

For some reason, the fact that affective changes occur which may accompany the loss of cognitive function or uncontrolled behavioral changes seems to be like waving a red flag in front of a bull. The pseudo-expert will immediately blame all of a patient's problems on *their reaction to the posttraumatic changes* rather than even accept the idea that the affective changes followed the injury. It should go without saying, but I'll say it anyway, that preinjury medical and psychosocial factors, as well as the possibility of litigation, can factor into the patient's problems. It remains the job of the physician to be able to factor these various aspects appropriately and not throw out the patient's medical problems because of a *presumption* of secondary gain and/or malingering.

In my experience, one of the major factors that cause litigation is the patients' feeling that they are not being treated fairly by their insurance company, which typically may refuse some, or all, medical care, and especially rehabilitation needed after an MTBI. When patients can't get care, "*who are they gonna call?*" Lawyers, not Ghostbusters. *How else can they hope to get care?* And then they are told that, because they have an attorney, they must be in it for the money. As we previously discussed, there are some attorneys who ARE in it for the money and do their clients an immense disservice. But there are good attorneys who want to help their clients by helping them obtain the necessary medical treatment.

The entire medical dance, post-injury, may begin in the emergency room, or at a patient's primary care physician's office. These professionals need to know how to prevent an MTBI from being magnified and lead to disabilities which may exceed those from the injury alone.[380,381]

Early recognition of an MTBI is obviously helpful. This should begin at triage in the emergency room, *if possible*. Remember that all pathophysiological damage does not take place in the first moments or even hours after an MTBI. It can occur over days, weeks, and, possibly, months. Therefore, it must be remembered that the initial examination may probably not give the entire story. It has been my experience that most physicians remember this. It is the "legal eagles" who, at deposition, will stupidly insist that there were "no signs of a brain injury in the emergency room." "Look, doctor, it doesn't say on the emergency room report that there's a brain injury found! So how can you say that the patient has a brain injury a year later?" Well, *duh*.

Physicians must learn and remember the facts. Prominent among which is the fact that in an emergency room, if triage does not reveal an obvious problem, the patient's observable medical difficulties are quickly dealt with most appropriately and the patient is released home, most typically with a sheet telling them what to do should there be signs of TBI. One study demonstrates this. A group of 129 patients were seen in an emergency room, all testing was negative and all were released home, none with the diagnosis of MTBI. At one month after injury, 32% of these patients had increased signs and symptoms consistent with MTBI.[382]

It is also important to realize that the classification and types of evaluations most useful for patients with possible MTBI (measurement of CBF, via SPECT or PET, evaluation for focal or general areas of hypometabolism) are not typically performed, nor are they typically paid for by the insurance industry.[383-385]

BOTTOM LINE

There remains a need to better define for patients, attorneys, and some physicians the term MTBI — in spite of the current, typically ignored, BISIG definition — as well as better define the associated features of the problem. There is a substantial group of patients who remain at least partially functionally disabled by MTBI which was never properly diagnosed or not given appropriate treatment.

There remains no question about the fact that MTBI may have persistent effects including affective, neurocognitive, and behavioral. There may also be comorbidities that may precede the injury or be secondary to the diathesis. Rehabilitation programs for such patients exist and should be utilized. They should include the patients' family/caregivers.[386-392]

Amazingly, (well, not really) one study analyzed medical claims data and found that follow-up check for MTBI sequelae was rare.[393]

As we will deal with in later chapters, some studies find that proper diagnosis and treatment with conventional therapies and early complementary neuroprotective agents were found to help patient's outcome.[394] Add to this proper education about posttraumatic signs and symptoms, along with reassurance that the problems are real, and the rate of return to work for MTBI patients is higher than if these things are not done.[395]

One last point before we move on. A Chinese group found that it might be better to further differentiate the diagnosis of MTBI. They felt that one way to do this is to look at mild head injury as patients having a GCS score of 15, with no acute radiological abnormalities. High-risk mild head injury was defined as patients with a GCS of 13 or 14, or a GCS score of 15 with acute radiographic abnormalities.[396] A good idea.

Let's talk about initial workup. Posttraumatic headache and vomiting may deserve more clinical attention than they currently receive as part of the "posttraumatic syndrome." These may, in some patients, be early markers for neurological deterioration, but admittedly in a small percentage of patients. Many patients who receive CAT scans in the emergency room may have abnormal but atypical findings which may increase the risk for misdiagnosis, including cerebral fat embolism or cervical vessel injury.[397-399]

To CAT scan or not to CAT scan during the initial emergency room evaluation? This subject has been debated quite a bit in the literature. Some feel that any loss of consciousness or posttramatic amnesia should be enough for a routine CAT scan. Others point out that abnormalities on CAT scan in patients with MTBI are common, but the need for neurosurgical intervention is not. The age of patients, particularly the more elderly and children under two, should probably be a reason for performing a CAT scan. As most MTBI patients have a GCS of 15, with the others having initial GCS scores of 13 and 14 and typically recovering in the emergency department to 15 before release, one cannot use this as the rule. Arrival GCS score and cranial soft tissue injury may be risk factors for intracranial hemorrhage. Early routine CAT scans are felt by some to be the most reliable and cost-saving procedures and, as we mentioned before, the usefulness of the CAT scan beats skull x-rays hands down.[299,371,400-406]

The Miller criteria (presence of headache, nausea, vomiting, and signs of depressed skull fracture and a GCS of 14) have been evaluated as primary criteria for screening patients for CAT scan, and appear to have come up short, especially if alcohol usage is involved.[407] It would appear to me that the most reasonable criteria would include: abnormal GCS, signs of basilar or depressed skull fracture, the presence of neurological deficit, progressive headache or vomiting, decreasing sensorium, and very young or very old ages. On the other hand, we can't forget that along with all this medicinal science is art. Many times a physician's gut feelings, which result from seeing hundreds or thousands of these patients, mean a lot more.

In the emergency room, a lot of things take place, usually with a feeling of controlled chaos. Many patients post injury have many initial physical, as well as some cognitive, complaints. Interestingly, one study found no significant statistical correlations between neuropsychological or neurological scores and the numbers of subjective complaints, indicators of personality disorders, or posttraumatic amnesia.[408] Again, while there are many initial physical complaints, a greater number of minor head and neck injuries, 70% in one study,[409] will resolve within weeks or months, leaving 30%, from that study to persist, a not uncommon theme.[410-412]

Another interesting study found that acute hypoglycemia could masquerade as head injury, and should be ruled out in the ER.[413]

Now that all that has been said, at least several times for effect and annotation, let's move on to the common neurological sequelae of MTBI.

A fact that belies the myth that MTBI is not a real problem, and will go away within one to three months, is the reality of organically based neurological problems that follow MTBI. Briefly, the most common (and a couple that aren't so common) are:

POSTTRAUMATIC EPILEPSY

- Both generalized tonic-clonic (grand mal) and partial complex seizures, the latter most common and secondary to a partial kindling effect after MTBI[414-416]
- Some of these seizures may manifest as intermittent behavior change (temporal lobe seizures without gross motor movement)
- Diagnosis can be difficult
- Treat the patient, not the test

POSTTRAUMATIC HEADACHE

- Posttraumatic migraine of various types, totally different from the more common posttraumatic migraine ("typical" migraine with aura and neurologically complicated migraine)[417]
  1. Acute confusional migraine[418]
  2. Transient global amnesia secondary to posttraumatic migraine[419]
  3. Posttraumatic migrainous hemiplegia[420]
  4. Changes in mental status secondary to posttraumatic migraine[421]
- Posttraumatic tension-type headache[422]

POSTTRAUMATIC VERTIGO

- Second only to posttraumatic headache in frequency after MTBI: can be secondary to soft-tissue or myofascial etiologies, or more central (brainstem or cerebellar) or peripheral etiologies (end organ or nerve)[423-424]
- Cervicogenic dizziness[425-428]

OTHER NEUROLOGICAL PROBLEMS

- Difficulties with the sense of smell and taste[429,430]
- Sleep disorders and difficulties with the sleep/wake cycle[431-434]
- Light and sound intolerance[435-438]
- Posttraumatic tremor[439]
- The syndrome of inappropriate ADH (antidiuretic hormone), also called diabetes insipidus, is well documented following an MTBI[440-443]
- Posttraumatic tinnitus is common[444,445]
- The posttraumatic delayed nonhemorrhagic encephalopathy following MTBI is not so common[446]

Now, to go over some of these problems, and others:

POSTTRAUMATIC SEIZURES

Over the years, I've seen grand mal and multiple forms of temporal lobe seizures in patients with mild and moderate TBI. The majority of patients with grand mal seizures developed this problem within 6 to 12 months. It may not occur for up to five years in other patients. One patient, with no prior history of seizures, had his first grand mal seizure one week post injury.

Particularly with temporal lobe seizures, evaluation with standard sleep/wake EEG is not particularly fruitful. In the last decade, the use of naso-temporal electrodes appears to have fallen out of favor, unfortunately.

A frequent clinical fact is that the patients may not be aware of having "seizures." They may report episodes of "lost time." Their spouses or significant others will report that the patient may be "zoning out" and having no recollection of it. True temporal lobe automatic behavior is less frequently seen or reported.

A major problem is the question of pseudo-seizures. This is particularly found in medico-legal cases, where it is more important to establish the relationship of the seizures to the mild or moderate TBI. As stated above, many patients will have negative standard EEGs. To the typical insurance company attorney, that's all that is needed to determine that the patient is malingering. Then, there are our friends, the bought and paid for doctors, who will state, no matter what the history, a negative EEG rules out the problem. It isn't real. One of the tenets I truly believe in when it comes to such cases, is: *Treat the patient, not the test result!* To put it nicely, you shouldn't be doing the test if you are not aware of specific indications for it. You don't do an EEG to evaluate the state of the union. You have to expect to find something that an abnormal EEG can help you treat. If the EEG is negative, does that mean that the patient is faking it? Absolutely not!

I have seen patients have grand mal seizures right in front of my eyes. I was there, I tested them for eye movements, muscle movements, and all the rest. Yet, a week later, their EEG is normal. And again, a month after that, it is normal. So, was I crazy? Was the patient faking? No. I placed the patient on anticonvulsant medications. The seizures stopped. In two cases, the patients took it upon themselves to stop their medications. The seizures returned. They went away again after the medication was restarted.

Now, with the MTBI population, you have to remember several important facts: First, don't use Phenytoin or Phenobarbital for seizures, as both medications can increase cognitive difficulty. Carbamazepine or Valproic Acid are my first line medications. Both of these medications, particularly Tegretol, will also help decrease emotional lability. This is obviously very helpful, as patients may activate a seizure focus from lack of sleep, stress, poor nutrition, not taking their medication, and so on. Stabilizing their mood is very helpful.

The typical patient with pseudo-seizures has a history of real seizures or a family member or close friend with real seizures (or, as I witnessed once, a neighbor with pseudo-seizures). So, you have to do your homework, clinically and historically.

Another patient was seen having four to six seizures a day. She was also on two to three times the normal dosages of *four* anticonvulsants at the same time. It didn't seem to occur to the clinicians seeing her that if she was on so much and so many different medications and was still having seizures, that *maybe there was a problem*!

The patient had been unconscious, after her trauma for a number of hours, five years before I saw her initially. Her seizure history went back five years. So, there probably was something there. So, I slowly weaned her off of one, then a second, and, finally, a third medication. She also saw a clinical psychologist to deal with some of the major stressors in her life. In the end, she was seizure-free on appropriate doses of one anticonvulsant. She was also able to easily comprehend that she was having pseudo-seizures for another reason, specifically to deal with other serious problems in her life. They stopped.

Another clinical problem is that of "rage attacks," which are typically not associated with altered consciousness, but the violence or aggressiveness is not goal-directed and appears purposeless. I have seen patients who claimed to have "rage attacks," in reality a form of partial complex seizure disorder, but with goal-directed actions. This is not the way it works. One patient intimidated his attorneys, his physicians, and others by the threat, and, on occasion, demonstrations of these "unconscious" seizures/rage attacks. This was unadulterated baloney. But he got away with it for over two years. Another patient got his way by threatening to have a rage attack, therefore he couldn't ride the bus or be with other people, but he could participate in his favorite pastime, large-scale card tournaments.

There appears to be an interictal syndrome of hyperirritability and aggressiveness that can be associated with, but not represented by, true seizure activity. This has been termed, by some, limbic instability, or irritability. Anticonvulsants may indeed help.

On the research side of things, the major causes of acute symptomatic seizures over a 49-year period in Rochester, Minnesota, were traumatic brain injury, cerebrovascular disease, drug withdrawal, and CNS infections.[447] The elevated risk of posttraumatic seizures varied, in another study, according to the severity of the injury and the time since the injury.[448]

Partial kindling effects may produce a model for the effects of subclinical electrophysiological dysfunction, which may produce partial seizure-like activity in the presence of neuropsychological and neurobehavioral dysfunction after minor TBI. Atypically, there were no stereotypical sequences. Testing was negative, yet the majority of the patients did well after starting on anticonvulsants.[449] After ambulatory EEG testing, it appeared that patients with an abundance of seizure-like behavioral symptoms, such as memory gaps, lost time, and even olfactory hallucinations, in the presence of relatively normal neuropsychological testing were "for real." Localized theta bursts found on the ambulatory EEG may have been diagnostic of an underlying neuro-electrical disorder.[450] Four years later, the same group of researchers found that episodic symptoms in children and adolescents after MTBI included staring spells, memory gaps, and temper outbursts. Anticonvulsant treatment revealed moderate to substantial improvement in 92% of the patients.[451] Evaluating groups of moderate and severe closed head injury patients, it was noted that early posttraumatic seizures were not related to the presence of intracerebral parenchymal damage, and did not increase the risk of mortality or outcome.[452,453]

The risk factors for early or late posttraumatic seizures are varied and include: primary convulsions, focal intracerebral hemorrhagic lesions, subcortical atrophy, impaired local CBF 3-12 months post injury, duration of coma, prolonged posttraumatic amnesia, depressed fracture, diffuse contusion, age, and penetrating injuries.[454-458]

An important consideration is prophylactic anticonvulsant usage. To me, leaving an MTBI patient without anticonvulsant medication until they have ictal symptoms is preferred. However, I will utilize Carbamazepine for behavioral problems earlier rather than later if the behavioral dysfunctions, including very labile emotionality and significant irritability, makes rehabilitation more difficult. Thus, patients on this medication for reasons other than seizures may not develop clinical signs of seizure activity because they are receiving anticonvulsant medication for "nonseizure" reasons.

Of course, the use of more than one medication (including non-anticonvulsants) can effect TBI patients. The use of fluvoxamine, a 5-HT reuptake inhibitor, has been found, in at least one reported case, to increase convulsive activity.[459]

The familiar neuron-specific enolase (NSE), a marker for brain injury, is increased in serum after a single seizure including complex-partial seizures as well as tonic-clonic seizures, and after an episode of status epilepticus. The latter is also associated with alterations in the BBB.[460,461]

In some patients with posttraumatic seizures and an associated lesion on CAT scan or MRI, the lesion may resolve or "disappear," with the patient continuing to have seizures.[462] This proves again, that patients with lice can also have ticks.

The psychogenic, or pseudo-seizures we discussed above, are more likely to occur after trauma. Sexual trauma is not significantly associated with psychogenic seizures.[463] Patients who have intractable seizures after mild TBI should be evaluated for pseudo-seizures as well as "real" seizures.[464]

It is important to remember that behavioral changes associated with epilepsy can occur during the ictal period, or during the inter-ictal period, especially in patients with partial complex seizures of temporal or frontal lobe or temporolimbic etiology.[465] This altered behavior may be more glaring in the TBI population.

While there are familial or genetic aspects to alcohol-associated seizures, the same has not been found to be true for posttraumatic seizures.[466] Rehabilitation outcomes in MTBI patients with posttraumatic seizures are not diminished if the seizures are controlled.[467] In a more moderate to severe group of TBI patients, worse outcomes in the patients who develop posttraumatic seizures during the first year post injury are found to be secondary to the effects of the brain injuries that caused the seizures rather than the seizures themselves.[468]

POSTTRAUMATIC AMNESIA

Clinically speaking, posttraumatic amnesia (PTA) is an important factor in the diagnosis of TBI. Its presence, or the lack thereof, is important information that must be looked for in the initial history. There is no necessity of this factor in the diagnosis of MTBI, but the duration of PTA may be a bellwether prognostically for the moderate and severe TBI patients.

Research has shown that PTA is a useful variable, particularly when age is also taken into account, in predicting specific functional rehabilitation outcomes.[469,470] When comparing coma patients with those who experienced PTA, both groups were noted to have a number of lesions in the central brain structures, but only PTA was related to the number of hemispheric areas in which the lesions were found.[471]

During the early phases of recovery from TBI, in patients who have had PTA, the level of functional cognition and the presence of agitation appear to be covariables. Testing revealed that cognition and agitation covary, with most of the variation being secondary to attentional difficulties.[472]

The basal forebrain appears to contribute to memory function by providing cholinergic innervation to some critical memory structures, including the amygdala and the hippocampus. It is probable that PTA may result from disconnection of pathways between the diagonal band nuclei and the hippocampal region, secondary to altered cholinergic tone in the hippocampus.[473] In a study of a patient with significant PTA, cerebral CAT scan and MRI were normal, while PET scan with (18F) FDG revealed a significant reduction of metabolism, bilaterally, in both the hippocampus and the anterior cingulate cortex, revealing the possible role in memory for past events for these areas.[474]

Various methods of testing for PTA recovery have been developed, including the Galveston Orientation and Amnesia Test (GOAT) and the Rivermead post-traumatic amnesia protocol, Orientation Group Monitoring system (OGMS).[475-477]

POSTTRAUMATIC CRANIAL NERVE DYSFUNCTION

Cranial nerve dysfunction is typically present on the first neurological evaluation. The most common problems include olfactory dysfunction as well as associated ageusia, and VIth nerve paresis, as it is the longest cranial nerve running through the skull. The latter problem may have spontaneous recovery.[478]

Olfactory problems are easily missed unless tested for specifically. The pathophysiology of traumatic anosmia may involve: injury to the neurofibrils which pass through the cribiform plate, olfactory bulb compression by hemorrhage and/or edema, injury to the central pathways of olfaction, abrasion of the olfactory bulbs by the cribiform plate, and injury to the nasal passages. Aside from anosmia, these problems may induce hyposmia (a decreased sense of smell), parosmia (changed perception or perversion of the sense of smell), or cacosmia (perception of an extremely offensive odor that does not exist). The latter is also part of a preseizure aura, and, without a history of trauma, a space-occupying lesion must be ruled out. Anosmia may have a late onset, after 3 or 4 weeks post injury, secondary to scarring or gliosis of the sensory tissue in the cribiform plate. Olfactory dysfunction has been well studied.[479,480]

Seventh cranial nerve dysfunction may induce loss of taste, as well as peripheral facial palsy.[481] In many cases, the lack of or changed perception of taste is secondary to anosmia, with or without seventh cranial nerve dysfunction. (Think of how tasteless food may be when you have severe nasal congestion secondary to an upper respiratory infection.) A good clinical question is whether or not the patient has started to use far more hot and spicy condiments than prior to the injury. Then, testing should occur as needed.

The vagus nerve may be affected post TBI in patients with severe injuries. This may lead to delayed gastric emptying, absent cardiac response to tracheal suctioning, high gastric residual volumes, and pulmonary edema in response to a urecholine challenge, all of which indicate autonomic nervous system dysfuncion.[482]

Ripping the roots of the cranial nerves related to vision (II-VII) out of the brainstem may occur in patients with severe head trauma from motor vehicle accidents. Their survival rate is typically nil.[483]

POSTTRAUMATIC VISUAL CHANGES

This topic will be dealt with in greater detail in part two.

Generally, patients who have had mild traumatic brain injuries may frequently show multiple types of visual dysfunctions, including oculomotor, binocular, accommodative, and visual field loss. MTBI patients must receive appropriate evaluations to provide both documentation of the problems and the development of necessary rehabilitative treatment.

Disorders of the visual system after MTBI have been studied.[484] The trochlear nerve (IV) is less frequently injured than the abducens (VI).[485] Lesions in the posterior medial temporal gyrus may induce visual motion perceptual changes.[486] Focal orbitofrontal lesions seen on MRI can result in a higher susceptibility to extraneous visual distraction.[487]

Visual problem solving appears to involve the right suprasylvian region in the ability to process and then act on visual information. There appears to be evidence that the right frontal lobe, particularly the ventral region, is important in providing a flexible approach to visual problem solving.[488] Interhemispheric communication, which can be compromised by TBI, is required for appropriate visual-spatial search abilities.[489]

There are various ways to anatomically evaluate visual changes. Visual-evoked cortical responses or potentials (VECPs) are demonstrably abnormal in patients post MTBI. The VECPs are also good objective assessments of visual system deficits and recovery.[490,491] A phased-array surface coil MRI of the orbits and optic nerves provides rapid and clear evaluations of lesions of the optic pathway.[492] SPECT may also show changes in rCBF in patients with a cortical visual impairment, in spite of normal MRI or CAT scan studies.[493]

As with most if not all aspects of physical disability in the presence of TBI, visual loss will be difficult to cope with, and the various behavioral, cognitive, and personality changes from the injury may make it more difficult for a survivor to adapt to new physical limitations.[494]

POSTTRAUMATIC DIZZINESS AND AUDITORY DYSFUNCTION

Dizziness (vertigo or lightheadedness) must be objectified as much as possible to allow for appropriate treatment. One of major causes of dizziness in MTBI and moderate TBI patients is myofascial. Trigger points in the sternocleidomastoid muscles are frequently found, and palpation will increase or induce the identical problem the patient has been describing. Physical therapy is one of the mainstays of treatment for this problem. In some patients Antivert may be helpful, but watch for its anticholinergic side-effects. Cervicogenic dizziness is also a common diagnosis.[495]

Patients who complain of head or neck pain post trauma may exhibit an increased reliance on visual input, as their vestibular orienting information systems may be dysfunctional secondary to cervical splinting or head tilting. A neuro-otological study comparing patients with dizziness post TBI who did and did not have pending litigation found that the litigation was not an issue. A specialized neurotological evaluation is commonly a necessary part of post-MTBI evaluations.[496,497]

Perilymphatic fistula, abnormal ruptures allowing peripymph to leak out of the inner ear and into the middle ear, are most commonly secondary to trauma. Diagnostic testing may include audiograms, electronystagmograms, electrocochleograms, and subjective and platform fistula testing. Surgical treatment involves repair of the oval and round windows in the ear. Persistent dizziness may occur, along with sensorineural hearing loss.[498,499] Care must be taken to verify the diagnosis, particularly in a TBI patient, before surgery is performed.

Benign positional vertigo may be secondary to MTBI and must be appropriately evaluated prior to treatment. A combination of medications as well as behavioral methods have been used for the treatment of BPV.[500]

Posttraumatic deafness from brainstem lesions to the inferior colliculi may be associated with normal BAERs.[501]

Electrical injury may induce permanent auditory dysfunction and brain damage, as seen in neurobehavioral testing as well as auditory testing.[502]

POSTTRAUMATIC MOVEMENT DISORDERS

Probably the most common movement disorder seen is tremor. However, this must be differentiated from benign essential tremor. The latter can be diagnosed simply by asking the patient what happens to the tremor after he or she has an alcoholic beverage. Typically, the tremor will stop for a while. Propranolol is one of the current treatment choices that may be considered for this problem in a patient with a TBI.

Posttraumatic movement disorders may be transient or persistent, and include tremor, dystonia to a disabling degree (secondary to damage to the basal ganglia and the thalamus with spillover effects to the hypothalamus, which can induce both autonomic instability as well as dystonic posturing), which is rare; hemiballismus, with SPECT-noted lesions in the region of the subthalamic nucleus of Louis; multifocal motor and vocal tics; and, in a small subgroup, ataxia. MTBI patients have, most typically, the least severe forms of movement disorders, but such problems are found in the MTBI population.[503-509]

Moderate to severe brain injury in young patients is associated with a longer latency to the start of movement disorders, as well as an increased tendency to develop generalized dystonia.[510]

In another study, the legal system was found to not adversely affect the outcome of posttraumatic movement disorders; it did not make them worse, either. Those patients with attorneys had more significant disability when compared to patients with movement disorders who did not have attorneys.[511]

POSTTRAUMATIC ENDOCRINE CHANGES

Posttraumatic endocrine changes may be seen in MTBI patients, but is typically more severe in moderate to severe TBI patients secondary to the trauma they receive. Evaluations should be performed when clinically warranted, and should include evaluation of function of the adrenocortical, gonadal, thyroid, and human growth hormone (hGH)-insulin systems. LH, FSH, prolactin, and hGH may be stimulated.

The endocrine abnormalities, if found, are not predictive of general outcome.[512,513] Diabetes insipidus has been seen after mild as well as severe TBI.[514]

Primary adrenal insufficiency may follow TBI. It can cause symptoms and signs from generalized weakness and fatigue to fulminant shock and death.[515] This disorder is rare, but an important one to remember.

While there is no apparent correlation between the severity of TBI and levels of testosterone, FSH, or LH, there is a high incidence of hypotestosteronaemia in the survivors of severe TBI. This may be more related to physiological stressors than disruption of the hypothalamic-pituitary-gonadal axis.[516]

POSTTRAUMATIC SEXUAL DYSFUNCTION

One of the areas that we, as clinicians, may need to work a bit harder on is helping patients with sexual dysfunction. The majority of these problems may be caused by stress, depression, and personality and behavioral changes experienced by both the patient and the patient's spouse or significant other.

After a TBI, whatever the level, a survivor's life is changed. Their perception of themselves is drastically altered. They may have increased irritability or flat out significantly labile emotionality. These problems will most certainly interfere with sexuality. Not to inquire about these aspects of a patient's life is to be remiss in our treatment and the total rehabilitation of TBI survivors.

Over the years, a number of my patients have gotten divorced post MTBI, with hyposexuality being one of major causes. Of course, it is not an isolated problem, there are many others, too.

I've seen only one patient with the Kluver-Bucy syndrome, which may be caused by ablation of the anterior temporal poles or hypothalamic injury, and which results in hypersexuality and hyperorality.[517,518] Her engagement was almost ruined by her sudden change from "demure" to hypersexual.

Endocrine disturbances, which are common with temporal lobe epilepsy in both sexes, may be associated with decreased libido and impotence, as well as reproductive and menstrual disorders.[519-521] The clinician needs to evaluate patients with sexual problems accordingly.

Two recent studies arrived at different conclusions. In one, 52 patients with a history of TBI were evaluated for the prevalence of sexual dysfunction and age, severity, and cerebral focus of injury. Patients with frontal lobe lesions reported more sexual satisfaction and function than the patients without frontal lobe injury. The time since the injury was inversely related to levels of sexual arousal: patients with more recent injuries in this study reported higher levels of arousal than the patients with older injuries. Right hemisphere lesions correlated with higher scores on reports of sexual arousal and sexual experiences.[522]

Another group looked at 92 TBI survivors with an elapsed time from injury ranging between 1 and 20 years. This study found that TBI frequently altered sexual functioning as well as desire. Decreased ability to achieve an erection, decreased ability to achieve orgasm, decreased sexual desire, and decreased frequency of intercourse were frequently reported. Many of the patients reported physiological sexual disturbances and diminished sexual ability.[523] Obviously, a lot more work needs to be done. TBI survivors need to be enabled to retain sexual functioning.

POSTTRAUMATIC CSF LEAK

In 20 years I've only seen two patients with CSF rhinorrhoea. Both were involved in significant motor vehicle accidents and had struck the steering wheel with their faces, both had broken noses. Surgery to repair the dural leaks was done on both. Neither developed meningitis.

There is also the question of prophylactic antibiotics. One study showed a greater incidence of meningitis in patients who were given antibiotics.[524]

As indicated, patients with significant facial trauma or periorbital hematoma appear to be at greater risk of dural tear and possible delayed CSF leakage.[525]

POSTTRAUMATIC FEVER

This problem is typically seen in the moderately severe and severe TBI patient. Fever may result from infection, thrombophlebitis, drug reaction, a defect in the central thermoregulatory system, or posttraumatic hyperthermia. All other possibilities of infection must be ruled out before the latter diagnosis is made.[526-528]

POSTTRAUMATIC BONE CHANGES

Heterotopic ossification is categorized by the formation of new bone in tissue that does not normally ossify. This complication is not uncommon in moderately severe and severe TBI patients with limited physical mobility. It should be noted that patients who have had a TBI demonstrate enhanced osteogenesis, most probably secondary to humoral factors, as the serum of these patients promotes *in vitro* growth of osteoblast cells.[529,530]

A BRIEF SURVEY OF OTHER CLINICAL PROBLEMS

- Urinary incontinence is seen in severely brain-injured patients, usually secondary to detrusor hyperactivity with synergic sphincter action. There is also a correlation between cerebellar and hemorrhagic infarctions and detrusor areflexia.[531,532]
- Stuttering can occur in MTBI patients. There is some correlation to stuttering and both neurogenic causes and psychogenic causes. Speech apraxia must also be ruled out.[533]
- Heart rate variability (HRV), a measure of the fluctuation around the mean heart rate, reflects both sympathetic and parasympathetic balance of the autonomic nervous system. Abnormalities of both time and frequency domains of HRV are present in TBI patients.[534] I have seen this problem in both moderate TBI survivors as well as MTBI patients, but more frequently in the former group. A cardiological consultation is a must.

None of the patients in my group had a prior history of known heart disease, including conduction difficulties.

- Spasticity, or increased muscle tonus, is relatively rare in MTBI patients. It may become a problem with moderate TBI patients, and is a problem in many severe TBI patients.[534,536] Treatment options must be carefully thought out. Oral Baclofen may increase cognitive deficits and increase sedation. Tizanidine is a useful therapy, but initial sedation and possible hypotension must be watched. Klonopin, a fifth-generation benzodiazepine, is more helpful and, once the sedation side-effects are gone, does not appear to functionally hinder cognition. In moderately severe and severe TBI patients, an intrathecal Baclofen pump may be needed.

- Some research has shown that head injury may be more common among patients with Alzheimer's disease. Head trauma may be a predisposing factor to Alzheimer's disease, particularly in patients without a known genetic contribution.[537]

- Aside from asking if head injury predisposes them to Alzheimer's disease, many patients ask if it will predispose them to a brain tumor. There is at least one reported case of a patient who, several years after sustaining a commotive left parietal trauma, developed symptoms of a tumor. CAT scan and MRI showed a large tumor, a mixed glioma that biopsy showed to be in continuity with the scar from the initial trauma.[538] Another interesting case report details a patient, with a large right parietal epidermoid cyst, who had a minor fall. The force of the fall was transferred by the cyst to the brain, and transdural herniation of the cyst contents to the brain parenchyma occurred. The patient suffered an MTBI.[539]

- During the course of an injury, physical damage may occur, causing musculoskeletal and myofascial problems. Not infrequently, posttraumatic temporomandibular joint disorders may occur.[540] These patients should have appropriate rehabilitation before being sent for surgery. They are best served by using a broad, transdisciplinary treatment protocol.

One thing about treating patients who have survived an MTBI is the diversity of the signs and symptoms, and the way the treatment team must think on its collective feet to meet all of the challenges found.

Treatment outcome is evaluated in a number of different ways, using different instruments, and will be discussed in a later chapter. In the meantime, a prospective study looking at the general health of MTBI patients one year post injury found that 50% of the patients continued to report sequelae. Outcome appeared to have no correlation to trauma severity. Patients with sequelae after one year had reported more symptoms at one week after trauma.[541] Other groups note that after moderately severe TBI, late social status and behavior, equated as quality of life, were related to the initial clinical findings.[542]

Another study of long-term health issues in TBI patients who lived in the community were assessed. A number of health-related issues were found, including neuroendocrine, neurological, and arthritic difficulties. The need for better patient education, as well as ongoing health screening for these patients, was indicated.[543]

The number of clinical aspects of MTBI is enormous. Understanding the patho-physiology makes many of the problems less difficult to treat. The cognitive/behavioral aspects are most important, and will be covered later.

6 Posttraumatic Headache

Posttraumatic headache (PTHA) follows acceleration/deceleration injuries ("whiplash") in as many as 90% of patients who experience a minor traumatic brain injury.[544] These headaches can be determined to be migraine, cluster, tension type, or, possibly, cervicogenic in nature. PTHAs may be secondary, also, to slip and fall accidents, violent altercations, and work-related injuries, aside from motor vehicle accidents. These headaches are frequently a part of the postconcussive syndrome, which, as previously noted, refers to a large number of signs and symptoms that may follow a blow to the head or an acceleration/deceleration injury, which may or may not induce a mild traumatic brain injury. They should be considered part of the PCS, not MTBI.

Up to 80% of patients with PTHA may enter remission within 6 months, leaving 20% of patients with chronic PTHA, lasting years in many cases.

Traumatic brain injury has been associated with many different pain problems, including PTHA. Of interest is the fact that MTBI and mild-moderate TBI patients express more complaints of PTHA than do moderate or severe TBI patients.[545] This population also has more complaints of cervical, shoulder, and low back pain in association with PTHA. Of concern is the ease with which these complaints may be ignored or considered to be "psychological" and secondary to depression.

It should also be remembered that simple concussion might be associated with PTHA, as well as vegetative and/or psychotic difficulties.[546,547]

More commonly, PTHA, the most common sequelae of head injury, is frequently associated with dizziness, irritability, and decreased concentration.[548] The chronic PTHA induces significant difficulties for the typical general practitioner, as well as the neurological specialist. This becomes especially true if there is evidence of de-novo migraine or cluster headache. The posttraumatic chronic pain syndrome may also be associated with increases of pain secondary to physical activity.[549]

A frequently asked question is why people who play various sports for a living, such as football players, wrestlers, and others, do not have high incidence of PTHA and/or MTBI. The answer is fairly simple: these people are physically very well conditioned, and when they play, they are always very prepared and always anticipate the possibility of physical contact/trauma. This differentiates them from the vast majority of people who are not even close to being in optimal physical condition, and who are injured unexpectedly, before they are even aware of the impending trauma.

Accumulated research has shown that when the head is free, rather than confined, it is more susceptible to an acceleration/deceleration injury. Almost 60 years ago, it was shown that in cats, less force was required to produce concussion when the head was free to move compared to when it was fixed or confined in place.[550] The concept of an acceleration/deceleration, or "whiplash," is important, as it involves a multitude of medical aspects. When an acceleration/deceleration injury occurs (most frequently from a rear-end motor vehicle accident), the physical or gravitational forces of a massive object such as a car striking another automobile are passed onto the most fragile and movable object not firmly secured in the automobile that was struck: the passenger. Even when the passenger is wearing a seatbelt, the head — essentially a ball at the end of a tether (the neck) — is thrown first forward, and then backwards when the tether can reach no farther and snaps back. If the head is turned at the moment of impact, the rotational forces are also very important to take into account, particularly when an MTBI is found.

There are many people involved in the insurance aspects of medicine, in addition to the medical and legal aspects, who make a good bit of money by testifying that such physical forces, especially when there was not a great deal of damage to a car, "could in no way cause any organic problems." Typically, such hired guns do not treat patients, which makes them purposely oblivious to the realities of the medical challenges found in these patients.

POSTTRAUMATIC MIGRAINE

Posttraumatic migraine, which may begin *de novo* — without a previous personal or family history of migraine — may have neurochemical similarities with MTBI. These may include increased extracellular potassium and intracellular sodium, calcium, and chloride; serotonergic changes; decreases in magnesium; increases in intracellular calcium; excessive release of excitatory amino acids; changes in catecholamine and endogenous opiod tonus; decreased glucose utilization; changes in neuropeptides; and abnormalities in nitric oxide formation and function.[551,552]

Migraine, including posttraumatic migraine, may be associated with a number of neurological symptoms or phenomena. This may include transient global amnesia, vestibular dysfunction, visual and auditory changes, and, possibly, an increased incidence of seizures.[551,553,554]

The trigeminovascular system is of great import in migraine.[551] In some children who develop posttraumatic neurological deterioration without focal lesions after minor head trauma, there may be an association with an "unstable trigeminovascular reflex," which induces the release of perivascular vasodilatory peptides which can contribute to cerebral hyperemia.[555]

Transient global amnesia (TGA) was initially attributed to bilateral temporal lobe seizure phenomena. More recently it has been attributed to migraine by some[551] and thought to be a totally separate disorder by others, possibly due to a different form of paroxysmal disorder in the brainstem.[556] TGA in the pediatric population is still felt to be secondary to ischemia of the temporo-basal structures induced by the MTBI and associated with a migrainous diathesis.[557]

Migraine equivalents, transient neurological symptomatology not associated with headache, are not uncommon; proper diagnosis is more difficult to the generalist, as well as the neurologist. In some, possibly more susceptible, individuals, minor, even trivial, head trauma can induce a migraine equivalent known as "footballer's migraine," as well as "posttraumatic cortical blindness." This particular migraine equivalent is certainly rare, but transient; total blindness may certainly be cause to call out a total, full court press workup.[558]

Other, more common, forms of transient neurologic disturbances associated with migraine are brainstem symptoms including vestibular difficulties, dizziness, disequilibrium, vertigo, and motion intolerance. These symptoms may also present as migraine equivalents, between migraine headache episodes or instead of the cephalic pain. Vertigo as a migraine equivalent may occur in about 25% of migraine patients, with the diagnosis being made, typically, by history of familial migraine, as all testing is typically negative. Migraine can also mimic Meniere's disease, with "vestibular Meniere's disease" being more frequently, but still not commonly, associated with migraine.[559,560]

Also, one should not forget the cervical causes of vertigo and dizziness, secondary to posttraumatic cervical and/or myofascial pathophysiology.

There is also a question of the possible relationship between posttraumatic migraine and posttraumatic benign encephalopathy. The latter, in children, may be associated with cortical blindness, brainstem disturbances, and seizure lasting from 5 minutes to 48 hours.[561]

Posttraumatic vertigo or dizziness is a very frequent accompaniment to MTBI. It may be secondary to peripheral, labyrinthine disturbance, or brainstem disturbance secondary to trauma, or it may be a migraine equivalent. The importance of this differential is most significant, possibly, when treatment is attempted. Clinically, this would be an important avenue of treatment to explore.

BOTTOM LINE

As indicated, trauma may induce the first migraine attack in a possibly susceptible patient, or increase the frequency, and possibly the severity, of preexisting migraine. The etiology of these changes may be secondary to neuronal/axonal and/or neurochemical abnormalities secondary to trauma.

Treatment is typically with valproic acid, an anticonvulsant medication. The use of beta-blockers such as propranolol is also useful. The use of a triptan for abortive care is also well tolerated if used appropriately.

Cluster headache has also been seen secondary to head trauma, again probably secondary to neuronal and/or axonal injury. Treatment, abortive or prophylactic, has been dealt with elsewhere.

POSTTRAUMATIC TENSION-TYPE HEADACHE

Posttraumatic tension-type headache, along with secondary analgesic rebound headache, is probably the most common primary headache disorder found after trauma.

The anatomy and physiology of the myofascial changes, associated sleep disorders, and other clinical aspects of tension-type headache have previously been written of in great (if not nauseating) detail.[562] Let us then slowly walk through Figure 6.1.

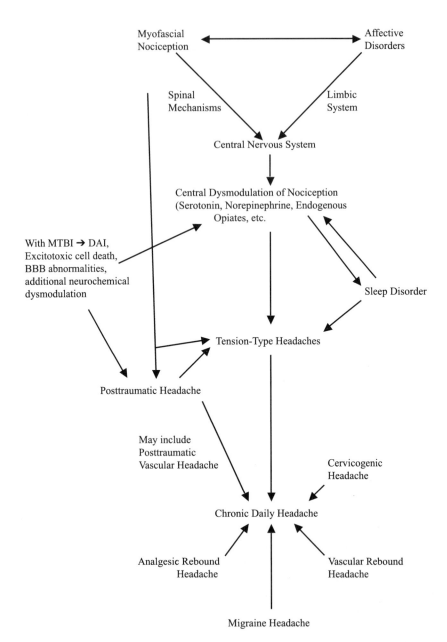

FIGURE 6.1 Chronic daily headache, including posttraumatic headache, with additional deficits from MTBI.

At the time of an injury such as an acceleration/deceleration injury, a slip and fall, or even, secondary to poor posture, sustained computer work, and so on, pain begins with myofascial nociception. For the sake of the fact that this text is about MTBI, let's focus on an acceleration/deceleration injury, or "whiplash." Let's talk about an MVA, a rear-end collision. The head, which may be rotated at the time of the impact, is the previously described ball at the end of the neck, or tether. It is thrown forward, stretching the cervical and upper back musculature. The head is then thrown backwards, possibly striking a headrest. Typically, this forward-and backward movement occurs more than once.

The musculature is not elastic. The sudden stretching will induce a reflex spasm, which is reinforced by the degree of the trauma. The spasmed muscles develop a diminished blood flow secondary to the degree of spasm-induced pressure on the smaller vasculature. This will induce muscle ischemia: a buildup of pain-inducing chemicals; metabolites of muscle work, such as lactic acid, bradykinin, serotonin, and prostoglandins which are algetic, that is, they stimulate nociceptive impulses. This, in turn, further reinforces the muscle spasm, again, reflexively. These nociception-enhancing chemicals appear to stimulate central mechanisms which, from continued stimulation, enhance reactive muscle contraction and the maintenance of the myogenic nociceptive cycle.[563,564]

Two important facts for later: there is a positive correlation between pericranial muscle tenderness and headache intensity, with the muscle pain being the source of nociception.[565] The pericranial muscles are innervated by sensory fibers in nerves from the second or third cervical roots and from the trigeminal nerve.[566]

Muscle fatigue, metabolic and neurochemical in nature, which is associated with chronic or prolonged (tonic) muscle spasm, may also be secondary to the depletion of epinephrine and norepinephrine, the peripheral sympathetic neurotransmitters (sympatheticopenia). Remember that the muscle spindle is directly affected by the sympathetic nervous system via the neurotransmitters, particularly norepinephrine. Prolonged and sustained peripheral sympathetic activity may lead to the depletion of norepinephrine at the synaptic receptors. Continuous afferent sympathetic input from myogenic nociception, including that from the buildup though ischemia of nociceptive metabolites, may result in sympatheticopenia.[567,568]

Three mechanisms of muscle pain are felt to be relevant to both acute and chronic tension-type headache via myogenic nociception which can be induced by: low grade inflammation associated with the release of algetic substances; short or long-lasting relative ischemia; and tearing of the ligaments and tendons, even microscopically, secondary to abnormal, sustained muscle tension/contraction.[566]

The above is typically followed by the development of a myofascial pain syndrome (MPS). The MPS is a localized or regional pain problem associated with small zones of hypersensitivity within skeletal muscle-trigger points. Trigger points in the muscles of the head, neck, and upper back may elicit headache as well as vertigo, tinnitus, and lacrimation. The MPS of the head and neck secondary to referred pain from trigger points may mimic other clinical conditions, including migraine, TMJ disorders, cervical neuralgias, TMJ disturbances, sinusitis, and a number of neurotological problems including vertigo, dizziness, tinnitus, and ear pain.[569-571]

The onset of the MPS on an acute basis may begin with one muscle and be associated with trauma, including an acceleration/deceleration injury or a slip and fall. It may also begin insidiously, in patients who work for hours typing into a computer. The MPS itself may be either active or latent, the latter associated with muscle dysfunction (decreased range of motion, shortened muscles) but no pain. In many patients the MPS "metastasizes" and involves associated musculature, becoming regional or involving multiple muscular regions.

Trigger points, when palpated, have consistent patterns of referred pain. They may shift between active — painful when palpated — and latent states.

Most importantly, continuous myogenic nociception from active trigger points appears to be the prime instigator of the central neurochemical nociceptive dysmodulation found in patients with chronic tension-type headache.

A LITTLE NEUROANATOMY AND NEUROCHEMISTRY

The central modulation of pain appears to originate in the brainstem and involves at least two systems. The "descending" inhibitory analgesia system appears to regulate the "gating" mechanisms of the spinal cord. This system includes the midbrain periaquaductal gray region, the medial medullary raphe nuclei, and the adjacent reticular formation, as well as dorsal horn neurons in the spinal cord.[572] The "ascending" pain modulation system originates in the midbrain and is projected to the thalamus.[573] Both systems utilize biogenic amines, opiod peptides, and non-opiod peptides.[572-574]

The ascending system appears to show more relevance to headache disorders. This system has projections from the brainstem to the medial thalamus which include large numbers of serotonergic and opiate receptors. The midbrain dorsal raphe nucleus, a serotonergic nucleus, projects to the medial thalamus and is associated with pain perception. Serotonergic projections to the forebrain are implicated in the regulation of the sleep cycle, mood changes, pain perception, and the hypothalamic regulation of hormone release.[575]

The endogenous opiate system (EOS) within the central nervous system may act as a nociceptive "rheostat" or "algostat," setting pain modulation to a specific level. As this level changes, an individual's pain tolerance may also change. Fluctuations in pain intensity may be interpreted as being secondary to fluctuations in the function of antinociceptive pathways.[576,577] Headache, along with other "nonorganic" central pain problems, are thought to be the most common expression of impairment of the antinociceptive systems.[578]

The EOS modulates the neurovegetative triad of pain, depression, and autonomic disturbances that are found in only two conditions: chronic tension-type headache (posttraumatic or otherwise) and acute morphine abstinence.[578] The EOS is also implicated as the primary protagonist in idiopathic headadche.[578,579] Reduced plasma concentrations of beta-endorphin have been found in idiopathic headache patients, including those with chronic (posttraumatic) tension-type headache.[580-583]

A primary relationship also exists between the EOS and the biogenic amine systems, which are intrinsic to both the pathophysiology of pain modulation and its treatment. Clinical and neuropharmacological information indicates that dysmodulated serotonergic neurotransmission probably generates chronic headache and head pain. It has also been noted that the ordinary, acute, or periodic headache may be the "noise" of serotonergic neurotransmission.[574]

Decreased levels of serotonin[584-586] (with good indications of an impairment of serotonergic metabolism in patients with chronic tension-type headache); Substance P, an excitatory neuropeptide;[587,588] and plasma norepinephrine[589] are found in chronic tension-type headache patients. The latter is also indicative of peripheral sympathetic hypofunction, which may also participate in the etiology or maintenance of central opiod dysfunction.[583] Platelet GABA levels are significantly increased in chronic tension-type headache patients. This may also act as a balance mechanism to deal with neuronal hyperexcitability, and may also be associated with depression.[590]

The opiod receptor mechanisms appear to be very susceptible to desensitization, or the development of tolerance. In chronic tension-type headache patients, opiod receptor hypersensitivity is marked, secondary to the chronically diminished secretion of neurotransmitters. This "empty neuron syndrome" may involve both autonomic and nociceptive afferent systems, as well as being latent, subpathological, or pathological with spontaneous manifestations.[591]

The EOS modulates the activity of monoaminergic neurons. A chronic EOS deficiency can provoke transmitter leakage of both opiod and bioaminergic neurotransmitters, and lead to neuronal exhaustion and "emptying," as well as compensatory effector cell hypersensitivity. The poor release of neurotransmitter along with cell/receptor hypersensitivity appears to be the most important phenomena of the hypoendorphin syndromes. It has also been concluded that chronic tension-type headache may result from dysmodulation of nociceptive impulses, with associated sensitized receptors.[592]

Chronic tension-type headache, including the chronic posttraumatic tension-type headache, may be, along with other chronic idiopathic headaches, a "pain disease" directly linked to central dysmodulation of the nociceptive and antinociceptive systems, either latent or pathological in nature. Research indicates that at least two arms of the main endogenous antinociceptive systems, the EOS and the serotonergic systems, are involved in the pathogenesis of chronic tension-type headache. This problem appears to be progressive, and the dysfunctions may result from neuronal exhaustion secondary to continuous activation of the systems.[582,591]

PATHOPHYSIOLOGY

To return to Figure 6.1, now most of the basics have been mentioned: continuous peripheral stimulation from myofascial nociceptive input from an MPS, with or without trigger points, may effectively trigger a change in the central pain "rheostat" associated with nociceptive input, secondary to the continuous need for pain-modulating antinociceptive neurotransmitters. The affective aspects of pain, including depression, anxiety, and fear, are secondary to changes in neurotransmitters such as serotonin and norepinephrine, and directly influence myofascial nociception, and further reinforce central neurochemical changes.

Between 4 to 6 and 12 weeks, changes in the central nervous system's central modulation of nociception can occur. Secondary to continuous peripheral nociceptive stimulation, in association with affective changes, the central modulating mechanisms will assume a primary rather than a secondary or reactive role in pain perception, as well as antinociception, shifting the initiating aspects of pain perception from the peripheral regions to the central nervous system. This intrinsic shift may make innocuous stimuli more aggravating to the pain-modulating systems, the "irritable everything syndrome." The already dysmodulated internal feedback mechanisms may react until central neurochemical mechanisms dominate, secondary to neurotransmitter exhaustion, and receptor hypersensitivity and abnormal biogenic amine metabolism/exhaustion occurs. These neurochemical changes may induce and/or exacerbate a sleep disorder (serotonergic in nature, from the nucleus raphe magnus) which, by itself, can perpetuate the central neurochemical dysmodulation which is primarily responsible for chronic tension-type headache.

Chronic posttraumatic tension-type headache, whether or not it is associated with an MTBI, has the same pathophysiological mechanisms. In the presence of an MTBI, other, significant pathophysiological changes occur which can potentiate or exacerbate the mechanisms described above. You may have noticed some of the similarities of the neurochemical pathophysiology discussed above with that of MTBI itself, discussed in Chapter 5.

In the face of dysmodulated neurochemical systems found in chronic tension-type headache, add direct myofascial trauma as an initiating event. The effects of diffuse axonal injury, which also affects the neurochemistry of the brain as neuronal degeneration and death occurs, can exacerbate the neurotransmitter pathophysiology. This may also explain the initiation of migraine, *de novo*, as brainstem trigeminovascular mechanisms may obviously be affected. Finally, excitotoxic injury, which leads to cell death from the overexuberant production of acetylcholine and glutamate, may also induce significant neuropathological "holes" in the primary neurotransmitter systems and exacerbate the headache pathophysiology.

Affective changes follow, with the additional problem of possible cognitive changes resulting from MTBI. The latter may make treatment more difficult.

Posttraumatic tension-type headache is the most common sequelae of an MTBI. It may also be associated with iatrogenic analgesic abuse. Before treatment or even diagnosis of cognitive deficits is attempted, inappropriate medications must be stopped and the headache ameliorated. Most commonly, for this to be done, the patient must be treated using an interdisciplinary headache treatment protocol. Please see the *Headache Handbook: Diagnosis and Treatment* for the details of this protocol.[562]

BOTTOM LINE

The neurochemical factors leading to the perpetuation of posttraumatic tension-type headaches appear to be further and more complexly involved than in chronic tension-type headache without associated MTBI. Treatment is most appropriately and cost-effectively performed in an interdisciplinary headache rehabilitation program. Tricyclic medications, GABAnergic medications, and NSAIDs are appropriate, while narcotics, Dilantin, barbiturates, and early-generation benzodiazepines are not.

One should not attempt to test for cognitive abilities in the presence of significant headache pain and depression. They must be treated before neuropsychological testing or the more functional speech/language and occupational therapy evaluations are done. While this was mentioned earlier, it is worth repeating:

Patients with MTBI who complain of headache do not appear to perceive their headache pain the same way a headache patient without an MTBI does. These patients know that they have headaches. On a scale of 0 (no pain) to 10 (worst pain imaginable — you couldn't tolerate it for a moment or two), individual patients, when first seen, will give you high numbers, e.g., 7 to 10, which is correlated to pathophysiological myofascial findings, including decreased cervical range of motion, muscle spasm, active trigger points, and more. As they go through treatment, you will see them regain appropriate physical functioning: normal cervical range of motion, amelioration of spasm and trigger points, etc., with a marked associated improvement of function. The patients' affect will be brighter, they will smile, have fewer if any pain behaviors, and resume doing the physical things they enjoy. Yet, when asked, they will continue to state that their headache pain is at the same level of 7 to 10 as when they were first seen. Whether they are perseverating or just unable to give an accurate subjective pain level (frontal lobe involvement), their stated pain levels may not change very much at all. Therefore, you must evaluate them on improvements in function, not by self-reported subjective decrements in headache pain levels.

The initial trauma may involve soft tissue injury to the scalp or face, which may be followed by an entrapment of a sensory nerve, or the sensory nerve may have been cut during the trauma via laceration. The entrapment may also occur during suturing of a laceration. Such entrapments may induce nerve, or neuropathic, pain. This is easily differentiated from other primary headache types. The pain is constant, burning, and relegated to the sensory distribution of the affected nerve. Anticonvulsant medications such as carbamazepine are best for the first-line treatment. In some cases, neurolytic procedures such as radiofrequency coagulation or cryoablation may be necessary. Both are good procedures, but have varying durations of benefit, most typically between 6 to 12 months.

Without question, injuries to the cervical spine and the superficial and deep structures of the neck (muscles, ligaments, bone, discs, or nerve roots) may occur. Cervical pain from trigger points in spasmed musculature as well as from cervical joint dysfunction may be referred to the head.

If the posttraumatic pain is suboccipital with lancinating, electrical-like shooting pain attributes, secondary to involvement of the occipital neurovascular bundle (the occipital nerve, artery, and vein), or secondary to prolonged muscle spasm/contraction or excessive vascular dilatation impinging on the greater occipital nerve of Arnold, this pain is known as "occipital neuralgia." It is always in the C_2 distribution at the back of the head. Indomethacin is the most effective treatment for this problem. Steroidal injections may also be utilized. Neuro-ablative procedures should be performed only when all other treatment has failed.

Preexisting arthritis or discogenic disease may also be exacerbated by the initial trauma. An appropriate neurological evaluation will help with these entities.

This now leads us to the third diagnosis, the one that is questioned by many and hailed by a few.

CERVICOGENIC HEADACHE

Just as the community of headache specialty physicians was rather hesitant (to be nice) to accept the fact that the musculature had a significant role in tension-type headache, the idea that headache can arise from the structures of the neck still has many detractors.

Dwyer, Aprill, and Bogduk[593] utilized fluoroscopic control to stimulate joints at segments C_{2-3} to C_{6-7} by distending the joint capsule with injections of contrast medium. They were able to show that each joint produced a clinically distinguishable, characteristic pattern of referred pain which enabled the construction of pain charts to be used in determining the segmental location of symptomatic joints in patients presenting with cervical zygapophyseal pain.

The diagnostic criteria for cervicogenic headache (CGHA) have been noted by several authors to differ a bit. Bogduk[594] defined them as referred pain perceived in any region of the head which was referred by a primary nociceptive source in the musculoskeletal tissues innervated by cervical nerves. Clinical features included: pain that was not lancinating and was dull or aching but could be throbbing, and located in the occipital, parietal, temporal, frontal, or orbital regions, unilaterally or bilaterally. There was some indication of cervical spine abnormality such as neck pain, tenderness, impaired cervical motion, aggravation of the headache by neck movements, or a history of cervical trauma.

Bogduk's diagnostic criteria included: identification by clinical examination, or by imaging of a cervical source of the pain found by valid antecedent studies to be reliably associated with the head pain, or complete relief of the head pain after controlled local anesthetic blockade of one or more cervical nerves or structures innervated by cervical nerves.

Sjaastad[595] also weighed in with specific criteria. He noted that cervicogenic headaches were one-sided, but could also be bilateral "unilaterally on two sides." The duration of a headache or exacerbation ranged from several hours to several weeks. Initially, the headache may be episodic, but can later become chronic-fluctuating. Symptoms and signs were referable to the neck, and included decreased range of cervical motion and mechanical precipitation of attacks. Autonomic symptoms such as nausea and photophobia are not marked, if present. A positive response to appropriate anesthetic blockade is considered essential. Sjaastad noted several Major Criteria:

1. Symptoms and signs of cervical involvement:
   a. Provocation of an irradiating head pain similar to the spontaneously occurring one:
      1. by neck movement and/or sustained awkward head positioning
      2. by external pressure over the upper neck or head on the side ipsilateral to the pain
   b. Restriction of cervical range of motion
   c. ipsilateral neck, shoulder, or arm pain of a vague, nonradicular nature or, on occasion, sharp arm pain in a radicular region

Symptoms and signs 1a-1c are listed in "order of importance." One or more of these must be present for the term "cervicogenic headache" to be used. Point 1a is itself sufficient criteria, but 1b and 1c are not. Point 2 is a necessary additional point.

2. Confirmation by diagnostic anesthetic blocks — necessary point
3. The pain is unilateral and does not shift from side to side.
4. Pain Characteristics:
   a. nonthrobbing pain, usually beginning in the neck
   b. episodes of varying duration
   c. fluctuating, continuous pain
5. Other characteristics of some importance:
   a. marginal or no effect from treatment with Indomethacin
   b. marginal or no effect from treatment with triptans or ergots
   c. female preponderance
   d. history of head or neck trauma

None of the single points under 4 or 5 are essential.

6. Other descriptions of less importance: various headache-related phenomena which are rarely present, and of only mild to moderate severity when present:
   a. nausea
   b. photo- and phonophobia
   c. dizziness
   d. blurred vision ipsilateral to the pain
   e. difficulty with swallowing
   f. fluid around the eye on the same side as the pain

The anatomical basis of CGHA is thought to be secondary to convergence in the trigeminocervical nucleus between nociceptive afferents from the field of the trigeminal nerve and the receptive fields of the first three cervical nerves. Headache appears to be secondary to structural problems in regions innervated by $C_1 - C_3$. These regions include the muscles, joints, and ligaments of the upper three cervical segments, as well as the dura mater of the spinal cord and the posterior cranial fossa and the vertebral artery.[596] Other anatomical causation has been identified and includes[597]:

1. Disrupted and/or ruptured cervical discs with irritation of the sympathetic sinu-vertebral nerves (in the disc) and nerve roots by mechanical and chemical means at single or multiple levels
2. Irritation of the articular branches to the cervical zygapophyseal joints derived from the medial branches of the cervical dorsal rami
3. Irritation of the peripheral branches and unmyelinated nerve structures to the muscle attachments at the spinous process of C_2 supplied by the C_2 and C_3 nerve roots: this includes the rectus capitis posterior, major obliquus capitis inferior major, semispinalis cervicis multifidus, semispinalis

capitis major and rectus capitis posterior minor and interspinal muscles at C_{1-2} and C_{2-3}

4. Pain from the end fibers of the greater tertiary occipital and sympathetic nerve structures with its C-fibers including the periosteum and suboccipital musculature (semispinalis capitis, rectus capitis posterior minor and major, trapezius, and occipitalis)

The treatment of CGHA begins with diagnostic anesthetic blocks that are typically mixed with long acting steroids such as hydrocortisone. This should temporarily relieve the CGHA for hours to days. If pain relief lasts for weeks to months, blocks should be repeated.

Once a specific targeted joint or disc is identified, the latter with discography if needed, a number of procedures have been utilized for treatment of CGHA. These include:

1. Neurolysis of the C_2 nerve root via decompressive surgery[598] as well as partial denervation of the suboccipital and paraspinal musculature[599]
2. Radiofrequency lesions to the muscle attachments of the spinous process at C_2[600,601]
3. Radiofrequency neurotomy of the sinu-vertebral nerves to the upper cervical disc, as well as to the outer layer of the C_3 or C_4 nerve root[602]
4. Radiofrequency denaturation of the occipital nerve[603-605]
5. Radiofrequency denaturation of the C_2 medial rami[606]
6. Cervical discectomy and fusion
7. C2 ganglionectomy[607]

The latter procedure is not often performed, while there remain proponents of radiofrequency lesioning versus the old cervical discectomy and fusion.

It is imperative to differentiate CGHA from both migraine headache and tension-type headache, as the treatments are completely different. Unfortunately, the literature in general argues the question of cervicogenic headache, although not the idea that headache may be associated with cervical pathology. It should be noted that the International Association for the Study of Pain (IASP) has recognized cervicogenic headache as a pain syndrome.[608] This criterion uses neck mobility as the major indicator of this diagnosis, but both tension-type headache and migraine have associated decrements in cervical mobility.

The different criteria for the diagnosis of CGHA make other previously recognized primary headache sufferers fall into the diagnostic hole. There appears to be too much overlap in the varying diagnoses. Likewise, patients with the diagnosis of CGHA may also fall into other diagnostic categories, or even multiple diagnostic categories.[609-611]

Not to be forgotten is the fact that the diagnosis specifically may follow an acceleration/deceleration injury or other cervical trauma.[612,613] This makes it imperative to consider the diagnosis of CGHA in patients with posttraumatic headache who do not show improvement following appropriate treatment for other diagnosed headache diatheses. On the other hand, clinically, CGHA appears to be found in less than 3% to 5% of the PTHA population.

MOVING RIGHT ALONG

If a posttraumatic headache patient also has an MTBI, the level of difficulty in making the diagnosis and treating that patient increases dramatically. Psychological factors are there; the neurochemical aspects of depression and anxiety, for instance, are well known. In the presence of an MTBI they become more difficult to tease out and deal with, as the patients may be dealing with pain as well as changes in cognition and behavior, including frontal lobe difficulties such as increased irritability and labile emotionality.

As previously noted (at least twice), you need to deal with headache and depression before evaluating the presence of an MTBI. This where your knowledge of neuropharmacology as well as neurorehabilitation will be really tested!

Another major problem facing patients and their treating physician(s) are the questions of medico-legal disability secondary to the posttraumatic headache syndrome, with or without the question of MTBI. Patients whose injuries involved a skull fracture, subdural hematoma, or severe lacerations, and whose gray matter is leaking out of their ears, *may* not have a problem in regard to disability. Unfortunately for the patients and their physicians, insurance problems do exist, beginning with getting approvals to treat a posttraumatic headache syndrome.

As noted earlier, some insurance companies deny that there are such things as MTBI or posttraumatic headaches. They have a number of paid clinicians to assure the legal system that this is so. They will try to prevent clinicians from even getting involved with treating these patients by refusing to pay them for treatment. *It does not matter* how devastating a patient's symptoms are, the patient will still face a difficult and totally unjustified legal battle just to get treatment approved, never mind the question of disability compensation.

The minions of the insurance companies are found both in clinical situations and legal ones. These "hired guns" make it as hard as possible for clinicians to do their jobs and treat patients appropriately. That's their job. Be prepared to deal with them.

It is interesting that the vast majority of patients with posttraumatic headaches, particularly those with headaches as part of a postconcussion syndrome, present the same way. Maybe they all spoke together on the Internet and planned it out? No, they are for real and are expressing the same symptomatology from the same causation (head trauma or acceleration/deceleration injuries). This is just like patients with chicken pox who initially present, clinically, in the same way.

Then there is the "M word," malingering. This is associated with the idea that settlement of litigation is all that is needed to put a stop to the posttraumatic headache syndrome. This is also a favorite theme of the insurance companies. True malingering is almost as rare as hens' teeth. There are published studies which demonstrate that legal settlement has nothing to do with the patients' symptoms ending or encouraging them to return to work.[614-617]

Chronic posttraumatic headache, with or without the other aspects of the post-concussion syndrome, are extremely common after head trauma and an acceleration/deceleration injury. These patients are very consistent in their presentations as well as in their descriptions of their symptoms and sequelae. This consistency is strong evidence that their problems are organic in nature and produced by the trauma.

Most patients with posttraumatic headache will have their headache resolve if they are given appropriate medical treatment. About 15% to 20% will have prolonged difficulties. Correct diagnosis and treatment may decrease this percentage. If the patient can get it.

7 Clinical and Neuropsychological Aspects: Things to Look For

One of the most telling problems involved in diagnosing and treating patients with an MTBI is that their affect may be "off." They may not act the way you, the clinician, may expect them to. Without a basic understanding of the possible problems you may encounter, you may be unsure if the patient is just "odd" or needs immediate psychiatric consultation.

One of the interesting phenomena is denial. Two former patients come immediately to mind. In one case, the patient, a 38-year-old male overachiever, was involved in an MVA with significant acceleration/deceleration injuries. He was an engineer at a local television station. After his injury, he, as well as his family members, noted significant deficits in his abilities to concentrate, short-term memory, and significant emotional lability. He came in for treatment, but after three weeks decided that there was nothing wrong with him. In spite of his family's objection, he left treatment. He could only get a job doing construction and, in the course of the first week of his employment, he became distracted when driving a forklift and drove it through a wall. He was fired. Several weeks later he came back to treatment, still in denial, but more open for treatment. We'll go through his history in detail in another chapter.

Another patient was a 46-year-old dentist. This gentleman experienced a slip-and-fall while on vacation. He had a short period of loss of consciousness. He returned to his practice and found himself unable to perform simple procedures such as filling a tooth. He told me about this, and he was asked to stop practicing for a while until we could sort things out. He persisted in practice. His office staff called me and reported that he had significant problems with doing procedures. He told me he would stop seeing patients. He had his first grand mal seizure while in his office. I started him on anticonvulsants and again strongly recommended that he stop seeing patients, which he claimed he would. To make a long story short (we'll go into it in detail in another chapter) he continued to see patients until I had to call the Dental Board, in his presence, and have his license suspended, as his danger of malpractice was very high. Still, he continued to see patients.

The man was very honest when continually confronted with the fact he shouldn't see patients. He stated, also repeatedly, that he knew he probably shouldn't but he thought that everything would "get back to normal" over time. Things were very complicated for almost a year. Finally, he was able to admit to being in denial of his deficits. His entire life, his sense of self was totally invested in his being a dentist. Not to practice dentistry was a devastating blow to his ego as well as his sense of self. I could understand this, but dealing with the medical and emotional aspects of his injury took a long, tortuous time until all the treatment goals were met.

There are a number of other things that the clinician must be cognizant of, in spite of not having any formal training psychologically or psychiatrically. So, in no particular order, some things to be aware of follow.

We have already spoken of the MTBI population as being part of a "Silent Epidemic." Another interesting thought is that the emotional risk factors that influence the outcome of an MTBI make them part of the "miserable minority." Preexisting personality traits that may make treatment more difficult include overachievement, grandiosity, and borderline personality traits, as well as dependency, narcissism, and perfectionism. These preexisting personality factors make treatment more difficult, and the question always arises, "Which came first, the personality issue or the TBI?"

Another significant problem is called "psychiatric disinhibition." Many of us with minimal psychopathology are able to deal perfectly well on a day-to-day basis, without any overt aspects of any psychiatric problems. A TBI, yes, even an MTBI, may disinhibit our ability to keep such problems under total control and essentially invisible. It is obviously difficult to determine which came first unless prior testing has been done, and even then it may be very difficult. However, it is easier to see in patients with minimal problems before an MTBI when, before your eyes, the difficulties become florid.

When looking at the patient reports of physical, affective, behavioral, and cognitive problems, which may exist for weeks, months, or even years after an MTBI, they exhibit neurobehavioral deficits. When looking at a group of patients evaluated for the associations between five sets of symptoms (memory problems, neurological problems, confusion, neurasthenia, and coordination), and five neurobehavioral areas (simple motor speed, response speed and attention, complex perceptual motor performance, visual memory, and learning), it was found that memory difficulties were the problems most frequently experienced by patients in association with performance deficits.[619]

There is evidence that MTBI may induce Axis I, or mood, psychopathology. One study found that prior to a TBI, the majority of patients with a diagnosis had substance use disorders. After TBI, the most frequent Axis I disorders included major depression and select anxiety disorders, including posttraumatic stress disorder (PTSD), panic disorder, and obsessive-compulsive disorder (OCD). Forty-four percent of patients had two or more Axis I diagnoses after TBI. Major depression and substance use disorders were more likely to remit after treatment than anxiety disorders.[620]

Other studies agree that (M)TBI is a risk factor for subsequent psychiatric disorders. Furthermore, post TBI, patients with depression and/or anxiety are more functionally disabled than others without these problems, which also make the patients perceive their impairments as more severe.[621,622] Loss of patients' sense of self is also commonly seen, and increases emotional difficulties.[623-625]

Interestingly, psychosocial disabilities associated with TBI appear to be more strongly associated with mood disorders than are physical disorders.[626]

In my experience, it has appeared to me that the realization of cognitive deficits post MTBI can be devastating to a patient. I am sometimes reminded of the panic and fear seen in the early Alzheimer's disease patients who are able to detect their accumulating deficits.

MTBI has been found to be the triggering event of the onset of pathophysiological changes as well as concomitant depression. Depression in the post-acute TBI patients may vary over time, peaking between one and three years after injury. Depression post brain injury appears to be enhanced in patients with mild differences between intelligence and impairment found on neuropsychological testing.[627-630]

Another problem I've encountered is that of the question of IQ loss. In highly intelligent people, testing may show a loss in the gross IQ score. The functional aspects associated with this loss are much less clear. One study found a mean loss of 14 points of Full Scale IQ using the WAIS-R. These patients also had personality dysfunctions including cerebral personality disorder, PTSD, and, in the majority of patients, a psychiatric diagnosis. The authors felt that the cognitive or IQ loss was secondary to an interaction between the TBI and distractions such as pain and emotional distress. They also noted the incidence of MTBI was underestimated.[631]

Personality disturbances after MTBI are well documented, and appear to be long lasting, according to some authors, and not as strongly associated to TBI according to others.[632-635]

One study looked at the relationship between MTBI and sexual abuse. The author found that patients with both problems exhibited more deficits in working memory, executive functioning, and memory than did members of patient groups with single diagnoses.[636] An unfortunate group of patients I have seen included some who became brain injured during a sexual assault, indicating the need to look a bit harder at these patients.

How MTBI patients cope with their losses is an important issue to evaluate. Early identification of those with the least amount of coping skills can expedite their treatment by having the psychologist begin dealing with coping skills as early as possible post injury. It is also known that patients who cope well are excellent "teachers" to those with similar problems who do not cope as well. This is a good reason for group therapy as an adjunctive treatment. Unfortunately, the insurance minions will not typically reimburse for this care.[637,638]

One of the most difficult patient types to deal with is the very needy patient with a borderline personality disorder. Research appears to indicate that TBI may be the cause, rather than the result, of a borderline personality disorder, and the more cerebral insults that have occurred, the more severe the borderline personality disorder becomes.[639,640] One of the more interesting aspects of this information is that in treating pain patients, those with borderline personality disorders may be the bane of a clinician's existence. Again, it was only after knowing about this apparent association, that my history and examination of these patients became even more inclusive.

Many patients post TBI become increasingly irritable and agitated. The definition of agitation was debated by the BI-SIG (Brain Injury Special Interest Group), a part of the American Academy of Physical Medicine and Rehabilitation. The physiatrists who were polled showed a great deal of variation in their definition of the characteristics that defined agitation. Most defined agitation during the acute recovery phase post TBI as posttraumatic amnesia along with an excess of behavior such as disinhibition, aggression, and/or emotional lability. Fewer felt the definition of delirium in the DSM-IIIR or DSM-IV to be appropriate.[641] Many patients initially fit this definition, at least in the post acute state. Emotional lability seems to endure a bit longer than agitation itself.

An important diagnosis to look for initially is an acute stress disorder (ASD). Research has found that MTBI is a precursor of ASD, particularly in patients with dissociative, reexperiencing, and avoidance symptoms.[642, 643] It is extremely important to determine the presence of ASD, as it must be dealt with using both psychotherapy and neuropharmacological treatments. If it is not adequately dealt with, treatment in general will suffer.

Things do get a bit stickier. One study shows that amnesia of the traumatic event results in less acute posttraumatic stress, intrusive symptoms, perceived injury, and fear of future risk. It was found that in spite of posttraumatic amnesia, a proportion of MTBI patients reported intrusive and avoidance symptoms.[644] In another study, an acute stress disorder was found in 14% of patients post MVA, and at one-month follow-up, 24% satisfied the criteria for PTSD. Six months post trauma, PTSD was found in 82% of patients who had been diagnosed with an acute stress disorder, and also in 11% of patients who had not previously been diagnosed with ASD.[645]

Patients who survived an MTBI were found to develop PTSD as often as those who did not report a TBI or cognitive symptoms.[646,647] In another study, it was felt that posttraumatic amnesia after a moderate TBI may protect against recurring memories and the development of PTSD. It was also felt that some patients with neurogenic amnesia may develop a form of PTSD without experiencing any reexperiencing symptomatology.[648] In spite of much clinical evidence to the contrary, another group felt that PTSD and MTBI were mutually exclusive disorders.[649]

Another group has determined that major depression and PTSD are independent sequelae following trauma, and both have similar prognoses and interact to increase dysfunction and distress.[650]

The obvious issue at hand is if a patient experiences posttraumatic amnesia, how can they develop the psychological stigmata that develops into a PTSD? If they can't remember the trauma, how can they be afraid of it? After all, they don't really remember what happened, so how can they be emotionally affected by it?

In clinical reality, it may be more frightening for a patient who last remembers driving a car and then nothing until they "come to" with physical injuries and cognitive complaints. As one patient told me, "It's like a black box. I was okay, then I wasn't, and something really bad happened to me. I may not remember what it was, but I'm afraid of it, as it must have been terrible to do these things to me." While he didn't remember the actual MVA, he remembered driving before the accident. He developed intrusive thoughts of car crashes, nightmares about car crashes, and a fear of driving. It might even have been worse for this gentleman, as the human imagination can frequently bring forth more frightening ideas than the reality, as frightening as that may have been.

Then, again, remembering the definition of MTBI, loss of consciousness or posttraumatic amnesia are not absolute prerequisites for the diagnosis. MTBI patients who experience a severe acceleration/deceleration injury frequently do remember their MVAs. This may explain a clinically increased number of MTBI patients with PTSD versus the more moderate to severe TBI injuries.

One author noted that it was a continuum of experience which represents the event; a "window" of real or imagined experience which may result from loss of consciousness and/or posttraumatic amnesia after a TBI which does not eliminate the possibility of the development of a PTSD. He raises the interesting question as to whether PTSD post TBI is a subclassification of PTSD.[651]

The question of substance abuse is important, as a good number of patients with TBI were under the influence of alcohol or drugs when they were injured. Substance abuse will make treatment more difficult, while it is difficult enough to determine the presence of substance abuse post injury. In the post-acute stages of rehabilitation, patients who were previously substance abusers may fall back on these self-destructive behaviors. During rehabilitation, it may be necessary to screen a patient for substance abuse if it is likely to have occurred; here, past history is extremely important.[652,653] So are the patient's living arrangements. I had one patient who went to live with his brother, who was also the neighborhood drug pusher. We were able to get him to move to an aunt's home in a different part of the city. Still other patients who finished rehabilitation developed more significant familial problems when they began to, or returned to, alcohol. Four patients come to mind who experienced marital separation or divorce secondary to alcohol. In two of these cases, the patients became more depressed by their deficits and began drinking to "deal with them." Pay attention to patients with histories of substance abuse, or possible propensities for it.

Speaking of relationship changes, research has shown up to 49% of a patient group undergoes divorce/separation during a five- to eight-year period post TBI.[654] This may have had to do with the actual difficulties of spousal role changes which, post TBI, are typically mostly losses.[655] Again, denial usually plays a role in the sundering of these relationships, as does the real and perceived difficulties of taking care of an injured person or being "injured" or "not whole anymore."[656,657] These perceptions by both patient and spouse or significant other need to be dealt with via family therapy, sometimes in addition to individual psychotherapy, to prevent the termination of the relationship. But, of course, insurance typically doesn't pay for this.

Speaking of insurance, one of their favorite tactics is to determine that a patient with an MTBI is malingering or faking the whole thing on a conscious basis. This has been dealt with earlier, along with references. However, one of the malicious minions of the insurance companies who has not, to my knowledge, ever identified a patient as having an MTBI or possibly even a moderate TBI, has determined that naïve subjects given symptom checklists and told to report symptoms of depression, PTSD, and MTBI can do so with a high degree of congruence. This is supposed to illustrate the ease with which actual patients can "fake" their illnesses.[658-660] (And someone actually pays for this!)

Finally, let's discuss some more interesting posttraumatic sequelae. One of the most common psychiatric entities seen in the MTBI patient is rapid cycling bipolar affective disorder. This is noted fairly easily if a clinician has frequent contact with the patient. Clinically, it appears to be associated in some patients with excessively labile emotionality. Carbamazepine is the treatment of choice. One study demonstrated that the etiology was possibly diffuse cerebral injury with a left frontotemporal predominance. The patient described also continued to experience this problem after cognitive recovery.[661]

A rare entity, but one I've seen, is the Kluver-Bucy syndrome, consisting of hyperphagia and hypersexuality. This patient had a short loss of consciousness, but her initial GCS was 15. She was diagnosed with an MTBI. This has also been noted to be part of a posttraumatic remission phase in more severely injured patients; it is associated with a favorable outcome in patients with traumatic disturbances of consciousness.[662]

As previously noted, obsessive-compulsive disorder (OCD) may occur after TBI, with questionable diffuse injury, possibly including the frontal regions, limbic areas, and basal ganglia.[663] This disorder may be particularly difficult to deal with; neuropharmacological treatments are improving for this entity.

The onset of pathological laughter and crying is typically associated with more severe injuries, as well as neurological abnormalities such as a pseudobulbar palsy.[664]

I have seen several patients with episodes of very violent visual hallucinations, as well as two who had what they described as totally horrible hallucinations. One MTBI patient experienced these problems along with psychotic symptomatology. Repeated EEGs were negative, as were structural studies. He needed a combination of an atypical neuroleptic and an anticonvulsant to become symptom free. There were no signs of frontal lobe seizures.[665]

Feelings of unreality and depersonalization were found in 60% of a group of 70 MTBI patients. Many of these patients also had diagnosed PTSD as well as vertigo. The feelings of unreality were not associated with cognitive impairment. The authors estimate the incidence of these problems to range from 13% to 67% of MTBI patients.[666] In my clinical experience, I would estimate approximately 20% of MTBI patients experienced these difficulties.

Perseveration as a possible frontal lobe problem is not uncommon in the MTBI population. The combination of perseveration and wandering, possibly associated with lesions in the frontal, temporal, or parietal lobes, as well as the subcortical motor regions, is noted with more severely injured patients. It is felt that attention and memory deficits are also involved in these behaviors.[667]

Problems with sustained arousal and attention are found in both MTBI and moderate TBI, typically more so in the latter group.[668,669] Typically, these factors are noted in initial evaluations in both speech/language and neuropsychological testing.

Finally, sleep disorders are not uncommon, particularly in those patients with posttraumatic pain or headache. This is more commonly associated with neurochemical changes (decreased serotonin, among others). Frequently there is an alpha wave intrusion into stage four, or delta sleep. The use of benzodiazepine sedative/hypnotics is not recommended for this patient population. There is a much more severe form of sleep abnormality associated with a posttraumatic apallic syndrome, with significant sleep fragmentation.[670] This can be seen in the severely injured TBI patient.

Obviously, we can go on and on, but I think we've briefly mentioned the most common difficulties that the clinician should recognize.

8 Interdisciplinary Evaluation of MTBI

All treatment should be functionally based, particularly the rehabilitation of an MTBI. After a patient's pain and depression have been ameliorated, and they continue to have complaints of cognitive deficits and proclaimed difficulties performing everyday tasks, it is time to perform an evaluation.

It is this author's experience that while functionality is the most important aspect of both evaluation and treatment, the first and expected evaluation is the neuropsychological evaluation. The problem is that while this test may give good information needed in developing a treatment plan, it is not functional. Not only is it not functional, it is not typically sufficient for designing a treatment protocol.

Even worse, it is often not felt to be "scientific," if one defines scientific as a test that gives a specific answer or information that implies definitive results. Am I speaking ill of the neuropsychological evaluation? Not at all. As long as I know the experience level of the tester is adequate and above, and that the tester is unbiased, I'm happy.

In neurology, as well as cardiology, hematology, and endocrinology, tests give answers you can typically take to the bank. Yes, there may be differing opinions, but the test comes out on paper and there is really only one way to read a result. It is either normal or abnormal, and books show how to decide that if a physician doesn't know. Either way, the expert knows what is right and what is wrong on the basis of factual, scientific knowledge.

Unfortunately, this "ain't necessarily so" when looking at the neuropsychological evaluation. Why is this? Probably because two different neuropsychologists who have two different biases, (one patient-oriented, for example, and one insurance-oriented) can look at the exact same data and obtain diametrically opposed diagnoses. One evaluator can find abnormalities that the other evaluator feels are fallacious. There are too many "weasel words" that can be used to twist interpretations. There are too many ways that the reality of "normal" and "abnormal" can be different depending on the circumstances of a legal case.

NEUROPSYCHOLOGICAL EVALUATION

Cognitive screening post MTBI remains quite variable with different methods of diagnosis, indications for testing, and utilization of results being used. A GCS score of 15 may absolutely be associated with a positive cognitive screen. Research has also indicated that there is significant variability in the recovery as well as the

0-8493-1955-2/00/$0.00+$.50
© 2000 by CRC Press LLC

response to treatment after MTBI. The use of early cognitive screening is also important to identify patients with MTBI who are more likely to have residual cognitive deficits after one month.[671-673]

It has also been found that during the first month after MTBI, some cognitive tasks, such as vigilance, may be unimpaired under normal conditions, but may be abnormal when task conditions require sustained effortful processing.[674] This is most commonly seen in areas of multitasking, where individual task performance may appear unimpaired unless the patient is attempting to perform more than one task simultaneously, as most of us do.

The neuropsychological evaluation is used to delineate cognitive and behavioral symptoms. It is used to help explain to a patient and their physician "what is wrong" when all other clinical tests have been normal.

The value of and need for a neuropsychological evaluation is frequently raised, as some clinicians do not understand this relatively new specialty. Another reason for this may be what some would consider the lack of definitive evidence after testing is finished. Raw data from a neuropsychological evaluation may frequently be subject to more than one interpretation, as noted above.

Cognitive impairment is frequently diffuse, with more prominent deficits in the areas of attention, information processing, memory, cognitive flexibility, and problem solving. It has been documented that neuropsychological testing may determine the presence of these changes in patients from one month to years post MTBI.[675-679] These tests are difficult to incorporate into a clinical office evaluation, and this may be one of many factors leading clinicians to fail to recognize these deficits, find no cognitive abnormalities in patients, and declare them "normal."[82,680,681]

Research has shown that when complaints of memory or other cognitive functions, along with irritability or fatigue, persist for more than a month post injury, a comprehensive neuropsychological evaluation should be performed.[682] It is important to determine the existence of deficits, for both the sake of the patient and for the rehabilitation process.

The formal neuropsychological testing procedures involve the neuropsychologist going over a patient's history and past records; a flexible test battery; process observations (how the patient takes the test, along with their reactions as they take it); input from outside observers, including family; and tests of mood and personality. After the tests are scored, patient feedback is given.

Process observations are an integral part of the neuropsychological testing. Every effort should be made to have the treating neuropsychologist administer the testing so these observations can be made, rather than having them just evaluate the raw testing data. It should be noted that a fixed battery of tests, such as the Halsted-Raytan or Luria-Nebraska, would not typically be sensitive to all the cognitive deficits sustained in an MTBI. A good neurological evaluation is flexible. Research, as well as clinical experience, has shown that measures of attention, concentration, speed, and efficiency of information processing are the most sensitive to neurologically-based, organic deficits post MTBI.[682] Attention and information processing are not by themselves specific to MTBI.

A specific hallmark of MTBI appears to be the breakdown of information processing, or the number of operations the brain can simultaneously perform. Slow thought processes, memory deficits, easy distractibility, and lack of attention after MTBI are thought to be secondary to attentional deficits, secondary to decreased ability to process information.[683] Gronwall has developed the paced auditory serial attention test (PASAT) which has been found to be extremely sensitive to MTBI.[684]

To repeat something important, anxiety may decrease concentration and complex mental processes, while depression can decrease cognitive functioning, particularly concentration, memory, and executive functions. These aspects of mood must be evaluated and taken into consideration when assessing neuropsychological testing.

There are other variables which can influence a patient's neuropsychological performance, including age, socioeconomic status, family dynamics, anxiety and depression, and the unconsciousness process of symptom magnification, litigation, drugs, alcohol, pain, and malingering.[682,685,686]

Kay[682] has written about the risk of dysfunctional response to MTBI, not testing, secondary to different personality aspects. He notes five personality styles, including those who are highly driven, possibly obsessive-compulsive, overachievers whose sense of self is tightly tied to intellectual achievement; and persons with tendencies toward grandiosity, with elements of narcissistic personality style, who tend to minimize and deny as well as hide their difficulties until their lives crumble around them before they will acknowledge their difficulties to others. He also notes persons who have suffered emotional deprivation as children, persons with strong tendencies toward dependency, and patients with "borderline" personalities.

Kay has also described several other things which need to be taken into account when evaluating a patient for MTBI, the first of which is "Individual Vulnerability." A significant number of variables will effect how a specific injury will effect a patient, and each person will have a specific level of vulnerability for each specific aspect. These include: neurological vulnerability, neurotransmitter balance, age, drug and alcohol abuse, family dynamics, previous central nervous system damage, personality structure, preexisting psychological problems, current levels of stress, and litigation.[682] The interaction of the neurological and psychological/psychiatric variables determines the individual vulnerability for any single individual post MTBI. These things must be taken into consideration when trying to account for the different outcomes seen in patients after similar injuries.

Kay also described the idea of the "shaken sense of self," which is seen, after an undiagnosed MTBI, as patients' loss of confidence in their abilities increases along with the decreased ability to predict or anticipate their performance in any given situation.

Failure to diagnose MTBI and at least discuss the anticipated cognitive and behavioral deficits with a patient, as well as other possible problems, can exacerbate psychological deterioration. If this occurs secondary to refusal to evaluate a patient for a potential MTBI, it becomes another form of iatrogenic exacerbation (see below).

With neurologically-based organic problems or "weak links" in the post-MTBI central nervous system, a patient will become more vulnerable to anxiety and depression. The presence of significant emotional dysfunction years after an MTBI is not evidence that organically-based neuropsychological problems do not exist. The primary or core organic deficits may be fueling and perpetuating the psychological overlay.

The measurement of a neuropsychological deficit is an important consideration. Two neuropsychologists may come to different conclusions when looking at the same raw data. One reason for this is, typically, that one of them administered the testing and was therefore able to perform direct observations regarding the way the patient took the test.

An even more important reason is that there are several methods that can be used to evaluate the neuropsychological test results. The first is done by comparing the results to normative comparison standards, therefore comparing patients to a large statistical group. This technique seems to find too frequently, in the MTBI patient, a lack of statistical significance for many patients who would be determined to demonstrate cognitive deficits if the second method, utilizing individual comparison standards, was performed. This entails determining specific measurement of deficits by comparing a patient's test results to his or her premorbid status, utilizing what Lezak has called the "Best Performance Method."[687] This technique uses test scores, other observations, and historical data. During the interpretation, the level of the best performance, be it the highest score or group of scores, serves as the best estimate of premorbid achievement, and becomes the standard against which all other aspects of a patient's current performance is compared. This methodology is more specific to the patient, and not a comparison of a single patient to very large statistical groups, which would be adequate for patients with moderate and severe deficits. If a patient was cognitively impaired, their least depressed ability found on testing, utilizing the best performance method, is felt to be the best representative of that person's original cognitive potential. Lezak also notes that a person's premorbid ability level can be reconstructed or estimated from many different kinds of behavioral observations and historical facts. But only if the clinician looks for them.

Another problem with neuropsychological testing is that it has not progressed to the level of specific determination of the majority of frontal lobe deficits. Behavioral problems, including psychiatric disinhibition, aggressive-violent behavior, and emotional lability are frequently seen and associated with frontal/temporal lobe damage and/or limbic system damage. This is not always picked up on neuropsychological testing, therefore giving the patient, his family, and his clinicians the wrong idea of what is going on with the patient's behavior.

Another important question is whether or not patients who have neuro-cognitive deficits that resolve within three to six months actually have the characteristic microscopic neuropathological changes found in acceleration/deceleration type injuries; or, do they have them, but in lesser severity or in areas of the brain which do not correspond to interpretation or even identification with present testing methods?

SOME OTHER ASPECTS

Impaired awareness of cognitive and behavioral sequelae post MTBI appear to be frequently found, with patient overestimation of functioning, as compared to family member ratings and other rating methods. The most common current method of obtaining this information is to compare a patient's self-ratings on questionnaires of functional abilities with ratings by relatives or clinical staff on the same questionnaire.[688,689]

As mentioned above, attentional deficits may not be easily found. One study showed a relative decline in processing speed in patients with MTBI as compared with control subjects, and that patients with MTBI show relatively subtle cognitive deficits which are primarily under conditions that require complex or controlled cognitive processing that exceeds their available cognitive resources. The attentional deficits apparent during dual task demands may represent decreased cognitive and, possibly, neural efficiency, which reflects an MTBI patient's subjective complaints and functional impairments.[690] MTBI may result in the slowing of very basic cognitive information processes.[691]

While possibly difficult to determine, TBI patients appear to have a working memory impairment secondary to a dysfunction in the central executive system, which may be related to executive function deficits that originate in the frontal lobes.[692] Insufficient attention to tasks can result in slips of action as automatic, unintended action sequences are inappropriately triggered. Such slips may arise in part from deficits in sustained attention, which is particularly likely to occur following frontal lobe and white matter injury.[693]

As briefly mentioned in an earlier chapter, SPECT findings have been found to predict neuropsychological test performance, while the obverse was not true. HMPAO SPECT may be a good complement to MRI or CAT scan by demonstrating brain dysfunction in morphologically intact brain regions, and providing some objective evidence for some of the impaired neuropsychological performance produced on testing.[334,694]

It has been felt that the effects of brain injury in young people would cause less impairment than in adults (the "Kennard Principle"). This is now being questioned, with possible clinical thought that damage to the rapidly developing brain can be more harmful than equivalent damage in an adult.[695]

In patients over 50 years of age, MTBI does not necessarily indicate a good prognosis, and it could be followed by very severe consequences.[696] Other studies also show that older adults show less complete recovery one year after TBI than younger adults, either because they have decreased reserves with which to deal with a brain injury, or because their physiological status creates a more destructive injury.[697] Another study found that the greater neuropsychological impairment found in older adults with TBI was most likely related to normal aging.[698]

Just to review, for those who are still wondering, the *executive functions* are important aspects of general functioning in the real world post injury, and are difficult things to evaluate with neuropsychological testing. Basically, intact executive functions allow a person to plan, initiate, follow through, and, at the same time, monitor the success of activities. These functions are based in the prefrontal areas of the frontal lobes. Frontal lobe injury in general may induce emotional disinhibition, emotional blunting, perseveration, affective lability, violent behaviors, and irritability. A lesion of the baso-medial frontal cortex may induce impairment in social judgment and sexual control. Injury to the dorsolateral frontal cortex may induce problems with the executive skills, and patients may not be able to plan, initiate, and execute a complex or even relatively simple task.

I will leave it to the chapter on neuropsychology in the second half of this book to get into more pertinent detail on neuropsychological testing and treatment.

As noted above, neuropsychological evaluation is not considered to be particularly functional in nature. On the other hand, both the Speech and Occupational Therapy evaluations are very functional in nature. I am almost always amazed by the lack of this knowledge by clinicians of both the medical and the neuropsychological classes.

If the neuropsychological evaluation is positive, then the more functional speech-language pathology and occupational therapy evaluations should be performed. Why wait? Because some of the "merry minions" of the insurance persuasion insist that a neuropsychological test be done first. One of the most idiotic situations I've run into was secondary to an insurance company's plan to deny care to the MTBI patient. They insisted that within the first six months post injury, a neuropsychological screen, not a full-fledged evaluation, must be done. This is despite research indicating that a full neuropsychological evaluation is done after a month or so if the patient has continuing complaints that warrant it.

The plan was this (believe me, this is true): I would order a full neuropsychological evaluation. I would be told by the insurance company person (or, more likely, the company the insurance company hired) that only a neuropsychological screen — a very abbreviated version of a full evaluation — could be done. So, wanting to help the patients, I would have a screen done. It would be positive. The company doing the insurance company's work, typically a "third-party administrator, or TPA," would have the screen results reviewed by one of their "bought-and-paid-for" neuropsychologists, who would opine that the neuropsychological screen was worthless (it was, too) and a full neuropsychological evaluation should have been done. Without that information, no treatment would be allowed. The problem was, the insurance company and the TPA wouldn't allow a full neuropsychological evaluation to be done. Checkmate. The patient couldn't receive care or even an appropriate evaluation within the most appropriate six-month post injury time period. The patient would develop a great deal of anxiety, depression, and symptom exacerbation while waiting for the end of the six-month period so a full evaluation could be done. Then, if the patients could keep it together and wait for six months (a good number just got disgusted and left before more care could be given, *the real reason for this run around*) the neuropsychological testing showed more depression and anxiety, which would "invalidate" the evaluation for neuropsychological purposes.

On occasion, I would be able to obtain a speech or occupational therapy evaluation that demonstrated significant functional deficits. Having escaped from having to pay for a neuropsychological evaluation, and therefore not being "officially" able to determine that a patient had an MTBI, the TPA did not care if occupational therapy or speech therapy was given on an occasional basis.

SPEECH-LANGUAGE PATHOLOGY EVALUATION

When an individual sustains an MTBI, their language-cognitive skills may be affected. As cognitive abilities and language are intrinsically and reciprocally related functionally, an impairment of language may disrupt one or more cognitive processes. The reverse is also true: cognitive deficits may disrupt language skills and abilities.[699]

The comprehensive cognitive/communication skills assessment performed by the speech-language pathologist (SLP) should include four basis areas: 1, how a person organizes information for processing and retrieval; 2, how a person codes and retrieves information; 3, how a person reasons and problem-solves; and 4, how language and cognitive deficits affect other areas of functioning.[700,701]

As noted above, some areas most frequently affected by an MTBI include short- and long-term memory; attention to tasks; ability to sequence information; problem solving (including deductive and abstract reasoning); reading comprehension; writing organization; grammar; and pragmatics, or social skills. These are far more functionally based than some of the information garnered by the neuropsychological evaluation. The focus of speech-language treatment is to help the patient relearn lost skills, or learn compensatory strategies to help compensate for any areas of deficit.

The SLP will identify and treat a patient's organizational and problem-solving abilities, visual and auditory attention, and areas of focused, selective, alternating, and divided attention. Assessment also involves interaction skills, including facial expression and tone of voice. Memory skills overlap into functional tasks such as reading and following directions. For this reason, the SLP will also evaluate various memory types (visual, auditory, delayed, remote, etc.) and help design and implement appropriate treatment strategies. Reading and writing skills are also evaluated for functionality by the SLP, who may need to devise compensatory strategies.

Pragmatic skills, the awareness of appropriate emotional, verbal, and nonverbal behaviors, are also evaluated. Functional pragmatic skills may effect a person's ability to socialize with family and friends, as well as job performance.

All of the cognitive aspects noted have a significant impact on a person's communication skills and his or her ability to function in the real world. The SLP works to teach patients how to relearn information or to incorporate strategies that compensate for deficits within their functional lives. It takes time and significant effort to generalize the use of compensatory strategies, including coordinated, continued guidance and encouragement from the SLP as patients go through trial-and-error periods to incorporate these new strategies and skills into their lives. The key to treatment success is practice in real-life situations. It is therefore common, if not mandatory, for treatment to take place in the community, not just at the clinical site.[702]

OCCUPATIONAL THERAPY EVALUATION

In a fashion similar to the SLP, the occupational therapist (OT) evaluates and treats on a functional basis. The OT evaluation involves identification of specific physical, cognitive, or perceptual deficits that may interfere with a patient's ability to perform functionally-oriented tasks. Treatment addresses the problems in individual or group treatments through the use of functional activities.[703,704]

The OT should evaluate various types of attention (sustained, selective, alternating, and divided). Deficits in divided attention or multitasking activities may make it very difficult for a patient to function at work, in a store, or at home.

Impaired multitasking is one of the most common and most devastating sequelae of an MTBI, forcing a person's abilities to function in the real world to be significantly downgraded. One cannot drive if multitasking abilities are impaired. Think about it.

Other aspects of an OT evaluation should include memory storage and recall of both auditory and visual information. The use of a day planner, for example, may be an appropriate functional compensatory strategy to deal with some memory deficits. Awareness of time and date may be impaired, as may be the ability to give and receive verbal and written directions. These aspects of cognition, which certainly impact on a patient's ability to work, and financial management, should be addressed in treatment.

Executive functioning is an important aspect of OT treatment, as are problem solving and abstract reasoning. The evaluation of situational problem solving, including safety and judgment issues, is very important. Difficulties with visual perception, poor tolerance or endurance, and upper extremity functioning are also part of the OT's purview. Activities of daily living (ADLs) are a key focus of OT evaluation and treatment, and should include personal hygiene, cooking, eating, dressing, parenting skills, and responsibilities in the home environment.

One of the most important responsibilities of the OT is the evaluation of a patient's vocational status. Work skills should be practiced through actual work tasks. Volunteer positions are utilized if actual work tasks cannot be obtained. Job interviewing skills should also be addressed and practiced.

Community reentry and leisure skills are addressed in individual and group treatments; pragmatics should be incorporated into these activities.

The OT treatment of the MTBI patient should emphasize the return to their previous roles and daily activities. This encompasses a patient's entire daily routine. As a member of the treatment team, the patient's input into the constantly evolving evaluation and treatment strategies is necessary and invaluable.

SOME FINAL NOTES ABOUT REALITY

The description of what and how various members of the MTBI treatment team should function is based on the treatment protocols the author has developed over 20 years. It works. Unfortunately, it is now more difficult to achieve the goals of patient independence.

The minions of the insurance companies will no longer pay for any form of group therapy. Many will no longer pay for care given outside of the treatment site. Little things, such as leisure activity evaluation and treatment aren't paid for. Remember the Therapeutic Recreational Therapist? That's a dying or dead breed, as insurance won't pay for their services.

Once, in court, where I was an expert witness, the opposing attorney, a known insurance "HO," couldn't find fault with anything in a patient's treatment for which I couldn't give him chapter, verse, and references. So, he spent most of his time arguing to the jury that the patient had been taken out of the clinic and that leisure activities such as bowling or going to the zoo had taken place.

I explained, as much as I was able, that 1, group activities in the real world are important for reasons discussed above — things like pragmatics, community reintegration, returning to a normal life, etc.; 2, think about the skills needed for something as simple as bowling: coordination, perception, focus, multitasking (being able to focus on bowling with noise, bright lights, and other distractions), and pragmatics — reactions to wining, losing, a poor throw, and so on; and 3, at least at that time, recreational therapy was part of the Commission on Accreditation of Rehabilitation Facilities (CARF) guidelines. None of this meant anything to this attorney, or if it did, it did not matter to him. His job was to prove that the patient had received inappropriate care, and he felt that this was amply demonstrated by recreational therapy. This particular minion of the insurance companies lost his case, but to me the point was made.

Recreational therapy and community reintegration don't sound like medicine, and, as the vast majority of people don't realize what rehabilitation entails, they are easy targets for the insurance companies and the legal eagles who work for them. The ability to provide the best care possible for MTBI patients is drawing to a close because of undisputed greed and a studied lack of caring.

We have discussed the concepts of iatrogenic- and nomogenic-induced exacerbation of symptomatology, that is, the lack or delay of treatment of patients with MTBI, mild–moderate TBI, or even the PCS or the PPCS can increase the psychosocial factors within the impairments/symptom complex. The lack of support by professionals, the restrictions imposed by some reimbursement sources, and skeptical loved ones (since the professionals say there is nothing wrong) frequently lead to anger, frustration, depression, and despair. The symptom complex may exacerbate, or increase. Some patients may become so dysfunctional that they are terminated from their jobs. This may continue, leading to a downward spiral of ever greater dysfunction.

Then, when some of these aspects are noted on evaluation, *it is the patient's fault*, never mind that the system is further disabling them. So, be aware, very aware, of a patient's history when making judgments.

9 Interdisciplinary Treatment of MTBI

DIMENSIONS OF BRAIN INJURY REHABILITATION

The essence of appropriate treatment is to take each patient as an individual with specific sequelae from an MTBI and develop a treatment plan that is both general and specific. Treatment must be functionally oriented and, therefore, must be evaluated by measures of functional improvement.

- Major treatment goals:
  1. Individualization of treatment
  2. Patient education
  3. Communication skills
  4. Family education
  5. Return to appropriate employment
  6. Posttreatment support as needed
- The interdisciplinary team
  1. Medical Director – experienced in diagnosis, treatment aspects, and neuropharmacological treatment
  2. Clinical and neuropsychology
  3. Occupational therapy
  4. Speech-language pathology
  5. Physical therapy
  6. Nurse-rehabilitation specialists
  7. Vocational specialists
  8. Family services
  9. Therapeutic recreation
  10. The patient and his or her family

Are all these people needed to help one survivor of an MTBI? It depends on each patient's specific needs. It also depends on several other things, unfortunately. These things include:

1. How focused you are in wanting to provide the patient the most appropriate rehabilitation, to take them to their maximal level of functioning

2. How well the patient's insurance company will reimburse the various aspects of treatment

3. How much you really care about patient outcome, supposedly the *sine qua non*, the essence of treatment accountability

Now we have to separate the doctors from the clinicians. As most of you know, managed care has managed to place upon the weary heads of the general practitioner the mandate that they must do everything for everyone — all patients — and to send a patient to a specialty consultation under penalty of financial or even more severe difficulties. Some doctors may take the same approach to the rehabilitation of the MTBI survivor, as well as the mild to moderately injured patient.

The majority of TBI is in the mild and mild-moderately severe categories. Most of the former, at least 70%, may do just fine in six months or so. The problem is, how do you know which seven out of ten MTBI patients that will be?

There already exists the nihilistic treatment viewpoint. Patients found to have suffered an MTBI are given acknowledgment and a pamphlet or two regarding the possible problems they may expect. They are then sent on their way, in the hopes that early education will prepare them for the life changes they may have to endure. Add to this the thinking of the minions of the insurance persuasion who have decided that there is no such thing as an MTBI, or, if there is such an animal, minimal treatment will do, because MOST MTBI patients will "magically get better without any help at all."

Then there is the all-pervasive PPO or TPA, whose hopefully high school-educated adjusters will determine for the physician how many physical therapy, occupational therapy, or speech therapy visits can be allowed, almost always in single digits. Worse, to my way of thinking, since these folks just follow a "cook-book" given to them by their employers, are the nurse case managers who have the authority, without the experience or education, to tell a patient and their family that they will receive no, or very limited, care, and who act as hatchet people for the insurance companies who employ them to do just that. They deny care, using their nursing license to do so, under their employer's banner. Is this my supposition? No way. Over the last ten years I've employed three nurses whom I've had the privilege to teach and work with in treating MTBI survivors. They quit working for me to join insurance company case management organizations. It is a tribute to them that all three lasted less than six months at their new jobs. After they left, they came back hoping to rejoin my clinical staff. The abuses of the system they had to participate in were just plain more than they could stomach and still look at their faces in a mirror without flinching. So they left the "cushy" world of the TPA or insurance case management organizations and returned to help the patients who needed help.

To Move On

- Vocational rehabilitation
  1. Work simulation
  2. Supported employment

3. Full vocational assessment
4. Physical/functional capacity evaluation

As will be discussed below, one of the measures of quality of life for the TBI survivor is the ability to return to work. Yet, many insurance companies won't pay for vocational services. (Depending on the state, vocational services after a work-related injury may or may not be paid for; it's rarer than hen's teeth in a motor vehicle medical liability insurance policy.)

The above paragraph may infer that the insurance companies won't allow vocational services. This is not true. They will tell you, the clinician, and even the patient, that it's allowed: they just don't have to or don't intend to pay for it. Typically, this is because it is not specifically written in the patient's insurance policy that he can receive that form of rehabilitation. If the patient can receive any form of rehabilitation at all is another question. Yeah, as if the typical person who buys automobile insurance is going to check for their ability to receive rehabilitation at all, never mind vocational rehabilitation.

A word of warning: never buy automobile insurance whose medical benefits are done via PPO. There are still some very good insurance policies without a PPO or TPA there to act as the forward guard in denying any needed treatment.

Medical consultants may be needed, including:

1. Neuro-otology
2. Neuro-ophthalmology
3. Optometry
4. Psychiatry
5. Primary Care
6. Dentistry
7. Audiology

There are typically several types of interested third parties:

1. Employer
2. Attorney
3. Insurance Representative
4. Case Manager
5. Other involved parties

It is best to remember that involvement doesn't always mean that the patient's best interests are always foremost in their minds. It is up to the Medical Director and the rest of the clinical staff to deal appropriately with these folk, most of whom, for better or for worse, have the right to obtain, legally, patient-oriented information.

The patient care overview therefore indicates that the patient, their family, and the treatment team, many times, need input from:

1. Medical consultants
2. Diagnostic services

3. Additional clinical services
4. Interested third parties

To recap a bit, the most common deficits seen in the MTBI population include:

1. Memory impairment
2. Irritability
3. Anxiety
4. Loss of self-esteem, the shattered sense of self
5. Behavioral and personality changes
6. Job loss/disruption
7. Lack of initiative
8. Difficulties with social interactions and family relationships
9. Reduced ability to concentrate
10. Poor control of impulses
11. Slowed information processing

And don't forget the most common medical problems:

1. Posttraumatic headache
2. Posttraumatic musculoskeletal pain syndromes
3. Vestibular disturbance
4. Visual disturbance
5. Fatigue

Other typical clinical problems, in no particular order, may include:

• Goal Setting	Attention	Procedural learning
• Planning	Concentration	Self-regulation
• Self-initiating	Memory	Endurance
• Self-monitoring	Information Processing	
• Disinhibition	Problem Solving	Motor and Sensory Changes
• Perseveration	Social Judgment	Impulse Control
• Flexibility	Emotional lability	Pragmatics
• Depression	Frustration	Aphasia/Dysphasia
• Irritability/Volatility		

So, why the heck would a full transdisciplinary treatment team be needed? I can't imagine. Can you?

During the patient evaluation stage, a preinjury profile is helpful. This would include:

• Educational history: school records, military records
• Social history: legal problems, living arrangements
• Vocational history: job and effectiveness

- Interpersonal history: marital status; number, types of friends
- Economic history: type of work, living environment, social programs utilized
- Psychiatric history: premorbid status

TREATMENT PARADIGMS

As noted above, patients should be evaluated as soon as possible. The typical patient has had posttraumatic headache or pain for weeks or months or longer, with depression and anxiety. Once all of the etiologies of a patient's problems can be determined, a quality treatment plan to deal with all of the issues can be devised. Pain and depression must be effectively treated early on.

While there are a number of different treatment paradigms and designs, emphasis here is placed on the patient with mild to mild-moderate TBI in the outpatient environment.

The single most important concept of treatment of a person with an MTBI is functionality. All forms of treatment, as well as evaluation, should be geared to this.

Over the last decade, we have seen the development of computer-oriented "cognitive rehabilitation," which is not a functional treatment. The use of a computer may enhance a patient's abilities in only specific areas of cognition, but these "treatments" most frequently do not generalize.[705, 706] Newer work with task performance in virtual environments is being developed, which should be very interesting.[707]

After a patient has been thoroughly evaluated by an interdisciplinary team, including neurology or physiatry, neuropsychology, speech-language pathology, and occupational therapy, an individualized treatment program or protocol is designed for the patient. For example, a "limited services" program consisting of several SLP and OT treatment sessions a week over the course of four to six weeks may satisfy a patient's needs. Other patients with more, or more severe, deficits may need a full interdisciplinary day treatment program. In this form of treatment, the patient is seen for treatment by the physician, the nurse rehabilitation specialist (who coordinates all care and interfaces more frequently with the patient and their family), SLP, OT, clinical or neuropsychologist, physical therapist (for continued pain and/or balance difficulties), and a vocational specialist who helps in the patient's return to work with appropriate accommodations, or the attainment of a new, more appropriate vocation. Therapeutic recreation has also commonly been used to help the SLP and OT in a more holistic approach to community reorientation and reintegration.

Important parts of treatment are the neuropharmacological aspects. There are a number of medications that should not be utilized for a patient with an MTBI, including narcotics, barbiturates (in analgesics or anticonvulsants), or Dilantin, all of which may increase cognitive dysfunction. The use of any psychoactive medications must be done carefully, but these medications may also be important and necessary to treatment to deal with affective and behavioral problems that may be hindering cognitive-oriented functional treatment.

The integration of therapeutic medication options in conjunction with a functionally oriented MTBI treatment program appears to enhance, and becomes synergistic in achieving, timely functional outcomes.[708] The use of such medications will necessitate careful and continuous patient medical management by the prescribing physician, who should also understand in detail the effects of these medications in the disrupted CNS found in the MTBI patient.

Research indicates that a holistic psychosocial rehabilitation program for post-acute TBI patients is effective.[709] Further, early intervention by a specialist TBI treatment team significantly reduces social morbidity and severity of postconcussional symptoms even six months post TBI.[710]

It has also been reported that after inpatient treatment for a TBI, survivors often experience mild to moderate regression in behavior and functional skills after they are discharged home. This also reiterates the importance of the high degrees of structure found in inpatient rehabilitation programs.[711] This was also found when there was a proliferation of inpatient pain management units, providing a "womb with a view," with patients typically showing regression upon returning to their homes. This illustrated the importance of a well-structured outpatient pain management program. The same facts have demonstrated the usefulness and importance of a highly-structured outpatient MTBI program, which is also far more cost-effective than an inpatient treatment program.

In reviewing a cross-section of mild and moderate TBI, it was noted that patients with increased severity of injury received more service seven to ten days post injury, but most service was given to mild TBI patients, in follow-up, to six months post injury.[712]

Other bits of interesting current knowledge indicate that, as one would expect, a patient's awareness of their deficits is a significant factor in the recovery process post TBI.[713] Improvement in functional performance can occur up to ten years after a TBI.[714]

It should come as no surprise, particularly to a clinician treating MTBI, that persons with MTBI may be influenced by their environment when performing household tasks.[715] This has been noted, clinically, by occupational therapists who appropriately treat persons with MTBI in their homes, as an extension of the outpatient clinical therapy. Home visits to evaluate activities of daily living and safety should be a part of each patient's treatment program.

Only the insurance companies and their associated legal minions underestimate the importance of leisure activities in the life of a patient who has survived a TBI. Quality of life issues certainly are impacted by the lack of leisure activities post MTBI. These may be dealt with via individual as well as group treatment protocols.[716] As helping patients to become independent in all aspects of their lives, including leisure activities, is one of the most important goals in therapy, it should not be forgotten.

An important aspect of functionality is the realm of motor skills. It has been found that motor deficits are present one year after MTBI; grip strength is more sensitive to recovery in the first year post MTBI, and finger tapping continues to be impaired one year post MTBI possibly secondary to its speed requirements.[717] Clinical evaluation and treatment by PT, as well as OT and TR (therapeutic recreation), are all important for the patient to regain maximal functionality. Other methods are being developed to enable patients to enhance motor control.[718,719] The benefits of exercise and physical conditioning to the TBI population are also felt to be important.[720-723]

As with all other branches of medicine, other types of treatment have been used for TBI. Craniosacral manipulation was found to be empirically useful in TBI patients, but iatrogenesis (adverse reaction) was found in low rates, but with significant problems.[724] The use of weak, complex pulsed magnetic fields was found to improve depression and decrease phobias while not changing physical symptomatology in MTBI patients.[725] Cranial electrical stimulation apparently decreased negative mood factors in MTBI without placebo effect or increased seizure activity.[726]

RECOMMENDED EVALUATION/TREATMENT GUIDELINES

The recommended guidelines below are for ambulatory patients who fit the diagnostic criteria of MTBI by the mild traumatic brain injury committee of the Brain Injury Interdisciplinary Special Interest Group of the American Congress of Rehabilitation Medicine, as noted earlier in this text. These patients will already have received an initial evaluation. Many times, the initial complaint is posttraumatic headache, pain or dizziness, or changes in behavior or emotional status with lability, or aggressive or violent behaviors. Changes in cognitive status may be volunteered by the patient, family, or significant other.

The patient should be asked about the neurovegetative triad of depression (sleep disturbance, loss of libido, changes in appetite). Talking with the spouse or significant other should be done at the time of the initial history, if possible. The patient's work status, including changes or problems, should be part of the history.

The neurological examination should include special attention to the cranial nerve examination for anosmia (loss of smell), aguisia (loss of taste), lateralization of hearing, and poor eye convergence. Pathological frontal lobe reflexes are commonly not evaluated by the examiner. Palmomental, jaw jerk, suck, snout, and glabellar should be checked. Balance should be evaluated, as should cerebellar functions. Sensory examination should include vibratory and positional testing.

As the patient describes their history, listen carefully for word-finding problems or variations in responses to questions.

A thorough musculoskeletal examination must be performed, particularly if the patient presents with a history of headache or other posttraumatic pain. It may be difficult to make an initial diagnosis of MTBI in the presence of pain or headache, although it may be highly suspect. Some patients have cognitive deficits so severe that they are very apparent. If the elements of pain and depression are primary, at least during the initial evaluation, the presumptive diagnosis of MTBI should be made a "rule out" and recommendations for its evaluation should be made.

As stated earlier, pain and depression should be treated as soon as possible, as they may figure significantly in the development of MTBI with persistent sequelae. Ideally, early intervention will decrease the chronic symptoms associated with pain and depression that can mask, initially, the cognitive and behavioral sequelae associated with MTBI.

If the patient is first seen within six weeks of their injury, their pain and depression may be relatively easily treated with appropriate therapy. If two or more months have passed, the patient may need treatment in an interdisciplinary headache or pain treatment program, as myofascial and affective changes along with sleep disorder and central neurochemical nociceptive changes have to be dealt with. Inappropriate treatment, or no treatment, will create much greater difficulties that will require more treatment, and more cost, in the future.

As stated several times in this text, functional gains or improvement in treatment must be carefully and closely monitored, as subjective pain complaints in a patient with MTBI may not change. Lack of improvement can be secondary to learned or perseverative behaviors or difficulty conceptualizing the pain rating scale.

Typically, after three or four weeks of pain treatment, the pain and at least a major component of any depression should be ameliorated. This is extremely important in the chronic patient before a concrete diagnosis of MTBI can be made. At that time, a neuropsychological evaluation can be done by a psychologist who has had specific specialty training in neuropsychological assessment; a weekend course is not sufficient. It is recommended that a psychologist familiar with the best performance method of determining cognitive deficits be used, as the results obtained will be more specific to the patient and provide the most treatment-oriented information if the presence of an MTBI is determined. This may also make the diagnosis more easily defensible in court, especially when many of the insurance minions don't approach cases in this way.

The neuropsychological evaluation should be performed as early as one month after injury — if the patient has no other significant problems such as pain or depression — if MTBI is clinically suspected.

At its best, the neuropsychological evaluation is not particularly functional. Problems that the patient may experience are hypothesized from any specific findings. Therefore, if the neuropsychological evaluation is positive, speech-language pathology and occupational therapy evaluations should be performed, as these evaluations supplement the neuropsychological evaluation with more functionally related information. In rare cases, these evaluations may need to be done first to demonstrate an unrequited need for a neuropsychological evaluation.

After all evaluations are finished, the interdisciplinary team meets and determines a specific, individualized treatment program. Patients with minimal difficulties need minimal treatment, which could encompass only several weeks. Other patients with more significant problems may require several months (8 to 12 weeks) of intervention. If job performance is affected, a job site evaluation and training in compensatory strategies may be required.

Often, treatment may involve retraining a patient to attend school. Many patients are students at the time of injury and have difficulty returning to school. Others will need to attend classes to train for another job or area of employment.

The typical full interdisciplinary outpatient MTBI treatment program will last between 8 and 12 weeks, depending on the deficits and individual needs of the patient. The patient will be treated by the physician, with neuropharmacological agents if needed; the psychologist or neuropsychologist; the speech-language pathologist and occupational therapists; biofeedback therapist if desensitization is needed; physical therapy for balance and continued pain problems; the therapeutic recreation specialist; and the vocational specialist.

Some common problems exist that clinicians should be aware of, if they have not yet encountered them. First, some of the minions of the insurance companies actually believe that the SLP and the OT perform identical services and therefore only one or the other should be used. Aside from the obvious absurdity of this notion, you must be certain that treatment documentation is excellent, with both the SLP and OT documenting everything they did in their specific purview. It is certainly true that both specialists can cross cover each other in some aspects, but OTs don't do speech training and SLPs typically don't do home visits for ADL activities. Don't be lulled into becoming sloppy in your documentation just because it doesn't make sense.

Another favorite tactic is to dismiss an injury because a patient may have had a previous psychological history. I've had a number of patients like this. One in particular had seen a psychotherapist years prior to her injury, for a limited time, to deal with issues of a divorce. She was therefore penalized because she had used the mental health system years prior to her injury; all of her cognitive and behavioral sequelae were directly linked to this single episode of psychotherapy many years predating her problems.

As an old professor of mine was fond of saying, "A patient with lice can also have fleas," or, to put it another way, even a schizophrenic can get hit by a truck. A past history of psychological problems *does not* mitigate against a diagnosis of MTBI. Frequently, the MTBI will exacerbate prior psychological problems (disinhibition), if any existed. Then the "friendly" insurance or legal folk will do their best to apportion a patient's psychological problems. They will find someone who will spout pseudo-erudite psychobabble which will state that 70% of the patient's psychological problems were preexisting, as if quantifying an intangible is anywhere near scientific.

Post MTBI psychological problems can be multifaceted. Sometimes, the only way to explain this is that the MTBI patient's psychological problems are like a black hole; everything that has or is going on emotionally/psychologically gets sucked in and comes out the other end, typically in an enhanced or modified form. To try to accurately identify which problems were solely preexisting an injury, and which were caused solely by the injury, and to demarcate the two types of problems is an exercise in futility. You have to treat what you find. When faced with a patient with a history of sexual abuse who has had an MTBI, you cannot reasonably ignore the former, as the latter may cause the patient to reinterpret the abuse using a mind exhibiting cognitive/behavioral changes. These patients may not think or understand or react to emotional interactions in the same way after an MTBI. To say it "ain't so" is to deny the complexity of the patient's problems and toady to the insurance folk who will use any excuse to not pay for an injury or various aspects of it.

Sometimes, to obtain appropriate care the patient needs to get an attorney, someone to fight for them outside of the medical arena. Yes, it's absurd, but that's the least of the things that can be said of managed care.

Third, as noted above, the thought of a person regaining the physical, social, cognitive, pragmatic, and community reentry skills that will enable them to be able to obtain some quality of life by correctly utilizing leisure activities rather than being forced to stay at home hiding behind the shades, is anathema to many insurance companies and the legal birds who work for them. They love to make that quite clear in the courtroom as they attempt to convince a jury of how absurd the idea of teaching leisure activities is, when they (the nonbrain-injured folk on the jury) don't get such goodies paid for by their insurance companies. I'm not making this up. This is how it is.

So, for the benefit of the Therapeutic Recreational therapists out there, and the clinicians who would use them appropriately, "Be careful out there."

A functionally-oriented treatment program will have a patient return to work by the middle of their treatment, so that work-related accommodations can be determined and implemented during the remainder of treatment. If a patient cannot return to their prior work, a volunteer position at a local facility may be obtained. Work-related skills are retaught in the clinic as well as on site.

Weekly or biweekly interdisciplinary team staff meetings should take place regularly. This is the optimal time for the treatment team to share information with the outside case manager, if the patient has one; the payer; and the patient. These meetings should not only include patient-specific information, but should be vehicles to inform other concerned individuals about the clinical and cognitive problems the patient is experiencing. It can be time used to explain why specific treatment protocols are being utilized. It is also a good time to present requests for compensatory equipment, etc.

Functionality is the key to the rehabilitation of the patient with an MTBI. The goal is to return the patient to his or her family, social systems, community, and vocation as smoothly as possible.

The psychological aspects of treatment are constantly changing. They encompass the patient as well as his or her family, significant others, and friends. Emotional lability or psychotic, aggressive, or frightening behaviors must be dealt with before they contribute to the dissolution of the family unit. For this reason, the psychologist must frequently work with the patient and the patient's family members.

Acute suicidal ideation must be dealt with immediately, as must any psychotic, aggressive, or violent behavior. In reality, many times the psychological problems mentioned are relayed to the psychologist by another member of the treatment team to whom the patient has spoken when they are too frightened or embarrassed to tell the psychologist or physician themselves.

The patient must be treated in the clinical setting, as well as be allowed to journey into the community with a feeling of safety by having their OT, SLP, and/or therapeutic recreational specialist accompany them. Treatment staff visits to a patient's home and work site are imperative for an evaluation in these settings to help the patient develop methods of generalizing specific skills and utilize compensatory strategies.

If the patient has visual-spatial deficits or significant driving phobia, a specialist needs to perform a driving evaluation. If a patient cannot drive safely, they must be taught how to use public transportation, both in the clinic and in the field, by actually doing so in the company of a therapist.

In terms of driving tests, cognitive function testing is not sufficient to predict driving performance. At least five factors must be evaluated and must be functionally effective for the patient to drive safely: higher order visual-spatial abilities, basic visual recognition and response times, anticipatory braking, defensive steering, and behavioral manifestations of complex attention. Standardized driving performance evaluations should be used.[727-730]

Group treatment is important and gives patients the message that they are not alone with their problems. It also enables them to learn from the experiences of other patients, which can be a very effective teaching tool. The importance of these group experiences cannot be understated. They are an important part of the therapeutic milieu that is developed by an experienced interdisciplinary MTBI treatment team. Just knowing that they are not the only ones with certain problems is important to patients.

Supervised group outings also give patients ways to obtain feedback on their abilities and deficits. Such feedback can come to a patient from a clinical staff member or other members of the patient group.

Constant medical supervision is necessary when dealing with neuropharmacological interventions and treatment for depression, anxiety, aggressive behavior, emotional lability, fast cycling bipolar activity, psychosis, and extreme fatigue, to name a few common problems. The use of psychoactive medications in an injury-disturbed or distorted physiological system — the brain — demands constant vigilance. Be careful to obtain from an HMO or PPO the ability to correctly monitor such medication usage. Being able to see a patient only once a month is a good reason to *not* use medications. On the other hand, to achieve an appropriate outcome, medications may need to be used. In a disturbed system, a patient's ability to tolerate a specific medication or its side-effects may be different than in the patient's premorbid state. For the patient's safety, as well as your own, seeing the patient at least weekly as you are trying new neuropharmacological treatments and/or ramping the dosages up or down is imperative. Sometimes you will need to see a patient several times a week. Your medical/clinical judgment is what is important here.

Some other issues of importance include:

PATIENT QUALITY OF LIFE

Patient performance on tests of cognitive speed, ability, and flexibility; complex attention; and memory during acute recovery periods may be useful in predicting how well a patient will behave in "real world" behavior and psychosocial outcomes.[731] Such test results are most useful in helping to determine the course of the individualized treatment a patient will receive.

The best definition of post-injury community integration is still being developed. It would appear to include, at the minimum, the idea that integration involves relationships with others, independence in the living situation, and activities to fill one's time. There appear to be at least nine indicators of a patient's ability to do these things: orientation, acceptance, conformity, close and diffuse relationships, living situation, independence, productivity, and leisure.[732]

Research has shown that employment was one of the strongest contributors to improved quality of life. Both functional independence and psychosocial variables must be dealt with to provide maximal quality of life.[733] The importance of return to work issues, as well as social pragmatics and other psychosocial variables worked on in clinical treatment, cannot be underestimated.

Treatment should never be given in a vacuum. It is important for both the clinical treatment team and the patient to develop and/or preserve a social network as post-treatment issues are dealt with.[734] Not so amazingly, others have found that rehabilitation programs should provide, in some cases, long-term assistance with community-based social integration, as well as more effective treatment strategies to develop these skills in TBI survivors.[735] Unfortunately, these things cannot occur overnight, leading to the necessity of the duration of treatment.

In another study, the majority of MTBI patients, regardless of age, recovered well according to the Glasgow Outcome Scale, and were capable of independent employment at the end of follow-up, which, in this case, was greater than five years.[736] No relationship was found between age at injury and preinjury education, and outcome. No specific descriptions of type and duration of treatment were given.

FAMILY ISSUES

Many studies have established that the burden of stress placed on family members and significant others of persons who have sustained a TBI is great. This can lead to significant depression in the caregiver, as well as increases in alcohol and other substance usage, including medication. Divorce/separation rates have been reported to approach 49% in one group within a 5- to 8-year period post injury.[737-744]

Stress levels were lessened in wives of TBI survivors who reported a lower level of financial strain, who felt their spouse had a relatively low level of psychopathology, and when the injury was relatively mild, based on the GCS. Other studies found that measures of injury severity, residual neurobehavioral dysfunction, and adequate social support for caregivers were reliable indicators of family function. Other information indicates that problems with cognition accounted for a significant amount of variance in life changes.[745-747]

Of interest is the finding that, contrary to what has been thought, there is typically general agreement between family members and patients regarding the patient's everyday problems.[748,749]

RETURN TO WORK

To quote directly from Hayden,[750] "1. Mild head injuries are common occurrences in the United States. 2. If not properly understood and managed, mild head injuries can be unnecessarily costly in terms of lost work days, financial expenditures, and human suffering. 3. If properly understood and treated, most victims of mild head injuries can return to productive lifestyles. 4. Factors that place persons at high risk for more severe symptoms and/or more lengthy recovery periods are easy to conceptualize."

In another study of an MTBI population, 45% of symptomatic individuals sought medical treatment for their condition. This study was one in which patients were given a brochure on MTBI and a follow-up phone call. The estimation that "most individuals" with MTBI will not use medical services is not sufficient, as the study did not go beyond three months post injury.[751]

The Centers for Disease Control notes that behavioral, economic, and psycho-social factors are important services utilized to improve function and can be expected to impact return to work after TBI.[752] As we are talking about the remainder of a person's life, the estimated mean cost of providing return-to-work services of $10,198 for the first year is not enormous. At the same time, it is difficult finding the resources to provide such care.[753,754]

Specific reasons for RTW (return to work) failure are not definitive. They have included the prediction aspects of the performance IQ score on the Wechsler Adult Intelligence Scale-Revised, as well as other predictive factors such as youth, functional limitations of visual and fine motor skills, and other work-related skills.[755-757]

On the other hand, it has been noted that being employed contributes to quality of life, social integration, a sense of well-being, and pursuit of leisure and home activities, whether the employment is full- or part-time.[758]

The author's experience is that not making an all-out effort to help a patient return to work is tantamount to wasting a life. The shattered sense of self we discussed above becomes even more distorted. There are always alternatives — volunteer positions and sheltered workshops are just two of them. To prevent a survivor of mild or mild to moderate TBI from maintaining social communication, increased confidence, and independence by working at *something*, if they cannot be a member of the "American work force" as we know it, will hasten the inevitable downward spiral that occurs cognitively, behaviorally, and psychosocially in MTBI patients.

OUTCOME INSTRUMENTS

One of the most difficult aspects of neurorehabilitation is trying to determine a patient's ability to benefit from rehabilitation, as well as quantifying the resulting increased functionality, if found. Various assessment tools which look at functional skills and outcomes exist; these include the Disability Rating Scale[759] (DRS), the Functional Independence Measurement (FIM),[760] and the Barthel Index,[761] to name a few. There are problems with many of these tools, particularly when looking at the MTBI population. In general, measurement tools have ceiling and floor limitations, meaning that they are not very sensitive to improvement among patients whose function is relatively high or very low. The FIM, which looks at basic ADL measures, is insensitive to progress of high-level patients who typically need speed and planning abilities to function in the community.[762] Appropriate measurement tools need to be sensitive to patient change during rehabilitation. Such tools are also not sensitive to low functioning patients.

The problem is obvious. If the assessment tool is insensitive to high- or low-level functioning patients, it may be very difficult to determine if progress is being made during rehabilitation. The *AMA Guide to the Evaluation of Permanent Impairment*[763] is not sensitive to such things, either, and no scientific studies have established the predictive validity of the system for its common use in establishing that the TBI survivor can work or what their needs might be for long-term care.

Global status ratings are important. They are typically not sensitive enough for clinical management or for planning rehabilitation treatment. The multidimensionality of assessment tools may be useful or not, depending on the overall experience of the interdisciplinary treatment team.

The majority of measures of independence in basic self-care, ADLs, and mobility were originally developed for the general rehabilitation population, but may be applicable to TBI patients with similar problems. The FIM, a general rehabilitation disability measure, is sensitive to improvement in inpatients with TBI, but not necessarily those in residential homes or community-oriented treatment programs. In spite of this, the FIM is the most widely used measure of disability. Clinicians use this tool to assess the degree of assistance needed by a TBI patient on a 7-point scale in 18 items. It is a general disability scale and has been used to assess TBI outcomes.[764] It is more sensitive to functional change during inpatient rehabilitation than the DRS. It must be remembered that the FIM was not designed for TBI. Its behavioral, cognitive, and community-related items do not appear to be adequate for TBI patients, particularly if they are comparatively high functioning.[765-770]

The Functional Assessment Measure (FAM) was made to be used in the Traumatic Brain Injury Model Systems project. It adds 12 items to the FIM, making the combined scale (FIM-FAM) more sensitive to TBI-specific problems. The additional items include more community functioning items such as car transfers and employability, which still appears to make it less useful in some of the higher-level MTBI patients and even mild-moderate TBI patients.[771]

We've mentioned the Glasgow Coma Scale many times in this text. It is felt to be a reliable prognosticator of patients' outcome. The GCS is based on three items: eye opening, best motor response, and verbal response. The highest score is 15, while the MTBI numbers range from 13-15. As we have discussed, the GCS may have varying reliability in the MTBI population.[772-774] The Glasgow Liege Scale was developed in 1982 and adds to the GCS items, including brainstem reflexes.[775]

The Glasgow Outcome Scale (GOS) rates global outcome. It has five points (from four, originally) which include death, vegetative state, severe disability, moderate disability, and good recovery. The GOS ratings have only weak correlations with neuropsychological performance, and, generally, limited sensitivity, as it may find patient levels of moderate disability and good recovery. Utilizing this measure, most severely injured patients with "good recovery" also have persisting neuropsychological deficits.[776-781] Another problem with the GOS is that there may be a great deal of subjectivity in the ratings. Finally, GOS ratings appear to plateau at six months, making it insensitive to patient gains after rehabilitation.[782,783]

Many other scales have been developed with good reliability for outcomes, but few, if any, appear to be specific to the MTBI population treated on an outpatient basis.[784-791]

A study performed by the U.S. Military found that the most effective way to save the costs of TBI patients is, primarily, to prevent them from occurring. Secondary and tertiary measures include evaluation and rehabilitation, where indicated, which should be "undertaken on a routine basis after TBI."[792]

One study looked at outcomes in cases of possible "compensation neurosis" post TBI. It was found that of 264 survivors who were not working at the end of litigation and who could be traced, 198 (75%) were not working an average of 23 months after their cases were ended.[793] One possible reason for this is the fact that MTBI to severe TBI patients who obtain attorneys have more severe deficits than those who do not.

One of the greater frustrations in treating the mild and mild-moderate TBI survivors for the last two decades was the lack of an outcome instrument that would meet the needs of the patients, particularly in demonstrating to the payers that successful rehabilitation had been provided. This frustration was found in other centers; in one, it was concluded that postacute traumatic brain injury rehabilitation aimed at retraining real-life functional abilities can lead to long-term improvements in independence.[794] To attempt to rectify this situation, in 1990 I began to develop a functional assessment scale (FAS), which has now been utilized for a decade. Fine tuning has been provided by the various members of the clinical treatment staff with whom I've been extremely fortunate to work. This scale, the HNRIC (Headache and Neuro-Rehabilitation Institute of Colorado) FAS, has been found to provide significant reliability over the decade it has been utilized. It is simple and provides a global assessment of the ADLs and community integration strategies needed by the mild and mild-to-moderate TBI patients we have treated in an outpatient facility.

The HNRIC FAS has 15 items, each with 5 levels. It is scored by the entire clinical treatment team, and takes approximately 10 minutes to complete. In practice, it was done when a patient was evaluated, and then monthly, with a final scoring when the patient was discharged. It was found to show an average 20% functional improvement (range 7% to 58%) for patients who completed their individualized rehabilitation programs.

The functional assessment scales included:

1. Medical Management
2. Vocational/Educational Functioning
3. Home Management/Consumer Skills
4. Money Management
5. Transportation
6. Self Care
7. Communication Skills
8. Interpersonal and Pragmatic Behaviors
9. Family Functioning and Social Network
10. Psychological Functioning
11. Neuropsychological Functioning
12. Neuromuscular Functioning
13. Pain
14. Fitness Scale
15. Leisure Activities

Each FAS item is rated 1 (lowest functioning) to 5 (independent functioning), or:

1. Significant Problems
2. Moderately Severe

3. Mild Difficulties
4. Minimal Difficulties
5. No Difficulties — Functionally Independent

The maximum total of 75 points is essentially equivalent to totally independent functioning with no medical/neuropsychological problems which would *interfere with normal functioning*. Therefore, the appropriate use of compensatory strategies is taken into consideration, as the scale does not indicate that no problems exist, just that patients have been able to compensate for them. Examples of parts of two items of the HNRIC FAS:

TRANSPORTATION

Dependent

The patient is able to use public transportation with moderate assistance/structure, or uses private transportation companies which provide close supervision, and the assistance of family members. The patient does not drive because of significant residual deficits.

More Independent

The patient may be appropriate for driving evaluation or drivers' training, or requires minimal assistance/structure to arrange for and use public transportation.

MONEY MANAGEMENT

Dependent

Consistently requires minimum-moderate structure/assistance for routine transactions, and moderate assistance for incidental expenses (doctor, insurance, broken appliance). Able to complete simple cash transactions accurately; maximum assistance for other aspects of personal finance.

More Independent

Able to independently complete routine transactions (monthly bills, budget, checks); requires minimal cues/structure for incidental expenses.

As the typical mild and mild to moderate TBI patient has an initial FAS score averaging 50 points (range 39 to 56), a 20% improvement can be substantial.

We have found the HNRIC FAS to be of substantial help as part of a systematic evaluation of the effectiveness and efficiency of the outpatient MTBI program. This is evaluated, generally, by: (1) comparing functional abilities of the patients from admission to discharge, (2) obtaining information from the patient and family members in follow-up regarding current status in the community, and (3) comparing efficiency measures (length of treatment, average charges) on all patients who have completed the program.

This ongoing internal quality assessment is an important aspect of a program's continuing function. While insurance companies mouth their requests for outcome data, they are more interested in costs. However, in determining program effectiveness as well as cost-effectiveness, continuous quality improvement is imperative.

CASE MANAGEMENT

There is very little literature regarding case management in patients with MTBI. This is not surprising given that case management is usually confined to "serious" or catastrophic cases.

Mattson,[795] in one of the few articles relating to MTBI and case management, stated:

> The expression "post-concussive rehabilitation" is almost an oxymoron for a case manager. The label "post-concussive syndrome" is often a catchword for a combination of seemingly unrelated psychological and physiologically perceived symptoms leading to disability. The handicap seems insurmountable. By the time the person reaches a case manager, there is often a generous measure of despair because current treatment is failing to ameliorate perceived problems or because the funder is crying "foul play" and is threatening to cut off reimbursement.

Mattson indicates the necessity of having a good clinical background and understanding of MTBI. She vividly describes the difficulties encountered by the patient and the treating staff when an MTBI is not identified and treated appropriately as early as possible.

The author has had the pleasure to work with excellent nurse case managers whose primary allegiance is to their patient in spite of the fact that the patient's insurance company may have hired them. Many of these nurses have fought as hard as the treatment staff to obtain appropriate care for patients. On the other hand, I have also had the misfortune to work with true nurse cash managers who believe it is their right to determine independently, or with the help of an insurance company IME, a patient's diagnosis and the necessity of treatment. The fact is that their job is denying care and therefore cutting costs, regardless of patient need. Some of them do it very well.

The case manager should be a knowledgeable facilitator, working with the medical treatment team to help a patient receive appropriate treatment. For this reason, they should have no preconceived allegiance to anyone but the patient they are asked to care for. The term "knowledgeable" must be accurate, otherwise the patient loses big time.

I have found it useful to have the treatment team's nurse rehabilitation specialists act as internal case managers. I have also found it best to have this nurse interact "nurse to nurse" with the external nurse case managers on a regular basis. The external nurse case managers are invited to all patient staff meetings where they can interact with the entire team.

INTERDISCIPLINARY TREATMENT STAFF NEEDS

A good bit has been written regarding physician stresses in this era of managed care, but little about the effects of stress on clinical treatment staff.

The reality is that clinical staff is subject to the same stressors secondary to managed care as physicians. When they can see that a patient needs care, but they are not "allowed" to administer it, they get frustrated. If they are not allowed to vent, they lose their clinical effectiveness and/or leave the facility hoping to find another place that "cares more about patients." The financial aspects of running an outpatient facility which hires such staff, but is subject to ever growing numbers of rules and treatment denials from payers, is a very difficult thing to accept for a clinical staff member. For this reason, a great deal of *pro bono* care has been provided at all facilities I have been connected with. That is a fiscally dangerous move, but keeping the clinical staff on top of their game and delivering appropriate patient care is even more important.

In the few studies on this subject, it was noted in one that nurses involved in the rehabilitation of TBI patients were thought to have more psychopathology than nurses treating nonTBI patients. This was found not to be true, while the need for nursing excellence in treating TBI patients has been emphasized.[796,797]

Another study dealing with decision making and attribution bias in a neurorehabilitation staff indicates that staff therapists made internal attributions for positive outcomes and external attributions for negative outcomes. Injury severity was not typically a factor in outcome unless the therapists were encouraged to make it one. The therapists accepted personal responsibility for positive outcomes, but not for negative outcomes.[798] This study did not take into consideration outside interference in rehabilitation, and the author has found no studies that included such information.

The responsibility for keeping excellent clinical staff happy and involved in the day-to-day exigencies of treating a patient with mild or mild to moderate TBI is given to the physician who "runs the team" on one hand, and to the owners of the establishment, hospital, or outpatient facility, who, on the other hand, must take into account the desire and need by clinical staff to help the patients they encounter.

CASE STUDIES

CASE ONE

AB was a 34-year-old right-handed female when I first met her. I had been contacted by the medical director of her PPO. The bottom line was that they had spent a great deal of money on AB, and they wanted it to stop. The patient had been placed in a psychiatric hospital three times in the previous eight months. She visited a hospital emergency room two to three times a month for complaints of pain during that same period of time. The PPO had spent an enormous amount of money over the prior five years. The medical director told me that I could do whatever I needed to do to "fix her."

The patient was literally carried into my office by her husband. History was pertinent for the fact that six years prior, AB had been working when a truck drove into the rear wall of the bar she tended, sending the bar itself onto her head. She was unconscious for at least six hours. She had developed seizures that were evidently difficult to stop. She was on four anticonvulsants, all of which were being given in massive dosages, at least twice the normal dosage levels. Her pain was severe, and had been diagnosed as posttraumatic headache. She was on four analgesics, two of which were narcotics, one of which contained a fast-acting barbiturate, and one of which was a non-steroidal anti-inflammatory. She had been subject to significant emotional lability, and twice she had been hospitalized for self-directed violence. She was on six different psychoactive drugs, antidepressants, anxiolytics, and tranquilizers. She was taking two other medications for hypertension. When first seen, she was on 16 different medications.

AB had been diagnosed with a moderate TBI and treated in a residential home after being released from the hospital after her initial injury. She met her husband during the first year after her injury, and they married soon afterward.

She was essentially homebound, unable to drive because of her seizures and other cognitive problems. Her social network was small.

Her initial neurological evaluation was pertinent for several frontal lobe release signs. She was drowsy, but otherwise neurologically intact.

The first thing that had to be done was to take her off of the incredible amount of medication she was taking. Because of her posttraumatic headaches, she was hospitalized for a three-day course of intravenous DHE-45 (dihydroergotamine) and metaclopramide. She was taken off of all pain medications, and while she was in the hosptial she was placed on clonidine for the autonomic signs of narcotic withdrawal. She was also placed on a long-acting barbiturate, from which she was weaned in two weeks. She was weaned from two of her anticonvulsants within the first week. The other two were slowly adjusted until she was on just one, carbamazepine, in normal levels. She was taken off of dilantin, gabapentin, and Phenobarbital.

When a patient still has seizures in spite of very high dosages of four anticonvulsants, it is necessary to wonder what kinds of seizures she was actually having. After working her up with an MRI and ambulatory EEG, it was felt that while she might have had posttraumatic seizures, she also had pseudoseizures. She was taught how to stop the pseudoseizures by herself, by placing pressure on the "great nerve of the neck." She stopped having seizures. When first seen, she and her husband had complained of three to five seizures a day.

The tranquilizers were phased out, as were the anxiolytics. The antidepressants were changed to more alerting medications, small dosages of specific serotonin reuptake inhibitors.

It took two weeks to stabilize AB on her new medication regime. She was no longer hypertensive, so those medications were also stopped. She was on four medications in total when she began treatment for her posttraumatic pain. She received physical therapy, psychotherapy, and biofeedback therapy, the latter to desensitize her from her anxiety triggers and teach her relaxation techniques. After three weeks of therapy, her headache, which was originally a constant 10 over 10, was ranging from 1 to 5 over 10. In another week, she had headache-free time.

After the initial three weeks of pain treatment, she received a neuropsychological evaluation, and then a speech-language and occupational therapy evaluation. There was no question that she had survived a TBI; she was considered a mild-moderate TBI patient.

The team met and designed a six- to eight-week treatment for AB. She was started in individual speech and occupational therapy, as well as group activities. She continued with psychotherapy with the neuropsychologist. During the second week of this treatment she came to see me, in tears. She had had a call from the psychiatrist who had hospitalized her three times in the prior eight months. This physician had told her that taking her off of so many medications was bad for her, and that she, the psychiatrist, would no longer see her. This upset AB.

Since the initial hospitalization, AB had not needed to visit any hospital ER. I received a call from the PPO medical director at the end of the third week of TBI treatment. On visiting with this doctor, I was told that the PPO would not pay for much of the therapy AB had been given despite of her significant gains. The CFO of the PPO, who negated the medical director's statements in front of him, offered to pay 50 cents on the dollar for the treatment already given. Her treatment was to be ended.

I requested twelve more hours of treatment so that we could finish at least part of our initial treatment plan. I was told by the CFO that that would not be reimbursed, in spite of the medical director's agreement that I could have the time to end AB's treatment appropriately.

The patient received the needed twelve hours of treatment. At the end of five weeks of TBI treatment, which had followed three weeks of pain treatment and medication management, AB was clear, coherent, seizure free, and on three medications in normal amounts: carbamazepine for seizures and emotional lability (200 mgs, tid); clonazepine, a fifth-generation benzodiazepine, useful for muscle relaxation and anxiolysis, with a sedative side effect, but clinically not found to hinder cognition like its earlier related medications, taken only at night (.5 mgs); and Zoloft, an SSRI antidepressant, 50 mgs in the morning. We followed her biweekly for her medications and emotional status.

During her treatment, AB had come to the office complaining of falling and striking her head on a coffee table in her living room. This was attended to in the general course of her therapy. Approximately three weeks after she finished her allowed treatment (plus the *pro bono* therapy) she returned to the office as an emergency patient, complaining of having fallen and striking her shoulder. Radiographs showed a fracture of the head of the shoulder.

Some things which had been bothering various members of the treatment team during the course of her treatment were brought to a head at this time. I was forced to push the patient verbally, who gave several differing stories as to the lack of presence of her husband. She finally admitted that he had been prone to fits of anger, particularly when she began to get better and become more independent. She had been physically abused by her husband, who had struck her head against furniture several times. Her shoulder had been injured when he pushed her against the wall; she was able to turn and take the force of the blow with her shoulder, rather than her head, fracturing the shoulder.

Social Services was called, and the patient was encouraged to report her husband to the police. She refused at first, but when she mentioned that he kept several firearms at their home, a girlfriend was called, and the patient and her friend were encouraged to stay in a hotel until the police talked with her husband.

After a very difficult time, AB and her husband were divorced. She developed pseudoseizures again, and we stopped them. Her Zoloft was stopped and she was started on amytriptyline. She overdosed on this medication, accidentally, she claimed, and had to be hospitalized as tricyclic overdose is potentially lethal. We were able to treat her by the good graces of the Victims of Violent Crimes, who paid for her treatment. Her PPO refused to help.

AB made it though the worst of this post treatment experience without needing additional medications or hospitalization (except for her accidental overdose), or seeking help in an ER. Her PPO told her that since she was not really a psychiatric patient, she would have to pay for her three most recent hospitalizations. I had to testify that they were the result of overmedication and poor diagnosis. After review, the PPO withdrew its demands for repayment.

Comments

The patient had originally been on not only very large numbers and dosages of medications, but at least half of them contributed to her poor cognition when she was initially seen. Although her minimally six hours of unconsciousness had helped her receive a diagnosis of TBI, the majority of her prior treatment did not fit the diagnosis.

AB's PPO had spent a minimum of $250,000 in the course of five or six years of her mismanaged care. Still, when less than $15,000 was warranted to end the reasons for the exceptional amounts of money spent on AB, they refused to pay the bill. This was just another PPO wanting something for nothing and ignoring its client's needs.

Case Two

WB, a 44-year-old right-handed woman, was involved in a motor vehicle accident in January 1995. There was no loss of consciousness, although the patient described striking the back of her head on the headrest, as well as an acceleration/deceleration injury. She was seen in initial consultation in March 1995. She had a significant cervical myofascial pain syndrome, her cervical range of motion being minimal on evaluation. She complained of significant memory and concentration difficulties, depression, and described a posttraumatic stress disorder (PTSD) with frequent flashbacks of her accident, and nightmares, and fear and anxiety when in a car and an extreme fear of driving.

WB was foreign born, but had been in the United States for 17 years and had attended college here. After four weeks of pain management, when her functional range of cervical motion had returned to normal, she was eager to deal with her cognitive deficits.

A neuropsychological evaluation was requested from the third-party administrator acting for her insurance company. The request was denied. After numerous attempts and six weeks later, approval was finally obtained and the neuropsychological evaluation was performed. The evaluation found deficits in attention, visual-spatial realms, comprehension, and more. A request for SLP and OT evaluations was made and denied. One month later we were allowed to do them. They were positive for significant functional deficits.

The neuropsychological test data and report were sent for a paper Independent Medical Evaluation (IME) by a psychologist. The IME psychologist stated, "She had no cognitive problems since English was her stated second language."

The patient's pain, which had been in remission, went into exacerbation as she became very "stressed" (her word) by her inability to receive necessary treatment. She complained of a different type of pain and numbness in her right arm. After examination, an electomyogram (EMG) and nerve conduction velocity (NCV) were ordered.

WB's husband wanted her to return to driving, as he could no longer take her to treatment and fulfill her needs to be taken other places. Because of her visual-spatial deficits and her fear of even being in an automobile, a driving evaluation was requested. The requests for the EMG/NCV and the driving evaluation were denied. Another month went by and approval for a three-week treatment program with SLP, OT, and psychology was given. In spite of the exacerbation of her pain, no further PT was approved. At the request of her husband, the payer was informed that in spite of the lack of medical approval, the patient had begun to drive. She continued to complain of significant anxiety, driving phobia, dizziness, and right-arm numbness, as well as continued cognitive problems. Requests were repeated for an EMG/NCV, a driving evaluation, and continued treatment, which had already been interrupted by two weeks, and were again denied. The physician wrote another letter stating that the patient should not be driving and that a driving evaluation was needed to determine, legally, if she was capable of driving.

A week later, in August, the patient had another IME, which stated that the original diagnosis made in April was correct. The physician concurred with a driving evaluation and an EMG/NCV. The patient's attorney was instrumental in choosing an impartial physician for the IME.

In early September 1995, approval was given for three physical therapy visits, three SLP visits, three OT visits, and two psychotherapy visits. On September 19, 1995, the recent IME, which had finally been reviewed by the payer, or TPA, and an EMG/NCV and driving evaluation were approved, along with another one to two weeks of treatment. However, at this time, the patient, feeling that she had been "jerked around" (again, her words) for five months, decided not to proceed with the driving evaluation or any other treatments. She stated, "They won't let me get what I need, so I give up."

In total, during the five-month period, WB had been approved for fewer than five weeks of treatment given in such a staggered fashion that the treatment team was unable to carry out its initial specific treatment plan. The exacerbation of her pain was also very problematic in terms of MTBI treatment. While a great deal of nonauthorized *pro bono* care was given, it could not make up for the ravages of time and the very significant exacerbation of the patient's psychological, physical, and cognitive complaints. The patient suffered increasing depression from this cycle or system of care.

In the end, the patient tired of the "run around" and left treatment. So, who "won?" The patient never finished her treatment or even took a driving test. She just dropped out of treatment. Her attorney indicated that she dropped her case as she wanted to "just move on with her life," in spite of her continued deficits.

Case Three

JD was a 46-year-old right-handed male who fell down a flight of concrete stairs. He experienced loss of consciousness lasting at least an hour. Two days later he returned to his work as a dentist. Three days later his staff heard a crash in the office kitchen and found JD having a grand mal seizure. Paramedics were called. The patient had no prior history of seizures. When the patient developed difficulties in performing basic dental procedures, which were caught by his employees, he came in for consultation.

Initial neurological examination revealed positive palmomental reflexes, bilaterally. Rapid alternating movements were slower on his dominant side. There was no tremor. He had a cervical myofascial pain syndrome, with decreased cervical range of motion and active trigger points which referred pain to the head.

An EEG was ordered. Anticonvulsants were not started at his request (actually, his statement was that he wouldn't take them) as the patient was also a pilot. We made a contract that he wouldn't attempt to fly again until we knew what was happening. He was started in physical therapy. Finally, he was asked to stop practicing until we could determine the extent of his problems. He agreed.

Several weeks later, JD's office staff called and stated that he had experienced another seizure. He had continued to work. His attendance at physical therapy was spotty. He was seen again two days later. At that time, we discussed the fact that he had to begin anticonvulsants. We also discussed the fact that he was working when he had been asked not to. He stated that he would have his father, a local dentist, cover for him.

It took several more months before JD began TBI treatment. During that time he continued to work, even though he would assure me that he would stop. He stated he was taking his anticonvulsant medication, but routine blood draws for levels were too low for this statement to be taken as total truth. He had become very depressed. He related that he had broken up with his fianceé. His work was his life, he noted, and not being able to work, or even do it correctly if he could, was very demeaning to him.

Finally, we met again and JD admitted continuing to work. We had been around and around with this problem, with some very heated arguments prior to that time. He admitted to filling a wrong tooth, as well as some other, fortunately, minor problems. This was verified by his office staff. We discussed the possibility of malpractice problems and the fact that he was not, at that time, capable of performing dentistry. We discussed alternatives such as teaching. He stated, "I know I was wrong, but I just thought everything would be all right again."

The State Board of Dentistry was called, with the patient present, and I explained that his license needed to be suspended for medical reasons. With JD's permission, I explained the problems and the treatment plan. As he was known to be an exceptional dentist and had worked with the State Board on a number of things, there was no problem at all.

JD began treatment and had a great deal of difficulty during speech and OT, frequently becoming very angry and throwing things around when he was not able to perform an exercise as well as he thought he should.

Treatment took five months because JD continued to show up irregularly. Even explaining that this was very detrimental to his care did not stop the problem. His attorney called and related that JD had married his fianceé several months previously. Although he was unsure, he felt that JD might have still been seeing patients.

JD and I had another long talk, with specific reference to not telling the truth regarding his marriage and his working. We again went over the possibility of significant medical malpractice issues if he worked, as his license had been suspended. He denied working, but stated that he had lied when he said he had broken up with his fianceé, and that he had indeed been married several months earlier. When asked why he wasn't straightforward about these things, he said, "My life has gone to hell, and she's the only good thing in it. I didn't want to get her involved with all these medical things. I wanted to keep both of these parts of my life separate." JD also stated that he had not told his wife about his diagnoses. He agreed to bring her in and have the two of them meet with the staff.

JD's wife was a wonderful woman who, much to his chagrin, had figured out that there was something going on, although she wasn't sure exactly what it was. The team went through all the various aspects of JD's problems and noted how far he had come. The plan, at the end of staffing, was for JD to enroll in school to obtain a real estate license, which was something he had wanted to do.

JD went through school, needing some help from the staff, and obtained his license. With his wife's help, he was able to finish working through the loss of his identity as a medical person and went on to have a successful career.

Comments

Denial is one of the most powerful problems seen in mild and mild-to-moderate TBI patients. In JD's case, unless outside intervention had been provided, he may have found himself with significant legal problems.

"A TBI does not make a person stupid." JD was and remains a highly intelligent man. His frustration and anger, leading to depression and a stubborn fight to maintain his major ego strength, his identity as a clinician, led to a number of problems, some of which could have been much worse. More than once, when dealing with JD, the author thought, "There but for fortune go I," which made it easier to continue dealing with JD, another professional who, through no fault of his own, had lost the major part of his identity.

Once JD's wife became formally involved, everything became easier. His attendance became excellent, there was never any question of whether or not he was taking his anticonvulsants, and, realizing that his "problem" wouldn't cause him to lose "the most important thing in my life," he was more able and willing to deal with the issues and push through them. Family interaction and alliance with the medical team was extremely important.

When all was finished, in spite of all the travel over rocky roads, JD had done very well indeed. It should be noted that because of the litigation coming from JD's slip and fall accident on the property of a hotel, his insurance would not pay for treatment. At the same time, any insurance company could have potential problems justifying treatment that took longer than needed secondary to the difficulties discussed above, particularly denial.

CASE FOUR

TB, a 34-year-old right-handed male, was involved in a motor vehicle accident in September 1991. He had been treated for pain prior to being evaluated for an MTBI approximately one year after his injury. He began treatment, but was fearful that his insurance company would not pay it. A lien was taken. After three weeks, TB, a highly-driven personality and overachiever with elements of grandiosity, decided to leave treatment. He wanted to return to work and did not feel that there was anything terribly wrong with him. He kept reminding the staff that he had been a member of Mensa before his motor vehicle accident.

TB's state of denial and minimization of his problems would not allow him to admit to his difficulties, which had been identified on neuropsychological, SLP, and OT evaluations.

He had been employed as a technical manager at a local television station before his accident. After the initial three weeks of treatment, he could only find a job doing construction. During his first week on the job he drove a forklift into a wall and was terminated. He returned to the clinic and asked to be placed back in treatment, which he was, although he continued to deal with large amounts of denial. After treatment he took a job at a computer store, where his physician ran into him. After TB said hello and went into another room to work, his co-workers, not knowing who the physician was, commented on how slow the man worked and that he "couldn't even think of two things at a time."

TB later went to work for a good friend who wanted him to do computer work, as well as simple bookkeeping. After five months, his friend let him go. The patient returned to the computer store, at a lesser salary, with an accommodation in place. He did not have to answer phones when he was working on a computer. He later took several courses and was promoted.

TB had been correct. His insurance company refused to recognize his injury. They attempted to prove that TB did not have an MTBI. In spite of significant pressure, he continued to work. His home life significantly deteriorated, with a bankruptcy; major surgery on his wife, who then had to stop working; and the birth of a baby with Down's syndrome. TB still could not perform his previous technical work. In spite of all of these personal setbacks, he continues to work and, in his words, "take everything one day at a time." He expresses significant regret for his cognitive losses.

Litigation was pursued and the case came to trial four years after TB finished treatment. His attorney, one of the really good guys, was alone at his table, with four attorneys, a legal assistant, and the original case adjuster sitting across the room. TB won two of three issues; the other had been thrown out by the judge.

The trauma of the trial induced TB's attorney to leave the practice of personal injury law. TB received less money than the amount of his four- to five-year-old medical bills, which were severely cut so that he could take home enough to help out his family.

Comment

In the end, in spite of winning a major lawsuit against a major insurance company, no one won anything. The patient had spent a number of years in legal limbo, with significant traumas added one onto another. His sense of self was not shattered, it was destroyed.

TB often spoke of the fact that in spite of his cognitive deficits, the insurance company seemed to take an unimaginably hard line, stating at one point that they didn't even believe that such a thing as an MTBI existed. If it wasn't for his family, he didn't believe he would have made it through the grief and turmoil. Yet, he kept working, doing the best he could do. For this reason, he should be considered successful.

CONCLUSIONS

An appropriate functional outcome after treatment is return to work, accomodated as needed; compensatory strategies utilized at home and work for safety as needed (such as remembering to turn off the stove); and good pragmatics in all 15 aspects of the previously discussed HNRIC functional assessment scale.

So, what is functional rehabilitation? When TBI survivors can, for example, safely, and by themselves, make a shopping list, drive safely or use the bus to go to the store, obtain the necessary items, pay the correct amount of money and recognize the correct change, safely drive home (remembering the directions unaided), and put the items in their proper places, when previously they could not, functional rehabilitation has been achieved. This is only one aspect, of course. Work-related functionality is necessary, as is appropriate functionality in a number of different spheres. Figure 9.1 is an algorithm of the evaluation and treatment recommendations.

BOTTOM LINE

The diagnosis and treatment of an MTBI is never done in isolation. Now, more than ever, it involves the combined efforts of physicians and other clinical specialists expert in dealing with MTBI in conjunction with the payer and their representatives. All members of this "team" must work in concert with one single idea in mind: to maximize the patient's functional independence.[702] There is no reason why this cannot happen. The proverbial playing field must be leveled, with all players working toward the same goal. Good judgment, good clinical skills, and the ability to be open to learning about a difficult clinical problem should be prerequisites for being a member of the treatment team.

The goal of clinical medicine is to help, to do no harm. Everyone participating in the care of a patient with MTBI must believe the same thing. Not to do so is an abrogation of everything we all hold so dear: the willingness, when one has the ability and the responsibility, to help those in need.

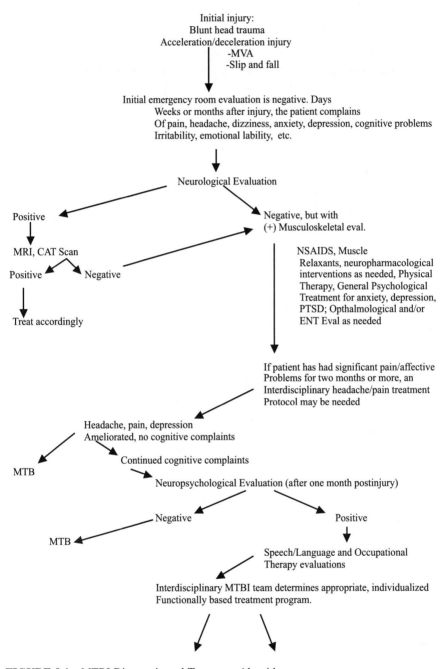

FIGURE 9.1 MTBI Diagnostic and Treatment Algorithm

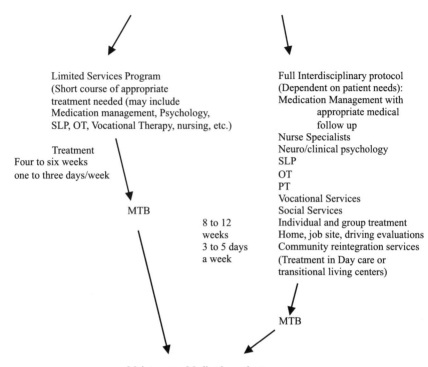

Limited Services Program
(Short course of appropriate
treatment needed (may include
Medication management, Psychology,
SLP, OT, Vocational Therapy, nursing, etc.)

Treatment
Four to six weeks
one to three days/week

MTB

8 to 12
weeks
3 to 5 days
a week

Full Interdisciplinary protocol
(Dependent on patient needs):
Medication Management with
        appropriate medical
        follow up
Nurse Specialists
Neuro/clinical psychology
SLP
OT
PT
Vocational Services
Social Services
Individual and group treatment
Home, job site, driving evaluations
Community reintegration services
(Treatment in Day care or
transitional living centers)

MTB

Maintenance: Medications, short
Courses of psychology, SLP, OT
Or vocational services needed to
Deal with new/ significant life/job
Change which the patient is unable
To deal with alone. Typically not
Something dealt with in treatment:
Issues of death of loved ones, leaving
Patient unable to cope, divorce,
Bankruptcy, etc.

FIGURE 9.1 cont.   MTBI Diagnostic and Treatment Algorithm

10 Neuropharmacological Treatment

Neuropharmacological treatment of patients who have sustained an acquired MTBI can sometimes be more of an art than a science. Each patient is different in specifics of the injury, pre- and post-injury medical conditions which may necessitate medication management, and in their ability to tolerate or deal with medication side effects. So, it is not likely that a "one prescription order" of medication will fit all patients. This chapter is meant to give the reader general guidelines, not to give specific information on what or how to prescribe a specific medication for a specific patient.

Clinicians need to use good judgment, particularly when utilizing medications that were originally tested or "normed" on patients with totally intact central nervous system physiological neuropharmacological homeostasis. This also means that what you may expect to happen in your "typical nonTBI patient" (if there is such a person) utilizing a specific medication may not carry over into the MTBI population. You may need to expect the unexpected.

I am attempting to write as clinically as possible, again, to decrease any aspects of "cookbookism." Drug dosages in this clinical population may be quite variable, so dosages are not indicated. The clinician needs to know enough about the medications to determine these for him or herself. The *Physician's Desk Reference* is a good place to have basic questions answered.

POSTTRAUMATIC EPILEPSY

As discussed earlier, early posttraumatic epilepsy in closed head injury occurs in possibly 4% of the TBI population. In survivors who also have a depressed skull fracture, the incidence is about 10%. There is an increased incidence of epilepsy in patients with penetrating head injury and/or mass lesions. Posttraumatic epilepsy may occur late after a TBI, anywhere from three months to five years, although most patients present within two years. Grand mal seizures are seen, while partial complex seizures are more frequently found.

Generally, anticonvulsant medications (ACMS) work by effecting pathologically changed neurons or seizure foci to prevent or reduce excessive discharges, or reduce the spread of excitation from a seizure foci and prevent detonation or kindling and disruption of function of normal groups of neurons.

Phenytoin is a membrane stabilizer. There is a concurrent diminution of cognitive status when this ACM is used, but it is possibly less than that of phenobarbitol.

Serum levels of phenytoin are increased by cimetidine and carbamazepine, and decreased by phenobarbitol. Serum protein binding has been correlated with albumin and is more variable in ICU and postacute patients than in controls. The initial high dosage requirements and subtherapeutic unbound plasma concentrations appear to be explained by increased metabolism, as the phenytoin dosage needed is typically reduced during convalescence.[799] There also appears to be an initial relationship between the presence of interleukin-6 and phenytoin plasma concentration.[800]

Phenobarbitol limits the spread of seizure activity and increases the general seizure threshold. It appears to increase the inhibitory effects of gamma-amino butyric acid (GABA) in the central nervous system. The use of this ACM in the TBI population demonstrates a decrease in cognitive status, as demonstrated on neuropsychological testing. Phenobarbital may have a prophylactic effect on late posttraumatic epilepsy, while phenytoin does not.[801] Serum blood levels may be increased with the use of phenytoin or valproic acid. It will also effect oral anticoagulant levels, as it decreases them secondary to enzyme induction.

Carbamazepine appears to reduce polysynaptic responses and blocks posttetanic potentiation. It is considered superior to phenytoin and phenobarbitol by virtue of a lack of perceived cognitive effects. Erythromycin can induce toxic carbamazepine levels, as can verapamil. Phenytoin and phenobarbital can decrease its serum levels. This ACM is also very useful when dealing with certain behavioral problems, as will be discussed below. As with phenobarbital, carbamazepine plasma levels are initially high, but later serum concentration decreases, which is an alteration of cabamazepine's pharmacokinetics.[802]

Valproic acid works in the internuncial neurons of the spinal cord, where it appears that levels of the inhibitory neurotransmitter GABA are increased. It does not appear to have any significant cognitive deficit effects. Salicylate can induce valproic acid toxicity. There is also a decreased initial plasma protein binding of valproate in the acute posttraumatic period. Multiple metabolic pathways for valproate appear to occur posttraumatically, with increases in the 6beta-hydroxycortisol to cortisol ratios, which suggests a nonspecific enzyme induction response to TBI.[803,804]

There are a number of new ACMS on the market, none of which has been specifically tested for their possible cognitive effects.

Gabapentin at low dosages may produce significant cognitive side-effects in the TBI patient. NonTBI patients frequently complain of feeling like they are "walking six inches above the ground" when starting to use this medication. I have not had an MTBI patient who wanted to stay on this medication for more than a day or two.

Midazolam has been used for the treatment of acute seizures or behavioral episodes post TBI.[805]

Tricyclic antidepressants (TCAs) may be associated with an increased incidence of seizures in severe TBI patients. Many patients with MTBI and/or moderate injury can take TCAs with very minimal risk, especially if they are concurrently taking carbamazepine. It should be remembered that TCAs might induce a seizure in .1 to 1% of nonTBI patients. Maprotiline and amoxapine may increase seizures in susceptible patients. Trazedone does not appear to be proconvulsive in normal doses, while bupropion should be avoided in patient with a TBI. The selective serotonin reuptake inhibitors (SSRIs) such as fluoxetine, paroxetine, and sertraline do not appear to be proconvulsive. Monoamino-oxidase inhibitors (MAOIs) do not lower the seizure threshold but can lead to hypersensitivity with certain foods — as does tyramine — or over-the-counter or other medications, and, in some cases, induce a seizure.

BEHAVIORAL CHANGES

Acquired MTBI may induce behavioral changes ranging from total behavioral suppression to aggression and psychiatric disinhibition, making the need for psychobehavioral medications an important part of treatment. As noted above, when used appropriately, these may further enhance the effectiveness of neurorehabilitation.

MAJOR TRANQUILIZERS

The major tranquilizers or neuroleptics — also known as antipsychotics — reduce emotion or affect as well as initiative. They may decrease agitation, restlessness, and aggressive, impulsive behaviors. They also decrease psychotic symptoms including hallucinations and delusions, as well as disorganized thinking.

These medications antagonize dopamine activity in the basal ganglia and limbic parts of the forebrain. They enhance turnover of acetylcholine, particularly in the basal ganglia. Major side-effects include the extrapyramidal syndrome (rigidity, nystagmus, and vermilliform movements of the tongue) and tardive dyskinesias.

When the more traditional types of neuroleptics are used, such as haloperidol, operant behavior may be diminished, but spinal reflexes remain unchanged. They may impair vigilance but not digit-symbol substitution, a test of intellectual functioning. They also may act as antiemetics, and may even normalize sleep disturbance.

Select areas of cognition have been found on serial testing to improve after antipsychotic agents have been discontinued.[806] In general, unless a patient has florid symptoms of psychosis, it would be a better idea to try one of the "newer" neuroleptics such as loxipine, risperidone, or clozapine, or the still newer atypical antipsychotics, which are still being released.[807,808] These medications tend to dull cognitive abilities, even in the MTBI population, and appropriate care should be taken.

MINOR TRANQUILIZERS

The minor tranquilizers, such as the early benzodiazepines, lorezepam, chlordiazepoxide, and so on, block arousal seen on EEG from the brainstem reticular formation. They have central depressant effects on spinal reflexes that appear to be secondary to their effects on the brainstem reticular formation. Central nervous system binding involves modulation of GABA as well as chloride ions.

These medications may be used as hypnotics, but they suppress stage four sleep (a commonly found problem associated with chronic headache or pain). They also carry significant potential for habituation and abuse. Alprazolam, an antianxiety/antidepressant agent, may be addictive in the MTBI population, as well as others.

Buspirone is distinct from benzodiazepines. It is nonsedating and nonaddictive. It is not a respiratory depressant, as are the earlier agents. It is effective in agitation associated with MTBI. It may be a mixed dopamine agonist/antagonist. It is a serotonin agonist (at the $5HT_{1A}$ receptor site). Buspirone also increases the activity of noradrenergic neurons in the locus ceruleus. There do not appear to be any cognitive side effects of buspirone.

When used in the MTBI population, buspirone is useful in decreasing anxiety, depression, irritability, inattention, and distractibility. It appears to be helpful to patients with mild movement disorders, akathesia and intention tremor. There appears to be a mild side effect profile.

It may take two or three weeks for a patient to develop a useful serum blood level. Depending on the initial need for the medication, in patients with an acute, severe anxiety reaction, it may be necessary to supplement buspirone for the first seven to ten days with a very controlled prescription usage of alprazolam. It does not appear to be very useful in patients with moderate-severe TBI.

ANTIDEPRESSANTS

Depression is a very frequent sequelae of survivors of MTBI, as it is associated with patients' increasing awareness of the type and degree of their deficits. Continued severe depression will interfere with cognitive remediation. As noted above, depression is also associated with pain, such as posttraumatic headache, which would also be associated with the initial injury. If depression is untreated or poorly treated, it can result in more functional disability and longer than expected or essentially ineffective rehabilitation, in- or outpatient.

There is no single antidepressant drug of choice. The reasons to use a particular antidepressant medication (ADM) depend on a patient's degree of agitation, the presence of a sleep disorder, low arousal or anergy, and so on. The particular side-effects of a medication may be an important consideration of its use. A tricyclic, in small doses, may be useful for a patient with a sleep disorder, while an SSRI with more alerting properties may be more useful for a patient with anergy. In other patients, the use of sedating medications may be contraindicated, as they may promote agitation secondary to the patients' fighting this side-effect, the "sundowner's syndrome."

There are various types of ADMs, including the tricyclics (amitriptyline, doxepin, imipramine, etc.), tetracyclics such as maprotiline, and others including the selective serotonin reuptake inhibitors such as fluoxetine. None may be more effective in TBI survivors, but they should be used before a trial of an MAOI. Also, their individual side-effect profiles are very important.

The majority of the ADMs potentiate the actions of biogenic amines in the CNS by blocking their reuptake at the synapse, the major means of their physiological inactivation. The TCAs have anticholinergic side-effects secondary to the inhibition of noradrenergic transport into adrenergic neurons, and from antagonism of muscarinic cholinergic and alpha-1 adrenergic responses to the autonomic nervous system neurotransmitters.

TCAs with the most serotonergic activity include amitriptyline and imipramine, and then, in order of decreasing serotonergic activity, desipramine and nortriptyline, followed by doxepine, and protriptyline. Desipramine and nortriptyline, have the most noradrenergic effectiveness. The TCAs with the most anticholinergic effects, in descending order, include amitriptyline, doxepine, imipramine, nortriptyline, and then desipramine and protriptyline.

Amitriptyline is useful in small doses in patients with sleep disorder, as the anticholinergic side-effects include sedation and dry mouth. It is the only medication which appears to physiologically "fix" the sleep architecture of pain-induced alpha intrusions into stage four sleep. Note that none of the TCAs have purely serotonergic actions.

Trazedone has mostly serotonergic activity, as do the SSRIs. Neither class has significant anticholinergic activity. Side-effects are again important. Several of the SSRIs, while perhaps more activating than the TCAs, have side effects that can include loss of libido, anorgasmia, and gastrointestinal side-effects.

Taking these things into consideration, patients with anergy or low arousal may be tried first on medications with higher arousal profiles, such as fluoxetine. Patients with concurrent pain problems should be tried on the more serotonergic medications, while TCAs in small dosages are helpful for sleep disorders, as their use will obviate any need for a sedative-hypnotic.

It is not harmful to utilize a small dose of TCA at night in addition to a small dose of SSRI in the morning. A problem with the potential for considerable harm is found in patients given high doses of both TCAs and SSRIs, as the Serotonin Syndrome may be induced. This syndrome may include significant cognitive changes, as well as nausea, headache, dizziness, and orthostatic hypotension. There is one reported case of a fluoxetine/trazedone combination related to sudden onset of dysarthria and speech blocking, which returned to normal when the fluoxetine was stopped.[809] Individually, trazedone has been used to manage aggression in TBI patients,[810] while fluoxetine has been used to treat emotional lability.[811]

In terms of specific TBI functions, amitriptyline is useful in the treatment of psychomotor agitation secondary to TBI recovery. Amitriptyline, imipramine, and nortriptyline decrease emotional incontinence (pathological laughing and crying) secondary to bilateral frontal lobe lesions. Venlafaxine has been used to treat TBI-induced obsessive/compulsive disorder.[812]

Increased risk of seizures in patients with a TBI may be seen in patients taking nonMAOI antidepressants, especially in patients with severe cognitive dysfunction. Overdosage of a TCA may be life threatening. As noted above, higher anticholinergic profiles may be useful for associated sleep disturbances, but at low doses, so as not to contribute to increased cognitive deficits secondary to sedation.

All ADMs may have the potential to cause orthostatic hypotension and cardiotoxicity. Fluoxetine and other SSRIs such as paroxetine and sertraline, as well as nortriptyline have fewer associated symptoms. Trazedone can cause priapism in males. Amoxapine is related to the neuroleptics and may cause similar side-effects.

The MAOIs do not have anticholinergic properties, and do not lower the seizure threshold. There is little if any sedation, and while they may have a stimulant effect on some patients, narcolepsy has been a reported side-effect. More importantly, the significant dietary and OTC medication restrictions secondary to the possibility of a hypertensive crisis make these medications potentially dangerous to use in the MTBI population, particularly in patients with TBI-induced impulsivity and cognitive impairment.

OTHER MEDICATIONS FOR BEHAVIORAL CONTROL

Lithium carbonate is useful in the treatment of mania and bipolar illness. It has serotonergic properties, and may be used with antidepressants or alone. Nonsteroidal anti-inflammatory mediations (NSAIDS) may increase serum lithium levels. Neurotoxicity may be seen if lithium carbonate is given with haloperidol, carbamazepine, or verapamil.

Carbamazepine is chemically related to the TCAs and blocks reuptake of norepinephrine. It is very useful in MTBI patients with episodic aggression, as well as fast-cycling mood disorder. Lithium does not appear to be very helpful with the fast cycling mood disorder. Carbamazepine is also useful in the treatment of emotional lability.

STIMULANTS

Methylphenidate is a mild CNS stimulant (sympathomimetic). It is dopaminergic in nature (via the prerelease of norepinephrine). In children with ADD, it improves behavior, concentration, and learning ability. It has been used in patients with neurologically-induced anergy, low arousal levels, and dense depression.[813-816] It may induce insomnia. Methylphenidate may safely be used in TBI patients with a high seizure risk.[817] Methylphenidate has a quick onset and a short half-life, and may increase serum levels of TCAs.

Dextroamphetamine has also been used to treat TBI patients and may enhance recovery and functional status during rehabilitation.[818]

L-dopa and its family of medications may increase mood, decrease apathy, and may induce a general alerting response with improvement in mental function and increased external interest. It may also induce hallucinations, paranoia, mania, anxiety, nightmares, depression, and organic brain syndrome with confusion or even delirium. Its use in TBI patients with severe cognitive deficits or high levels of impulsivity may be contraindicated unless tight controls are in place.

Another dopaminergic medication, amantadine hcl, increases release of dopamine from central neurons and delays its reuptake. Although it was initially used as an anti-viral agent, amantadine may be very useful in the treatment of fatigue in TBI patients, as well as patients with multiple sclerosis. It may also induce hallucinations, confusion, and nightmares when used with anticholinergic agents.

AGGRESSION

There are three basic paradigms of aggression. Predatory aggression is associated with little or no autonomic nervous system (ANS) arousal, no increased irritability, and unpredictable, goal-directed behavior. Affective aggression is associated with ANS arousal, and may escalate in relation to provocation. Nondirected aggression has no target or provocation; sympathetic arousal occurs but is short-lived. The patient may be amnestic, lethargic, and/or remorseful.

Acetylcholine (Ach) is an activating agent. It is distributed throughout the CNS and enhances all forms of aggression, especially predatory aggression. TBI from severe acceleration/deceleration injury can lead to the lunging and biting behaviors of this paradigm.

The primary mediators of affective aggression are catecholamines, including norepinephrine (NEP) and dopamine (DA). The locus ceruleus is the primary site of NEP-releasing neurons. NEP increases arousal and attention. DA, especially in the region of the ventral mesencephalic tegmental area of the frontal dopaminergic systems, is implicated in the origin of affective aggressive behaviors. DA also enhances vigilance and is associated in the etiology of psychotic states seen with agitation.

Nondirected aggression has been associated with a partial-complex seizure disorder, a "human dyscontrol syndrome."

Serotonergic systems are inhibitory to affective and predatory aggression. Lesions of the raphe nuclei enhance both types of aggression. Human studies show an inverse relationship between cerebrospinal fluid (CSF) 5HIAA — the major metabolite of serotonin — and aggressive behavior.

GABAnergic systems inhibit aggressive behavior.

TBI can alter an individual's adaptive control of aggression secondary to psychiatric disinhibition, the human dyscontrol syndrome.

The goals of treating aggression in the TBI population in general would include decreasing excitatory neurotransmitters, Ach, NEP, DA, and anabolic steroids; increase inhibitory neurotransmitters, serotonin and GABA; and control abnormal CNS electrical activity.

Decreasing Ach will decrease predatory aggression. Anticholinergic medications may be used, particularly shortly after injury, including scopolamine and benztropine mesylate (Cogentin). A good cognitive baseline is needed, as anticholinergic medications may have a detrimental effect on memory.

Control of NEP and DA is complex, as both pre- and postsynaptic mechanisms are involved. Postsynaptic blockade may be performed with beta-adrenergic receptors, using propranolol, nadolol, or metoprolol. Neuroleptics block postsynaptic DA receptors, but their extended use is problematic. Presynaptic ANS receptor binding agents may be used, such as the alpha-2 agonist clonidine, which decreases NEP activity. ADMs may also help in "down regulation" of NEP.

Limbically active ACMs, including carbamazepine and valproic acid, are the medications of choice for nondirected aggression associated with partial complex seizures.

Sodium valproate has also been found to be effective in treating destructive and aggressive behaviors in TBI patients without seizure disorders. Various affective disorders including depression and mania may be treated effectively with valproic acid.[819]

Anabolic steroids may be antagonized by medroxyprogresterone.

Enhancement of serotonergic activity decreases affective aggression. Fluoxetine, which prevents the presynaptic reuptake of serotonin, and trazedone, a competitive $5HT_1$ and $5HT_2$ receptor blocker, are both useful. Buspirone, a $5HT_A$ agonist, is also effective in the treatment of aggression in the TBI population.[820]

Lithium enhances serotonin, and is useful in treating aggression. Benzodiazepines are GABAnergic and good in emergency/acute problems. However, they may decrease cognition and be habituating, significant limitations for long-term use. Valproic acid is effective in treating TBI-induced agitation and associated mood disorders, as is carbamazepine.

FRONTAL LOBE SYNDROME

The frontal lobe syndrome typically includes problems with impulsivity, perseveration, disinhibition, and amotivation, as well as attention, planning, and problem-solving difficulties. These symptoms may respond to dopaminergic agents, including amantadine, l-dopa/carbidopa and bromocriptine. One drug or a combination of two may be successful. Side-effects must be carefully screened and the medication levels or types changed as necessary.[821-823]

The amotivational syndrome, a part of the spectrum of frontal lobe dysfunction, appears to be secondary to posttraumatic dysfunction of the mesolimbic/mesocortical dopaminergic systems, which give rise to various deficits in reward responsiveness and frontal cognitive function. Both bromocriptine and amantadine have been used successfully in treating this problem. Bromocriptine has also been used to treat performance difficulties on clinical measures of executive function and multitask performance, and has been found to work well for dysexecutive syndromes secondary to prefrontal damage.[824-826]

ANALGESICS

Analgesic medications may be necessary to treat posttraumatic musculoskeletal pain syndromes, with the exception of posttraumatic headache. In the latter instance, chronic intake of analgesic medications, including OTC drugs and narcotic and/or barbiturates containing analgesic can induce an analgesic rebound headache syndrome. Immediately post injury, analgesics are appropriate for the first seven to ten days.

When possible, the use of nonnarcotic analgesics such as the NSAIDS is appropriate. GI side-effects may make these medications inappropriate. The use of the new COX 2 inhibitors, such as celecoxib, is very helpful in these patients. This family of NSAID has far fewer GI side-effects.

The use of muscle relaxants which do not have significant sedative effects, such as carbamethacol and tizanidine, are good adjunctive therapies when used together with an NSAID. The concurrent use of physical therapy is frequently also indicated. Tizanidine may have initial sedative side-effects, as well as possible hypotension, and must be adjusted carefully to avoid potentiation of these problems.

The acute use of narcotics may induce cognitive difficulties secondary to sedation. When tolerant to the dosage, narcotics are relatively free of neuropsychological effects. Naltrexone, a narcotic antagonist, has been used for the postconcussion syndrome. Codeine and propoxyphene have been used for akethesias. The use of narcotic agonist/antagonists for short periods of time does not appear to effect neuropsychological performance. Both narcotics and narcotic agonist/antagonists (such as butorphanol) can be addicting, so care must be used when giving them to patients with cognitive deficits post TBI.

OTHER DRUGS

Some studies have found an increased utilization of other drugs in the TBI population. The use of many of these drugs is decidedly detrimental to the TBI patient.

Alcohol enhances the potential for recurrent TBI via falls and motor vehicle accidents. It can lower the seizure threshold, as well as enhance TBI-related cognitive and behavioral changes, and suppress neuronal recovery. PostTBI patients appear to be more susceptible to the acute and chronic CNS effects of alcohol. Alcohol may also interfere with various medications, including antidepressants, anxiolytics, benzodiazepines, anticonvulsants, neuroleptics, and lithium.

Caffeine is a stimulant. Excessive use may lower the seizure threshold, and increase weight loss and aggression. It is a xanthine, an adenosine antagonist. Adenosine is a purinergic neurotransmitter with modulatory effects on other neurotransmitter systems, including serotonin, NEP, and DA. The stimulant effects of caffeine come from the release of purinergic tone. Carbamazepine is an adenosine agonist.

Drug and alcohol abuse is seen in a statistically greater than "normal" percentage of patients with one or more TBI.

The use of THC (tetrahydrocannabinol), the main psychoeffective agent in marijuana, affects short-term memory, new information acquisition, and performance of complex cognitive tasks. It may induce anxiety, panic states, dysphoria, depersonalization, and disassociation. The related "amotivational syndrome" is also not helpful to TBI patients with frontal lobe symptoms of indifference and poor motivation.

Cocaine has toxic effects similar to amphetamines. It can induce seizures, including status epilepticus. It may induce severe aggressive behavior, irritability, rage, impulsive behavior, and toxic psychosis. It may also be associated with vasculitis, cerebral vasculopathy, and increased cerebral vascular fragility.

The use of hallucinogens effects serotonergic transmission with mixed agonist/antagonist actions. Phencyclidine may induce psychosis, disrupt learning and memory, and increase aggression. It may also be neurotoxic to specific neurons. Like PCP, LSD and mescaline may induce cerebral vasospasm, hypoxia, and cell death.

There should be no need for a *bottom line* here. The use of these drugs in an already disrupted physiological system will further induce neurological and cognitive decline. They should be avoided in survivors of TBI.

The treatment of heterotopic ossification (myositis ossificans traumatica) and spasticity, seen in the moderate-severe TBI patient, is beyond the scope of this text.

POSSIBLE TREATMENT

The usefulness of donepezil hydrochloride (Aricept), an acetylcholinesterase inhibitor approved for the treatment of cognitive deficits in Alzheimer's disease, in the treatment of MTBI is still under investigation.[827] Acetylcholinesterase is an enzyme that metabolizes, or breaks down, acetylcholine. By inhibiting this enzyme, it is hoped that a greater concentration of Ach in the brain will enhance memory and learning. Other, possibly similar, medications appear to be in the pharmaceutical "pipeline."

Physostigmine, as well as scopolamine, has also been used in experimental and clinical studies with results that may be difficult to determine.[828] Most of this research has been performed in experimental TBI preparations on mice or rats who were pretreated with one of the medications. There is a paucity of human research.

One of the great difficulties in developing a new treatment for TBI is that the typical TBI population is so different, in spite of having the same nominal diagnosis. There are great differences between MTBI patients. These would be magnified in the moderate and severe TBI patients who are commonly also being treated for multiple traumas, and are, therefore, on multiple medications, with or without induced hypothermia or barbiturate coma. There are few ways to ensure the "purity" of a statistical sampling of patients. This certainly makes the development of new treatments difficult.

Another major factor would be the need to utilize multiple centers, most if not all of which would already have their own protocols. Just how does one perform a controlled study?

In attempting to create new treatments, it would appear to this author that there might be several paths to investigate. First, as is being done now, we know that acetylcholine is important in memory, so trying to enhance its CNS tonus would be appropriate, much the same way a patient with Parkinson's disease is treated by increasing CNS dopamine. Secondly, we know that there are several distinct problems/issues that will affect the diagnosis and treatment of the TBI patient.

As has been stated earlier in this text, the damage produced by a TBI does not end when the patient reaches the hospital emergency room. Diffuse axonal injury and apoptosis will continue for days, weeks, or even months. This may mean that we first have to find a better way to stage these patients, with specific treatment dependent on timing post injury.

During the time between the actual trauma and the end of the neurophysiological/neurochemical damage/neuronal death, it would appear that the CNS is essentially more vulnerable to injury, or rather continued injury. One aspect of this problem is the idea that there is increased need for glucose post injury, while at the same time, there is hypoperfusion, which means that there is a difference between the CNS's needs and the ability of the body to achieve them on a metabolic basis. Would it be possible to increase perfusion to the injured regions? PET scans can show the exact regions of increased glucose need, while a SPECT scan can demonstrate cerebral perfusion, as can magnetic resonance angiography (MRA).

Third, there are other, newer areas of investigation which are looking at antioxidant medications, the effects of CNS trauma on the immune system, and neurotrophic factors. All are exciting, all are possible, but a lot of work must proceed first — including the admission by some that there *is* such a thing as an MTBI.

BOTTOM LINE

The use of psychoactive medications in the neuropharmacological treatment of patients with MTBI or moderate and severe TBI is, as noted, more of an art than a science. Experience is the best teacher.

Neuropharmacological medications are important adjuncts to the treatment of a patient with an MTBI. Their proper use will make total neurorehabilitation easier by helping the patient to be able to concentrate on cognitive remediation as well as behavioral interventions. It will also make the task more cost-effective. To treat a survivor of an acquired MTBI with only medications, as some purported doctors recommend, is to do a significant disservice to the patient and those who do their best to help them.

References

1. Erichson, JE, On concussion of the spine: *Nervous Shock and Other Obscure Injuries of the Nervous System and Their Clinical, Medical, and Legal Aspects*, Longmans, Green, and Co., London, 1882.
2. Trimble, MR, *Posttraumatic Neurosis- From Railway Spine to Whiplash*, John Wylie & Sons, New York, 1881.
3. Page, H, *Injuries of the Spine and Spinal Cord Without Apparent Mechanical Lesion*, J & A Churchill, London, 1885.
4. Denny-Brown, D, Russell, WR, Experimental cerebral concussion, *Brain*, 64(93), 1941.
5. Groat, SA, Simmons, JQ, Loss of nerve cells in experimental cerebral concussion, *J. Neuropath and Exp. Neurol.*, 150, 1959.
6. Wechsler, IS, Trauma and the nervous system, *JAMA*, 104:519, 1935.
7. Oppenheimer, DR, Microscopic lesions of the brain following head injury, *J. Neurol. Neurosurg. Psych.*, 31:299, 1968.
8. Reusch, J, Intellectual impairment and head injuries, *Am. J. Psych.*, 100:480, 1944.
9. Gronwall, D, Wrightson, P, Delayed recovery of intellectual function after minor head injury, *Lancet*, I:605, 1974.
10. Gronwall, D, Wrightson, P, Cumulative effects of concussion, *Lancet*, I:995, 1975.
11. Levin, HS, Grossman, RG, Behavioral sequelae of closed head injury, *Arch. Neurol.*, 35:720, 1978.
12. Gorman, WF, Whiplash: Fictive or factual, *Bulletin Am. Acad. Psych. and Law*, 7:245, 1979.
13. McNab, I, The whiplash syndrome, *Clin. Neurosurg.*, 20:232, 1974.
14. Toglia, JU, Acute flexion-extension injury of the neck, *Neurology*, 26:808, 1976.
15. Povlishock, JT, Becke, DP, Cheng, CLY, Vaughan, GW, Axonal change in minor head injury, *J. Neuropath. Exp. Neurol.*, 42:225, 1983.
16. Kay, T, Harrington, DE, et al., Definition of mild traumatic brain injury, *J. Head Trauma Rehabil.*, 8(3):86, 1993.
17. Zasler, ND, Mild traumatic brain injury: medical assessment and intervention, *J. Head Trauma Rehabil.*, 8(3):13, 1993.
18. Annegers, DW, Grabow, JD, Kurland, LT, et al., The incidence, causes and secular trends of head trauma in Olmsted County, Minnesota, 1935-1974. *Neurology*, 30:919, 1980.
19. Kalsbeek, WD, Mclaurin, RL, Harris, BS, et al., The National Head and Spinal Cord Injury Survey: major findings, *Neurosurgery*, 53:S19, 1980.
20. Klauber, RK, Barret-Connor, E, Marshall, LF, et al., The epidemiology of head injury: a prospective study of an entire community, San Diego County, California 1978. *Am. J. Epidemiology*, 113:500, 1981.
21. Cooper, K, Tabaddor, K, Hauser, WA, et al., The epidemiology of head injury in the Bronx, *Neuroepidemiology*, 2:70, 1983.
22. Desai, B, Whitman, S, Coonly-Hoganson, R, et al., Urban head injury, *J. Natl. Med. Assoc.*, 75:875, 1983.
23. Jagger, J, Levine, J, Jane, J, et al., Epidemiological features of head injury in a predominantly rural population, *J. Trauma*, 24:40, 1984.

24. Whitman, S, Coonley-Hogason, R, Desai, B, Comparative head trauma experience in two socioeconomically different Chicago area communities: a population study, *Am. J. Epidemiol.*, 119:570, 1984.

25. Kraus, JF, Black, MA, Hessol, N, et al., The incidence of acute brain injury and serious impairment of a defined population, *Am. J. Epidemiol.*, 119:186, 1984.

26. Willer, B, Abosh, S, Dalmer, E: Epidemiology of disability from traumatic brain injury, in Wood, R, (Ed.), *Neurobehavioral Sequalae of TBI*, Taylor & Francis, London, 1990.

27. Wong, PP, Dornan, J, Schentag, CT, Statistical profile of traumatic brain injury: a Canadian rehabilitation population, *Brain Injury*, 7:283, 1993.

28. Kraus, JF, Epidemiology of Head Injury, in Cooper, PR, (Ed.), *Head Injury*, Williams & Wilkins, Baltimore, 1993.

29. Kraus, JF, McArthur, DL, Epidemiologic aspects of brain injury, *Neurol., Clin.*, 14:435, 1996.

30. Stewart, DP, Kaylor, J, Koutanis, E, Cognitive deficits in presumed minor head-injured patients, *Acad. Emerg. Med.*, 3:21, 1996.

31. Gabella, B, Hoffman, RE, Marine, WW, Stallones, L, Urban and rural traumatic brain injuries in Colorado, *Ann. Epidemiol.*, 7:201, 1997.

32. Traumatic Brain Injury - Colorado, Missouri, Oklahoma, and Utah, 1990–1993, *MMWR Morb. Mortal. Wkl. Rep.*, 46:8, 1997.

33. Traumatic Brain Injuries kill or disable 4000 a year in Oklahoma, *J. Okla. State Med. Assoc.*, 85:37, 1992.

34. Diamond, PT, Brain injury in the Commonwealth of Virginia: an analysis of Central Registry data, 1988–1993, *Brain Inj.*, 10:413, 1996.

35. Thurman, DJ, Jeppson, L, Burnett, CL, et al., Surveillance of traumatic brain injuries in Utah, *West J. Med.*, 165:192, 1996.

36. Warren, S, Moore, M, Johnson, MS, Traumatic head and spinal cord injuries in Alaska (1991–1993), *Alaska Med.*, 37:11, 1995.

37. Van Balen, HG, Mulder, T, Keyser, A, Towards a disability-oriented epidemiology of traumatic brain injury, *Disabil. Rehabil.*, 18:181, 1996.

38. Wong, PP, Dornan, J, Schentag, CTG, Ip, R, Keating, M, Statistical profile of traumatic brain injury: a Canadian rehabilitation population, *Brain Inj.*, 7:283, 1993.

39. Wallace, GL, Stroke and traumatic brain injury (ma'i ulu) in Amerika Samoa, *Hawaii Med. J.*, 52:234, 1993.

40. Liko, O, Chalau, P, Rosenfeld, JV, Watters, DA, Head injuries in Papua New Guinea, *P. N. G. Ned. J.*, 39:100, 1996.

41. Annoni, JM, Beer, S, Kesselring, J, Severe traumatic brain injury-epidemiology and outcome after 3 years, *Disabil. Rehabil.*, 14:23, 1992.

42. Ceviker, N, Baykaner, K, Keskil, S, Cengel, M, Kaymaz, M, Moderate head injuries in children as compared to other age groups, including the cases who had talked and deteriorated, *Acta Neurochir. (Wein)*, 133:116, 1995.

43. Moscato, BS, Trevisan, M, Willer, BS, The prevalence of traumatic brain injury and co-occurring disabilities in a national household survey of adults, *J. Neuropsychiatry Clin. Neurosci.*, 6:134, 1994.

44. Tate, RL, McDonald, S, Lulham, JM, Incidence of hospital-treated traumatic brain injury in an Australian community, *Aust. N. Z. J. Public Health*, 22:419, 1998.

45. Hillier, SL, Hiller, JE, Metzer, J, Epidemiology of traumatic brain injury in South Australia, *Brain Inj.*, 11:649, 1997.

46. Wrightson, P, Gronwall, D, Mild head injury in New Zealand: incidence of injury and persisting symptoms, *N. Z. Med. J.*, 111:99, 1998.

47. Nell, V, Brown, DS, Epidemiology of traumatic brain injury in Johannesburg - II. Morbidity, mortality and etiology, *Soc. Sci. Med.*, 33:289, 1991.

48. Johansson, E, R"onnkvist, M, Fugl-Meyer, AR, Traumatic brain injury in northern Sweden. Incidence and prevalence of long-standing impairments and disabilities, *Scand. J. Rehabil. Med.*, 23:179, 1991.

49. Ingebrigtsen, T, Mortensen, K, Romner, B, The epidemiology of hospital-referred head injury in northern Norway, *Neuroepidemiology*, 17:139, 1998.

50. Chiu, WT, Yeh, KH, Li, YC, et al., Traumatic Brain Injury registry in Taiwan, *Neurol. Res.*, 19:261, 1998.

51. Barnfield, TV, Leathem, JM, Incidence and outcomes of traumatic brain injury and substance abuse in a New Zealand prison population, *Brain Inj.*, 12:455, 1998.

52. McGuire, LM, Burright, RG, Williams, R, Donovick, PJ, Prevalence of traumatic brain injury in psychiatric and non-psychiatric subjects, *Brain. Inj.*, 12:207, 1998.

53. Viano, D, von Holst, H, Gordon, E, Serious brain injury from traffic related causes: priorities for primary prevention, *Accid. Anal. Prev.*, 29:811, 1997.

54. Gennarelli, TA, Champion, HR, Copes, WS, Importance of mortality from head injury in immediate survivors of vehicular injuries, *International Research Council on Biokinetics of Impact*, 167, 1992.

55. Sacks, J, Holmgreen, P, Smith, SM, et al., Bicycle associated head injuries and deaths in the United States from 1984 through 1988. How many deaths are preventable, *JAMA*, 266:3016, 1991.

56. Zentner, J, Franken, H, L"obbecke, G, Head injuries from bicycle accidents, *Clin. Neurol. Neurosurg.*, 98:281, 1996.

57. Sosin, DM, Sacks, JJ, Motorcycle helmet use laws and head injury prevention, *JAMA*, 267:1649, 1992.

58. National Highway Traffic Safety Administration, *U.S. Department of Transportation: Traffic Safety Facts 1994*, Washington DC, U.S. Department of Transportation, 1994.

59. Frankowski, RF, Descriptive epidemiologic studies of head injury in the United States, 1974–1984, *Adv. Psychosom. Med.*, 16:153, 1986.

60. U.S. Department of Health and Human Services: Injury Prevention, Meeting the Challenge, *Am. J. Prevent. Med.*, 5(Suppl):1, 1989.

61. Blyth, CS, Mueller, F, Football injury survey: Part I: when and where players get hurt, *Physician Sportsmed.*, Sept: 45, 1974.

62. Rutherford, G, Miles, R, Overview of sports related injuries to persons 5-14 years of age, Washington, DC, U.S. Consumer Product Safety Commission, 1981.

63. Corsellis, JAN, Bruton, CJ, Freeman-Brown, D, The aftermath of boxing, *Psychol. Med.*, 3:270, 1973.

64. Mawdsley, C, Ferguson, FR, Neurological disease in boxers, *Lancet*, 1:795, 1963.

65. Sparade, FR, Gill, D, Effects of prior alcohol use on head injury recovery, *J. Head Trauma Rehabil.*, 4:72, 1989.

66. Rimel, RW, Jane, JA, Bond, MR, Characteristics of the head injured patient, in Rosenthal, M, Griffith, ER, Bond, MR, Miller, JD, (Eds.), *Rehabilitation of the Adult and Child with Traumatic Brain Injury*, FA, Davis, Philadelphia, 8, 1990.

67. Lindenbaum, GA, Carroll, SF, Daskel I, et al., Patterns of alcohol and drug abuse in an urban trauma center: the increasing role of abuse, *J. Trauma*, 29:1654, 1989.

68. Binder, LM, Persisting symptoms after mild head injury: a review of the postconcussive syndrome, *J. Clin. Exp.*, 8(4):323, 1986.

69. Bohnen, N, Jolles, J, Neurobehavioral aspects of postconcussive symptoms after mild head injury, *J. Nerv. Ment. Dis.*, 180(11):683, 1992.

70. Bohnen, N, Twijnstra, A, Jolles, J, Post-traumatic and emotional symptoms in different subgroups of patients with mild head injury, *Brain Inj.*, 6(6):481, 1992.

71. Sturzenegger, M, DiStefano, G, Radanov, BP, Schnidrig, A, Presenting symptoms and signs after whiplash injury: the influence of accident mechanisms, *Neurology*, 44:688, 1994.

72. Anderson, SD, Postconcussional disorder and loss of consciousness, *Bull. Am. Acad. Psychiatry Law*, 24:493, 1996.

73. Karzmark, P, Hall, K, Englander, J, Late-onset post-concussional symptoms after mild brain injury: the role of premorbid, injury-related, environmental, and personality factors, *Brain Inj.*, 9:21, 1995.

74. Gasquoine, PG, Postconcussion symptoms, *Neuropsychol. Rev.*, 7:77, 1997.

75. Landy, PJ, neurological sequelae of minor head and neck injuries, *Injury*, 29:199, 1998.

76. Barrett, K, Ward, AB, Boughey, A, et al., Sequelae of minor head injury: the natural history of post-concussive symptoms and their relationship to loss of consciousness and follow-up, *J. Accid. Emerg. Med.*, 11:79, 1994.

77. Szymanski, HV, Linn, R, A review of the postconcussion syndrome, *Int. J. Psychiatry Med.*, 22:357, 1992.

78. Chambers, J, Cohen, SS, Hemminger, L, et al., Mild traumatic brain injuries in low-risk patients, *J. Trauma*, 41:976, 1996.

79. Bohnen, N, Van Zutphen, W, Twijnstra, A, et al., Late outcome of mild head injury: results from a controlled postal survey, *Brain Inj.*, 8:701, 1994.

80. Mayou, R, Bryant, B, Outcome of "whiplash" neck injury, *Injury*, 27:617, 1997.

81. Cicerone, KD, Kalmar, K, Does premorbid depression influence post-concussive symptoms and neuropsychological functioning? *Brain Inj.*, 11:643, 1997.

82. Leininger, BE, Gramling, SE, Farrell, AD, et al., Neuropsychological deficits in symptomatic minor head injury patients after concussion and mild concussion, *J. Neurol. Neurosurg. Psychiatry*, 53:293, 1990.

83. DiStefano, G, Radanov, BP, Course of attention and memory after common whiplash: a two year prospective study with age, education and gender pair-matched patients, *Acta Neurol. Scand.*, 91:346, 1995.

84. Parker, RS, Rosenblum, A, IQ loss and emotional dysfunctions after mild head injury incurred in a motor vehicle accident, *J. Clin. Psychol.*, 52:32, 1996.

85. Jacobson, J, Gaadsgaard, SE, Thomsen, S, Henriksen, PB, Prediction of post-concussional sequelae by reaction time test, *Acta Neurol. Scand.*, 75(5):341, 1987.

86. Barrett, K, Buxton, N, Redmond, AD, et al., A comparison of symptoms experienced following minor head injury and acute neck strain (whiplash injury), *J. Accid. Emerg. Med.*, 12:173, 1995.

87. Gimse, R, Tjell, C, Bjorgen, IA, Saunte, C, Disturbed eye movements after whiplash due to injuries to the posture control system, *J. Clin. Exp. Neuropsychol.*, 18:178, 1996.

88. Heikkila, HV, Wenngren, BI, Cervicocephalic kinesthetic sensibility, active range of cervical motion, and oculomotor function in patients with whiplash injury, *Arch. Phys. Med. Rehab.*, 79:1089, 1998.

89. Rubin, AM, Woolle, SM, Dailey, VM, Goebe, JA, Postural stability following mild head or whiplash injuries, *Am. J. Otol.*, 16:216, 1995.

90. Soustiel, JF, Hafner, H, Chistyakov, AV, et al., Trigeminal and auditory evoked responses in minor head injuries and post-concussion syndrome, *Brain Inj.*, 9:805, 1995.

91. Otte, A, Ettlin, TM, Nitzsche, EU, et al., PET and SPECT in whiplash syndrome: a new approach to a forgotten brain? *J. Neurol. Neurosurg. Psychiatry*, 63:368, 1997.

92. Bicik, I, Radonov, BP, Schafer, N, et al., PET with 18fluorodeoxyglucose and hexamethylpropylene amine oxime SPECT in late whiplash syndrome, *Neurology*, 51:345, 1998.

93. Kant, R, Smith-Seemiller, L, Isaac, G, Duffy, J., Tc-HMPAO SPECT in persistent post-concussion syndrome after mild head injury: comparison with MRI/CT, *Brain Inj.*, 11:115, 1997.

94. Evans, RW, The postconcussion syndrome and the sequelae of mild head injury, *Neurol. Clin.*, 10(4):815, 1992.

95. Young, B, Sequelae of head injury, Wilkins, RH, Rengachary, SS, (Eds.), *Neurosurgery*, McGraw-Hill, New York, 1691, 1985.

96. Alves, WM, Jane, JA, Post-traumatic syndrome. in Youmans, JR, (Ed.), *Neurological Surgery*, 3rd Ed., WB Saunders, Philadelphia, 2230, 1990.

97. Brenner, C, Friedman, AP, Merrit, HH, Denny-Brown, DE, Post-traumatic headache, *J. Neurosurg.*, 1:379, 1944.

98. Hoganson, RC, Sachs, N, Desai, BT, Whitman, S, Sequelae associated with head injuries in patients who were not hospitalized: a follow-up survey, *Neurosurgery*, 14:315, 1984.

99. Jones, RK, Assessment of minimal head injuries: Indications for in-hospital care, *Surg. Neurol.*, 2:101, 1974.

100. Brenner, DN, Gillingham, JF, Patterns of convalescence after minor head injury, *J. R. Coll. Surg.*, Edinburgh, 19:94, 1974.

101. Symonds, D, Concussion and its sequelae, *Lancet*, 1:1, 1965.

102. Oddy, M, Humphrey, M, Uttley, D, Subjective impairment and social recovery after closed head injury, *J. Neurol. Neurosurg. Psychiatry*, 41:611, 1978.

103. Rimel, RW, Jane, JA, Minor head injury: management and outcome, in Williams, RH, Rengachary, SS, (Eds.), *Neurosurgery*, McGraw-Hill, New York, 1608, 1985.

104. Ritchie, WR, Recovery after minor head injury. Letter to the Editor, *Lancet*, 2:1315, 1974.

105. Rutherford, WH, Merrett, JD, McDonald, JR, Sequelae of concussion caused by minor head injuries, *Lancet*, 1:1, 1977.

106. Rutherford, WH, Merrett, JD, McDonald, JR, Symptoms at one year following concussion from minor head injuries, *Injury*, 10:225, 1978-79.

107. Berrol, S, Terminology of post-concussive syndrome, *Phys. Med. Rehabil: State of the Art Reviews*, 6(1):1, 1992.

108. Alexander, MP, Mild traumatic brain Injury, Pathophysiology, natural history and clinical management, *Neurology*, 45:1253, 1995.

109. Elson, LM, Ward, CC, Mechanisms and pathophysiology of mild head injury, *Semin. Neurol.*, 14:8, 1994.

110. Gentilini, M, Michelli, P, Shoenhuber, R, et al., Neuropsychological evaluation of mild head injury, *J. Neurol. Neurosurg. Psychiatry*, 48:137, 1985.

111. Dikmen, SS, McLean, A, Temkin, N, et al., Neuropsychological outcome at one month post injury, *Arch. Phys. Med. Rehabil.*, 67:507, 1986.

112. McLean, A, Dikmen, SS, Temkin, N, et al., Psychosocial functioning at one month after head injury, *Neurosurgery*, 14:393, 1984.

113. Stuss, DT, Stethem, LL, Hugenholt, H, et al., Reaction time after traumatic brain injury, Fatigue, divided and focused attention and consistency of performance, *J. Neurol. Neurosurg. Psychiatry*, 52:742, 1989.

114. Levin, H, Mattis, S, Ruff, R, et al., Neurobehavioral outcome following minor head injury: a three center study, *J. Neurosurg.*, 66:234, 1987.

115. Dikmen, SS, Temkin, N, Armsden, G, Neuropsychological recovery: relationship to psychosocial functioning and postconcussional complaints, in Levin, HS, Eisenberg, HM, Benton, AL, (Eds.), *Mild Head Injury*, Oxford University Press, New York, 2290, 1989.

116. McFlynn, G, Montgomery, F, Fenton, GW, Rutherford, W, Measurement of reaction time following minor head injury, *J. Neurol. Neurosurg. Psychiatry*, 48:137, 1984.

117. Gronwall, D, Wrightson, P, Cumulative effects of concussion, *Lancet*, 1:995, 1974.

118. Ewing, R, McCarthy, D, Gronwall, D, et al., Persisting effects of minor head injury observable during hypoxic stress, *J. Clin. Neuropsychol.*, 2:147, 1980.

119. Stuss, DT, Ely, P, Hugenholtz, H, et al., Subtle neuropsychological deficits in patients with good recovery after closed head injury, *Neurosurgery*, 17:41, 1985.

120. McLean, A, Temkin, NR, Dikmen, SS, et al., The behavioral sequelae of head injury, *J. Clin. Neuropsychol.*, 5:361, 1983.

121. Jones, JH, Viola, SL, LaBan, MM, et al., The incidence of post minor traumatic brain injury syndrome: a retrospective survey of treating physicians, *Arch. Phys. Med. Rehabil.*, 73(2):145, 1992.

122. Katz, RT, DeLuca, J, Sequelae of minor traumatic brain injury, *Am. Fam. Physician*, 46(5):1491, 1992.

123. McSherry, JA, Cognitive impairment after head injury, *Am. Fam. Physician*, 40(4):186, 1989.

124. Wrightson, P, Gronwall, D, Time off work and symptoms after minor head injury, *Injury*, 12(6):445, 1989.

125. Boll, TJ, Barth, J, Mild head injury, *Psychiatr. Dev.*, 28(5):509, 1983.

126. Harrington, DE, Malec, J, Cicerone, K, Katz, HT, Current perceptions of rehabilitation professionals toward mild traumatic brain injury, *Arch. Phys. Med. Rehabil.*, 74(6):579, 1993.

127. Middelboe, T, Anderson, HS, Birket-Smith, M, Friss ML, Minor head injury: impact on general health after one year. A prospective follow-up study, *Acta Neurol. Scand.*, 85(1):5, 1992.

128. Cicerone, KD, Psychological management of post-concussive disorders, *Phys. Med. Rehabil.: State of the Art Reviews*, 6(1):129, 1992.

129. Russell, WR, Recovery after minor head injury, (letter), *Lancet*, ii: 1315, 1974.

130. Alves, WM, Natural history of post-concussive signs and symptoms. *Phys. Med. Rehabil.: State of the Art Reviews*, 6(1):21, 1992.

131. Mateer, CA, Systems of care for post-concussion syndrome, *Phys. Med. Rehabil.: State of the Art Reviews*, 6(1):143, 1992.

132. Alexander, MP, Neuropsychiatric correlates of persistent postconcussive syndrome, *J. Head Trauma Rehabil.*, 7(2):60, 1992.

133. Radanov, BP, DI, Stefano G, Schnidrig, A, et al., Role of psychosocial stress in recovery from common whiplash, *Lancet*, 338:712, 1991.

134. Ettlin, TM, Kischka, U, Reichmann, S, et al., Cerebral symptoms after whiplash injury of the neck: a prospective clinical and neuropsychological study of whiplash injury, *J. Neurol. Neurosurg. Psychiatry*, 55:943, 1993.

135. Schoenhuber, R, Gentilini, M, Anxiety and depression after mild head injury: a case control study, *J. Neurol. Neurosurg. Psychiatry*, 51:722, 1988.

136. Zasler, ND, Neuromedical diagnosis and management of post-concussive disorders, *Phys. Med. Rehabil.: State of the Art Reviews*, 6(1):33, 1992.

137. Krapnick, JL, Horowitz, MJ, Stress response syndromes, *Arch. Gen. Psychiatry*, 38:428, 1981.
138. Weingartner, H, Cohen, RM, Murphy, DL, et al., Cognitive processes in depression, *Arch. Gen. Psychiatry*, 38:42, 1981.
139. Leininger, BE, Kreutzer, JS., Neuropsychological outcome of adults with mild traumatic brain injury, Implications for clinical practice and research, *Phys. Med. Rehabil.: State of the Art Reviews*, 6(1):169, 1992.
140. Wells, CE, Pseudodementia, *Am. J. Psychiatry*, 136:895, 1979.
141. Fenton, GW, The postconcussional syndrome reappraised, *Clin. Electroencephalogr.*, 27:174, 1996.
142. Taylor, AE, Cox, CA, Mailis, A, Persistent neuropsychological deficits following whiplash: evidence for chronic mild traumatic brain injury? *Arch. Phys. Med. Rehabil.*, 77:529, 1996.
143. Greiffenstein, MF, Baker, WJ, Gola, T, Motor dysfunction profiles in traumatic brain injury and postconcussion syndrome, *J. Int. Neuropsychol. Soc.*, 2:477, 1996.
144. Mathiesen, T, Kakarieka, A, Edner, G, Traumatic intracerebral lesions without extracerebral haematoma in 218 patients, *Acta Neurochir. (Wien)*, 137:155, 1995.
145. Sripairojkul, B, Saeheng, S, Ratanaler, S, et al., Traumatic hematomas of the posterior cranial fossa, *J. Med. Assoc. Thai*, 81:153, 1998.
146. Koc, RK, Akdemir, H, Oktem, IS, et al., Acute subdural hematoma: outcome and outcome prediction, *Neurosurg. Rev.*, 20:239, 1997.
147. Massaro, F, Lanotte, M, Faccani, G, Triolo, C, One hundred and twenty-seven cases of acute subdural haematoma operated on, Correlation between CT scan findings and outcome, *Acta Neurochir. (Wien)*, 138:185, 1996.
148. Wong, CW, Criteria for conservative treatment of supratentorial acute subdural haematomas, *Acta Neurochir. (Wien)*, 135:38, 1995.
149. Vaz, R, Duarte, F, Oliveira, J, et al., Traumatic interhemispheric subdural haematomas, *Acta Neurochir. (Wien)*, 111:128, 1991.
150. Lee, KS, Doh, JW, Bae, HG, Yun, IG., Relations among traumatic subdural lesions, *J. Korean Med. Sci.*, 11:55, 1996.
151. Firsching, R, Heimann, M, Frowein, RA, Early dynamics of acute extradural and subdural hematomas, *Neurol. Res.*, 19:257, 1997.
152. Borzone, Mk, Rivano, C, Altomonte, M, Baldini, M, Acute traumatic posterior fossa subdural haematomas, *Acta Neurochir. (Wien)*, 135:32, 1995.
153. Riesgo, P, Piquer, J, Botella, C, et al., Delayed extradural hematoma after mild head injury: report of three cases, *Surg. Neurol.*, 48:226, 1997.
154. Shigemori, M, Tokutomi, T, Hirohata, M, et al., Clinical significance of traumatic subarachnoid hemorrhage, *Neurol. Med. Chir. (Tokyo)*, 30:396, 1990.
155. Kakarieka, A, Braakman, R, Schakel, EH, Clinical significance of the finding of subarachnoid blood on CT scan after head injury, *Acta Neurochir. (Wien)*, 129:1, 1994.
156. Taneda, M, Kataoka, K, Akai, F, et al., Traumatic subarachnoid hemorrhage as a predictable indicator of delayed ischemic symptoms, *J. Neurosurg.*, 84:762, 1996.
157. Gaetani, P, Tancioni, F, Tartara, F, et al., Prognostic value of the amount of posttraumatic subarachnoid haemorrhage in a six month follow up period, *J. Neurol. Neurosurg. Psychiatry*, 59:635, 1995.
158. Medele, RJ, Stummer, W, Mueller, AJ, et al., Terson's syndrome in subarachnoid hemorrhage and severe brain injury accompanied by acutely raised intracranial pressure, *J. Neurosurg.*, 88:851, 1998.
159. Mlay, SM, Delayed intracranial haematomas, *East Afr. Med. J.*, 67:717, 1990.

160. Meyer, CA, Mirvi, SE, Wolf, AL, et al., Acute traumatic midbrain hemorrhage: experimental and clinical observations with CT, *Radiology*, 179:813, 1991.
161. Kurth, SM, Bigler, ED, Blatter, DD, Neuropsychological outcome and quantitative image analysis of acute haemorrhage in traumatic brain injury: preliminary findings, *Brain Inj.*, 8:489, 1994.
162. Birbamer, G, Gerstenbrand, F, Aichner, F, et al., Imaging of inner cerebral trauma, *Acta Neurol. (Napoli)*, 16:114, 1994.
163. Ezzat, W, Ang, LC, Nyssen, J, Pontomedullary rent. A specific type of primary brainstem traumatic injury, *Am. J. Forensic Med. Pathol.*, 16:336, 1995.
164. Hashimoto, T, Nakamura, N, Richard, KE, Frowein, RA: Primary brainstem lesions caused by closed head injuries, *Neurosurg. Rev.*, 16:291, 1993.
165. Goscinski, I, Kwaitkowski, S, Cichonski, J, Moskala, M, Posttraumatic brainstem haematoma, *Acta Neurochir. (Wien)*, 134:16-20, 1995.
166. Zarkovic, K, Jadro-Santel, D, Grcevic, N, Distribution of traumatic lesions of corpus callosum in "inner cerebral trauma," *Neurol. Croat.*, 40:129, 1991.
167. Vuilleumier, P, Assal, G, Complete callosal disconnection after closed head injury, *Clin. Neurol. Neurosurg.*, 97:39, 1995.
168. Tokutomi, T, Hirohata, M, Miyagi, T, Abe, T, Shigemori, M, Posttraumatic edema in the corpus callosum shown by MRI, *Acta Neurochir. Suppl. (Wien)*, 70:80, 1997.
169. Primus, EA, Bigler, ED, Anderson, CV, et al., Corpus striatum and traumatic brain injury, *Brain Inj.*, 11:577, 1997.
170. Yang, DN, Townsend, JC, Ilsen, PF, Bright, DC, Welton, TH, Traumatic porencephalic cyst of the brain, *J. Am. Optom. Assoc.*, 68:519, 1997.
171. Van Zomeren, AH, ten Duis, HJ, Minderhoud, JM, Sipma, M, Lightning stoke and neuropsychological impairment: Cases and questions, *J. Neurol. Neurosurg. Psychiatry*, 64:763, 1998.
172. Aoki, N, Oikawa, A, Sakai, T, Symptomatic subacute subdural hematoma associated with cerebral hemispheric swelling and ischemia, *Neurol. Res.*, 18:145, 1996.
173. Schmidt, RH, Grady, MS, Loss of forebrain cholinergic neurons following fluid-percussion injury: implications for cognitive impairment in closed head injury, *J. Neurosurg.*, 83:496, 1995.
174. Rogers, RD, Sahakian, BJ, Hodges, JR, et al., Dissociating executive mechanisms of task control following frontal lobe damage and Parkinson's disease, *Brain*, 121 (pt 5):815, 1998.
175. Coolidge, FL, Griego, JA, Executive functions of the frontal lobes: psychometric properties of a self-rating scale, *Psychol. Rep.*, 77:24, 1995.
176. Minderhoud, JM, van Zomeren, AH, van der Naalt, J, The fronto-temporal component in mild and moderately severe head injury, *Acta Neurol. Belg.*, 96:31, 1996.
177. McCarthy, G, Nobre, AC, Bentin, S, Spencer, DD, Language-related field potentials in the anterior-medial temporal lobe: I. Intracranial distribution and neural generators, *J. Neurosci.*, 15:1080, 1995.
178. Stuss, DT, Alexander, MP, Hamer, L, et al, The effects of focal anterior and posterior brain lesions on verbal fluency, *J. Int. Neuropsychol. Soc.*, 4:265, 1998.
179. Crowe, SF, Dissociation of two frontal love syndromes by a test of verbal fluency, *J. Clin. Exp. Neuropsychol.*, 14:327, 1992.
180. Smith, ML, Leonard, G, Crane, J, Milner, B, The effects of frontal- or temporal-lobe lesions on susceptibility to interference in spatial memory, *Neuropsychologia*, 33:275, 1995.
181. Ferreira, CT, V'erin, M, Pillon, B, et al, Spatio-temporal working memory and frontal lesions in man, *Cortex*, 34:83, 1998.

182. Godefroy, O, Rousseaux, M, Divided and focused attention in patients with lesion of the prefrontal cortex, *Brain Cogn.*, 30:155, 1996.
183. Bechara, A, Tranel, D, Damasio, H, Damasio, AR, Failure to respond autonomically to anticipated future outcomes, *Cereb. Cortex.*, 6:215, 1996.
184. Burgess, PW, Shallice, T, Bizarre responses, rule detection and frontal lobe lesions, *Cortex*, 32:241, 1996.
185. Viallet, F, Vuillon-Cacciuttolo, G, Legallet, E, et al, Bilateral and side-related time impairments in patients with unilateral cerebral lesions of a medial frontal region involving the supplementary motor area, *Neuropsychologia*, 33:215, 1995.
186. Duncan, J, Burgess, P, Emslie, H, Fluid intelligence after frontal lobe lesions, *Neuropsychologia*, 33:261, 1995.
187. Zihl, J, Hebel, N, Patterns of oculomotor scanning in patients with unilateral posterior parietal or frontal lobe damage, *Neuropsychologia*, 35:893, 1997.
188. Rushworth, MF, Nixon, PD, Renowden, S, et al., The left parietal cortex and motor attention, *Neuropsychologia*, 35:1261, 1997.
189. Maeshima, S, Uematsu, Y, Ozaki, F, et al., Impairment of short-term memory in left hemispheric traumatic brain injuries, *Brain Inj.*, 11:279, 1997.
190. Barontini, F, Maurri, S, Isolated amnesia following a bilateral paramedian thalamic infarct. Possible etiologic role of a whiplash injury, *Acta Neurol. (Napoli)*, 14:90, 1992.
191. Wood, DM, Bigler, ED, Diencephalic changes in traumatic brain injury, *Brain Res. Bull.*, 38:545, 1995.
192. Sakas, DE, Bullock, MR, Patterson, J, et al., Focal cerebral hyperemia after focal head injury in humans: a benign phenomenon? *J. Neurosurg.*, 83:277, 1995.
193. Kelly, DF, Kordestani, RD, Martin, NA, et al, Hyperemia following traumatic brain injury: relationship to intracranial hypertension and outcome, *J. Neurosurg.*, 85:762, 1996.
194. Kelly, DF, Martin, NA, Kordestani, RD, et al, Cerebral blood flow as a predictor of outcome following traumatic brain injury, *J. Neurosurg.*, 86:633, 1997.
195. Chan, KH, Miller, JD, Dearden, NM, Intracranial blood flow velocity after head injury: relationship to severity of injury, time, neurological status and outcome, *J. Neurol. Neurosurg. Psychiatry*, 55:787, 1992.
196. Marion, DW, Darby, J, Yonas, H, Acute regional cerebral blood flow changes caused by severe head injuries, *J. Neurosurg.*, 74:407, 1991.
197. Bouma, GJ, Muizelaar, JP, Choi, SC, et al, Cerebral circulation and metabolism after severe traumatic brain injury: the elusive role of ischemia, *J. Neurosurg.*, 75:685, 1991.
198. Lee, JH, Martin, NA, Alsina, G, et al, Hemodynamically significant cerebral vasospasm and outcome after head injury: a prospective study, *J. Neurosurg.*, 87:221, 1997.
199. Romner, B, Bellner, J, Kongstad, P, Sjoholm, H, Elevated transcranial Doppler flow velocities after severe head injury: cerebral vasospasm or hyperemia? *J. Neurosurg.*, 85:90, 1996.
200. Brown, JI, Moulton, RJ, Konasiewicz, SJ, Baker, AJ, Cerebral oxidative metabolism and evoked potential deterioration after severe brain injury: new evidence of early posttraumatic ischemia, *Neurosurgery*, 42:1057, 1998.
201. Le Roux, PD, Newel, DW, Lam, AM, et al, Cerebral arteriovenous oxygen difference: a predictor of cerebral infarction and outcome in patients with severe head injury, *J. Neurosurg.*, 87:1, 1997.
202. Newell, DWS, Aaslid, R, Stooss R, et al., Evaluation of hemodynamic responses in head injury patients with transcranial Doppler monitoring, *Acta Neurochir. (Wien)*, 139:804, 1997.

203. Shiina, G, Onuma, T, Kameyama, M, et al., Sequential assessment of cerebral blood flow in diffuse brain injury, by 123I-iodoamphetamine single-photon emission CT, *AJNR Am. J. Neuroradiol.*, 19:297, 1998.

204. McLaughlin, MR, Marion, DW, Cerebral blood flow and vasoresponsivity within and around cerebral contusions, *J. Neurosurg.*, 85:871, 1996.

205. Junger, EC, Newell, DW, Grant, GA, et al., Cerebral autoregulation following minor head injury, *J. Neurosurg.*, 86:425, 1997.

206. Strebel, S, Lam, AM, Matta, BF, Newell, DW, Impaired cerebral autoregulation after mild brain injury, *Surg. Neurol.*, 47:128, 1997.

207. Marmarou, A, Barzo, P, Fatouros, P, et al., Traumatic brain swelling in head injured patients: brain edema or vascular engorgement? *Acta Neurochir. Suppl. (Wien)*, 70:68, 1997.

208. Lang, DA, Teasdale, GM, Macpherson, P, Lawrence, A, Diffuse brain swelling after head injury: more often malignant in adults than children? *J. Neurosurg.*, 80:675, 1994.

209. Kazan, S, Tuncer, R, Karasoy, M, et al, Post-traumatic bilateral diffuse cerebral swelling, *Acta Neurochir. (Wien)*, 139:295, 1997.

210. Childers, MK, Rupright, J, Smith, DW, Post-traumatic hyperthermia in acute brain injury, rehabilitation, *Brain Inj.*, 8:335, 1994.

211. Albrecht, RF II, Wass, CT, Lanier, WL, Occurrence of potentially detrimental temperature alterations in hospitalized patients at risk for brain injury, *May. Clin. Proc.*, 73:629, 1998.

212. Marion, DW, Penrod, LE, Kelsey, SF, et al., Treatment of traumatic brain injury with moderate hypothermia, *N. Engl. J. Med.*, 336:540, 1997.

213. Dietrich, WD, The importance of brain temperature in cerebral injury, *J. Neurotrauma.*, 9 Suppl 2:S475, 1992.

214. Servadei, F, Nanni, A, Nasi, MT, et al., Evolving brain lesions in the first 12 hours after head injury: analysis of 37 comatose patients, *Neurosurgery*, 37:899, 1995.

215. Thatcher, RW, Camacho, M, Salazar, A, et al., Quantitative MRI of the gray-white matter distribution in traumatic brain injury, *J. Neurotrauma.*, 14:1, 1997.

216. Gale, SD, Johnson, SC, Bigler, ED, Blatter, DD., Nonspecific white matter degeneration following traumatic brain injury, *J. Int. Neuropsychol. Soc.*, 1:17, 1995.

217. Cervos-Navarro, J, Lafuente, JV, Traumatic brain injuries: structural changes, *J. Neurol. Sci.*, 103 Supple:S3, 1991.

218. McD. Anderson, R, Opeskin, K, Timing of early changes in brain trauma, *Am. J. Forensic Med. Pathol.*, 19:1, 1998.

219. Parizel, PM, Ozsarla, K, Van Goethem, JW, et al., Imaging findings in diffuse axonal injury after closed head trauma, *Eur. Radiol.*, 8:960, 1998.

220. Oehmichen, M, Meissner, C, Schmidt, V, et al., Axonal injury- a diagnostic tool in forensic neuropathology? A review, *Forensic Sci. Int.*, 95:67-83, 1998.

221. Abou-Hamden, A, Blumbergs, PC, Scott, G, et al., Axonal injury in falls, *J. Neurotrauma.*, 14:699, 1997.

222. Blumbergs, PC, Scott, G, Manavis, J, et al., Topography of axonal injury as defined by amyloid precursor protein and the sector scoring method in mild and severe closed head injury, *J. Neurotrauma.*, 12:55, 1995.

223. Christman, CW, Grad, MS, Walker, SA, et al., Ultrastructural studies of diffuse axonal injury in humans, *J. Neurotrauma.*, 11:173, 1994.

224. Geddes, JF, Vowles, GH, Beer, TW, Ellison, DW., The diagnosis of diffuse axonal injury: implications for forensic practice, *Neuropathol. Appl. Neurobiol.*, 23:339, 1997.

225. Vaz, R, Sarmento, A, Borges, N, et al., Ultrastructural study of brain microvessels in patients with traumatic cerebral contusions, *Acta Neurochir. (Wien)*, 139:215, 1997.

226. Castejon, OJ, Morphological astrocytic changes in complicated human brain trauma. A light and electron microscopic study, *Brain Inj.*, 12:409, 1998.

227. Castejon, OJ, Valero, C, Diaz, M, Light and electron microscope study of nerve cells in traumatic oedematous human cerebral cortex, *Brain Inj.*, 11:363, 1997.

228. Castejon, OJ, Electron microscopic analysis of cortical biopsies in patients with traumatic brain injuries and dysfunction of neurobehavioral system, *J. Submicrosc. Cytol. Pathol.*, 30:145, 1998.

229. Castejon, OJ, Valero, C, Diaz, M, Synaptic degenerative changes in human traumatic brain edema. An electron microscopic study of cerebral cortical biopsies. *J. Neurosurg. Sci.*, 39:47, 1995.

230. Crooks, DA, Scholtz, CL, Vowles, G, et al., Axonal injury in closed head injury by assault: a quantitative study, *Med. Sci. law*, 32(2):109, 1992.

231. Imajo, T, Diffuse axonal injury: its mechanism in an assault case, *Am. J. Forensic Med. Pathol.*, 17:324, 1996.

232. Ramsay, DA, Shkrum, MJ, Homicidal blunt head trauma, diffuse axonal injury, alcoholic intoxication and cardiorespiratory arrest: a case report of a forensic syndrome of acute brainstem dysfunction, *Am. J. Forensic Med. Pathol.*, 16:107, 1995.

233. Engel, S, Wehner, HD, Meyermann, R, Expression of microglial markers in the human CNS after closed head injury, *Acta Neurochir. Suppl. (Wien)*, 66:89, 1996.

234. Fukuda, K, Aihara, N, Sagar, SM, et al, Purkinje cell vulnerability to mild traumatic brain injury, *J. Neurotrauma.*, 13:255, 1996.

235. Povlishock, JT, Traumatically induced axonal injury: pathogenesis and pathobiological implications, *Brain Pathol.*, 2:1, 1992.

236. Povlishock, JT, Jenkins, LW, Are the pathobiological changes evoked by traumatic brain injury immediate and irreversible? *Brain Pathol.*, 5:415, 1995.

237. Bernstein, L, Garzone, PD, Rudy, T, et al., Pain perception and serum beta-endorphin in trauma patients, *Psychosomatics*, 36:276, 1995.

238. Pasaoglu, H, Inci Karakucuk, E, Kurtsoy, A, Pasaoglu, A, Endogenous neuropeptides in patients with acute traumatic head injury, I: cerebrospinal fluid beta-endorphin levels are increased within 24 hours following the trauma, *Neuropeptides*, 30:47, 1996.

239. Stachura, Z, Kowalski, J, Obuchowicz, E, et al., Concentration of enkephalins in cerebrospinal fluid of patients after severe head injury, *Neuropeptides*, 31:78, 1997.

240. Markianos, M, Seretis, A, Kotsou, A, Christopoulos, M, CSF neurotransmitter metabolites in their clinical state, *Acta Neurochir. (Wien)*, 138:57, 1996.

241. Karakucuk, E, Pasaoglu, H, Pasaoglu, A, Oktem, S, Endogenous neuropeptides in patients with acute traumatic head injury, II: Changes in the levels of cerebral spinal fluid substance P, serotonin and lipid peroxidation products in patients with head trauma, *Neuropeptides*, 31:259, 1997.

242. Murdoch, I, Perry, EK, Court, JA, et al, Cortical cholinergic dysfunction after human head injury, *J. Neurotrauma.*, 15: 295, 1998.

243. Ziegler, MG, Morrissey, EC, Marshall, LF, Catecholamine and thyroid hormones in traumatic injury, *Crit. Care Med.*, 18:253, 1990.

244. Tang, YP, Noda, Y, Nabeshima, T, Involvement of activation of dopaminergic neuronal system in learning and memory deficits associated with experimental mild traumatic brain injury, *Eur J. Neurosci.*, 9:1720, 1997.

245. Peterson, SR, Jeevanandam, M, Harrington, T, Is the metabolic response to injury different with or without severe head injury? Significance of plasma glutamine levels, *J. Trauma*, 34:653, 1993.

246. Peterson, SR, Jeevanandam, M, Holaday, NJ, Lubhan, CL, Arterial-jugular vein free amino acid levels in patients with head injuries: Important role of glutamine in cerebral nitrogen metabolism, *J Trauma*, 41:687, 1996.

247. Goodman, JC, Valadka, AB, Gopinath, SP, et al., Lactate and excitatory amino acids measured by microdialysis are decreased by pentobarbital coma in head-injured patients, *J. Neurotrauma.*, 13:549, 1996.

248. Brown, JI, Baker, AJ, Konasiewicz, SJ, Moulton, RJ, Clinical significance of CSF glutamate concentrations following severe traumatic brain injury in humans, *J. Neurotrauma.*, 15:253, 1998.

249. Baker, AJ, Moulton, RJ, MacMillan, VH, Shedden, PM, Excitatory amino acids in cerebrospinal fluid following traumatic brain injury in humans. *J. Neurosurg.*, 79:369, 1993.

250. Sinz, EH, Kochanek, PM, Heyes, MP, et al, Quinolinic acid is increased in CSF and associated with mortality after traumatic brain injury in humans, *J. Cereb. Blood Flow Metab.*, 18:610, 1998.

251. Cornford. EM, Hyman. S, Cornford. ME, Caron. MJ. Glut1 glucose transporter activity in human brain injury, *J. Neurotrauma.*, 13:523, 1996.

252. Jacobs, A, Amino acid uptake in ischemically compromised brain tissue, *Stroke*, 26:1859, 1995.

253. Koiv, L, Merisalu, E, Zilmer, K, et al., Changes of sympatho-adrenal and hypo-thalamo-pituitary-adrenocortical system in patients with head injury, *Acta Neurol. Scand.*, 96:52, 1997.

254. Lenzen, J, Hildebrand, G, Laun, A, et al., Function tests on the neuroendocrine hypothalamo-pituitary system following acute midbrain syndrome, with special reference to computer tomographical and magnetic resonance imaging results, *Neurosurg. Rev.*, 16:183, 1993.

255. Woolf, PD, Cox, C, Kelly, M, et al., Alcohol intoxication blunts sympatho-adrenal activation following brain injury, *Alcohol Clin. Exp. Res.*, 14:205,1990.

256. Altura, BM, Memon, ZS, Altura, BT, Cracco, RQ, Alcohol-associated acute head trauma in human subjects is associated with early deficits in serum ionized Mg and Ca. *Alcohol*, 12:433, 1995.

257. Ferguson, RK, Soryal, IN, Pentland, B, Thiamine deficiency in head injury: a missed insult? *Alcohol*, 32:493, 1997.

258. Robertson, CS, Goodman, JC, Narayan, RK, et al, The effect of glucose administration on carbohydrate metabolism after head injury, *J. Neurosurg.*, 74:43, 1991.

259. Gross, H, Kling, A, Henry, G, et al., Local cerebral glucose metabolism in patients with long-term behavioral and cognitive deficits following mild traumatic brain injury, *J. Neuropsychiatry Clin. Neurosci.*, 8:324, 1996.

260. Ertel, W, Keel, M, Stocker, R, et al., Detectable concentrations of Fas ligand in cerebrospinal fluid after severe head injury, *J. Neuroimmunol.*, 80:93, 1997.

261. Waterloo, K, Ingebrigtsen, T, Romner, B, Neuropsychological function in patients with increased serum levels of protein S-100 after minor head injury, *Acta Neurochir. (Wien)*, 139:26, 1997.

262. Ingebrigtsen, T, Romner, B, Serial S-100 protein serum measurements related to early magnetic resonance imaging after minor head injury, Case report, *J. Neurosurg.*, 85:945, 1996.

263. Marmarou, A, Intracellular acidosis in human and experimental brain injury, *J. Neurotrauma.*, 9 Suppl 2:S551, 1992.

264. Clark, RS, Kochanek, PM, Obrist, WD, et al., Cerebrospinal fluid and plasma nitrite and nitrate concentrations after head injury in humans, *Crit. Care Med.*, 24:1243, 1996.

265. Clark, RS, Carcillo, JA, Kochanek, PM, et al., Cerebrospinal fluid adenosine concentration and uncoupling of cerebral blood flow and oxidative metabolism after severe head injury in humans, *Neurosurgery*, 41:1284-92, 1997.

266. Kochanek, PM, Clark, RS, Obrist, WD, et al., The role of adenosine during the period of delayed cerebral swelling after severe traumatic brain injury in humans, *Acta Neurochir. Suppl. (Wien)*, 70:109, 1997.

267. Smirnova, IV, Salazar, A, Arnold, PM, et al., Thrombin and its precursor in human cerebrospinal fluid, *Thromb Haemost.*, 78:1473, 1997.

268. Marti, HH, Gassmann, M, Wenger, RH, et al., Detection of erythropoietin in human liquor: Intrinsic erythropoietin production in the brain, *Kidney Int.*, 51:416, 1997.

269. Vazquez, MD, Sanchez-Rodriguez, R, Osuna E, et al., Creatine kinase BB and neuron-specific enolase in cerebrospinal fluid in the diagnosis of brain insult, *Am. J. Forensic Med. Pathol.*, 16:210, 1995.

270. Ross, SA, Cunningham, RT, Johnston, CR, Rowlands, BJ, Neuron-specific enolase as an aid to outcome prediction in head injury, *Br. J. Neurosurg.*, 10:471, 1996.

271. Yamazaki, Y, Yada, K, Morii, S, et al., Diagnostic significance of serum neuron-specific enolase and myelin basic protein assay in patients with acute head injury, *Surg. Neurol.*, 43:267, 1995.

272. Adle-Biassette, H, Duyckaerts, C, Wasowicz, M, et al., Beta AP deposition and head trauma, *Neurobiol. Aging*, 17:415, 1996.

273. Sherriff, FE, Bridges, LR, Sivaloganathan, S, Early detection of axonal injury after human head trauma using immunocytochemistry for beta-amyloid precursor protein, *Acta Neuropathol. (Berl.)*, 87:55, 1994.

274. McKenzie, KJ, McLellan, DR, Gentleman, SM, et al., Is beta-APP a marker of axonal damage in short surviving head injury? *Acta Neuropathol. (Berl.)*, 92:608, 1996.

275. Graham, DI, Gentleman, SM, Lynch, A, Roberts, GW, Distribution of beta-amyloid protein in the brain following severe head injury, *Neuropathol. Appl. Neurobiol.*, 21:27, 1995.

276. Gentleman, SM, Greenberg, BD, Savage, MJ, et al., A beta 42 is the predominant form of amyloid beta-protein in the brains of short-term survivors of head injury, *Neuroreport*, 8:1519, 1997.

277. Pleines, UE, Stover, JF, Kossman, T, et al., Soluble ICAM-1 in CSF coincides with the extent of cerebral damage in patients with severe traumatic brain injury, *J. Neurotrauma.*, 15:399, 1998.

278. McKeating, EG, Andrew, PJ, Mascia, L., The relationship of soluble adhesion molecule concentrations in systemic and jugular venous serum to injury severity and outcome after traumatic brain injury, *Anesth. Analg.*, 86:759, 1998.

279. Munno, I, Damiani, S, Lacedra, G, et al., Impairment of non-specific immunity in patients in persistent vegetative state, *Immunopharmacol. Immunotoxicol.*, 18:549, 1996.

280. Bednar, MM, Gross, CE, Howard, DB, Lynn, M, Neutrophil activation in acute human central nervous system injury, *Neurol. Res.*, 19:588, 1997.

281. Kossman, T, Stahel, PF, Morganti-Kossmann, MC, et al., Elevated levels of the complement components C3 and factor B in ventricular cerebrospinal fluid of patients with traumatic brain injury, *J. Neuroimmunol.*, 73:63, 1997.

282. Ross, SA, Halliday, MI, Campbell, GC, et al., The presence of tumour necrosis factor in CSF and plasma after severe head injury, *Br. J. Neurosurg.*, 8:419, 1994.

162 Minor Traumatic Brain Injury Handbook: Diagnosis and Treatment

283. Cinat, M, Waxman, K, Vaziri, ND, et al., Soluble cytokine receptors and receptor antagonists are sequentially released after trauma, *J. Trauma*, 39:112, 1995.
284. Mathiesen, T, Edner, G, Ulfarsson, E, Andersson, B, Cerebrospinal fluid interleukin-1 receptor antagonist and tumor necrosis factor-alpha following subarachnoid hemorrhage, *J. Neurosurg.*, 87:215, 1997.
285. Quattrocchi, KB, Frank, EH, Miller, CH, Severe head injury: effect upon cellular immune function, *Neurol. Res.*, 13:13, 1991.
286. Quattrocchi, KB, Frank, EH, Miller, CH, et al., Suppression of cellular immune activity following severe head injury, *J. Neurotrauma.*, 7:77, 1990.
287. Kossman, T, Hans, V, Imhof, HG, et al., Interleukin-6 released in human cerebrospinal fluid following traumatic brain injury may trigger nerve growth factor production in astrocytes, *Brain Res.*, 713:143, 1996.
288. McKeating, EG, Andrews, PJ, Signorini, DF, Mascia, L, Transcranial cytokine gradients in patients requiring intensive care after acute brain injury, *Br. J. Anaesth.*, 78:520, 1997.
289. Kossman, T, Han, V, Imhof, HG, et al., Intrathecal and serum interleukin-6 and the acute-phase response in patients with severe traumatic brain injuries, *Shock*, 4:311, 1995.
290. Kossman, T, Stahel, PF, Lenzlinger, PM, et al., Interleukin-8 released into the cerebrospinal fluid after brain injury is associated with blood-brain barrier dysfunction and nerve growth factor production, *J. Cereb. Blood Flow Metab.*, 17:280, 1997.
291. Stahel, PF, Kossmann, T, Joller, H, et al., Increased interleukin-12 levels in human cerebrospinal fluid following severe head trauma, *Neurosci. Lett.*, 249:123, 1998.
292. O'Sullivan, ST, Lederer, JA, Horgan, AF, et al., Major injury leads to predominance of the T helper-2 lymphocyte phenotype and diminished interleukin-12 production associated with decreased resistance to infection, *Ann. Surg.*, 222:482, 1995.
293. Kraus, JF, Nourjah, P, The epidemiology of mild, uncomplicated brain injury, *J. Trauma*, 28:1637, 1988.
294. McAllister, TW, Neuropsychiatric sequelae of head injuries, *Psychiatr. Clin. North Am.*, 15:395, 1992.
295. Lynch, R, Traumatic head injury: implications for rehabilitation counseling, *Appl. Rehabil. Counsel*, 3:32, 1983.
296. Minor head injury becomes a "silent epidemic", *News AFT*, 28:345, 1983.
297. Mohanty, SK, Thompson, W, Rakower, S, Are CT scans for head injury patients always necessary? *J. Trauma*, 31:801, 1991.
298. Shackford, SR, Wald, SL, Ross, SE, et al., The clinical utility of computed tomographic scanning and neurologic examination in the management of patients with minor head injuries, *J. Trauma*, 33:385, 1992.
299. Stein, SC, Omalley, KF, Toss, SE, Is routine computed tomography scanning too expensive for mild head injury? *Ann. Emerg. Med.*, 20:1286, 1991.
300. Ross, SP, Ros, MA, Should patients with normal cranial CT scans following minor head injury be hospitalized for observations? *Pediatr. Emerg. Care*, 5:216, 1989.
301. Stein, SC, Ross, SE, Mild head injury: a plea for routine early CT scanning, *J.H. Trauma*, 33:11, 1992.
302. Stein SC, Ross SE, The value of computed tomographic scans in patients with low-risk head injuries, *Neurosurgery*, 26:638, 1990.
303. Servadei, F, Ciucci, G, Morchetti, A, et al., Skull fracture as a factor of increased risk in minor head injuries. Indication for a broader use of cerebral computed tomography scanning, *Surg. Neurol.*, 30:364, 1988.

304. Servadei, F, Ciucci, G, Pagano, F, et al., Skull fracture as a risk factor of intracranial complications in minor head injury. A prospective CT study in a series of 98 adult patients, *J. Neurol. Neurosurg. Psychiatry*, 51:526, 1998.

305. Jeffries, RV, Lozada, L, The use of the CAT scanner in the management of patients with head injury transferred to the regional neurosurgical unit, *Injury*, 13:370, 1982.

306. Besenski, N, Brzovic, Z, Prpic-Vuckovic, R, et al., CT detection of minimal brain lesions in closed cerebral trauma, *Neurol. Croat.*, 41: 33, 1991.

307. Tatalovic-Osterman, L, Jadro-Santel, D, Besenski, N, Diagnostic possibilities of closed head injuries of acceleration type using computed tomography, *Neurol. Croat.*, 40:231, 1991.

308. Besenski, N, Broz, R, Jadro-Santel, D, et al., The course of the traumatizing force in acceleration head injury: CT evidence, *Neuroradiology*, 38 Suppl 1:S36, 1996.

309. Kido, DK, Cox, C, Hamill, RW, et al., Traumatic brain injuries: Predictive usefulness of CT, *Radiology*, 182:777, 1992.

310. Jeret, JS, Mandell, M, Anziska, B, et al., Clinical predictors of abnormality disclosed by computed tomography after mild head trauma, *Neurosurgery*, 32:9, 1993.

311. Gibson, TC: Skull X-rays in minor head injury. A review of their use and interpretation by casualty officers, *Scott Med. J.*, 28:132, 1983.

312. Rosenorn, J, Duus, B, Nielson, K, et al., Is a skull X-ray necessary after milder head trauma? *Br. J. Neurosurg.*, 5:135, 1991.

313. Levin, HS, Williams, DH, Eisenberg, HM, et al., Serial MRI and neurobehavioral findings after mild to moderate closed head injury. *J. Neurol. Neurosurg. Psychiatry*, 55:255, 1992.

314. Doezma, D, King, JN, Tandberg, D, et al., Magnetic resonance imaging in minor head injury. *Ann. Emerg. Med.*, 20:1281, 1991.

315. Fumeya, H, Ito, K, Yamagiwa, O, et al., Analysis of MRI and SPECT in patients with acute head injury, *Acta Neurochir. Suppl. (Wien)*, 51:283, 1990.

316. Evans, RW, Mild traumatic brain injury, *Physical Med. and Rehabil. Clinics N. AM.*, 3:427, 1992.

317. Yokota, H, Kurokawa, A, Otsuka, T, et al., Significance of magnetic resonance imaging in acute head injury, *J. Trauma*, 31:351, 1991.

318. Levin, HS, Amparo, E, Eisenberg, HM, et al., Magnetic resonance imaging and computerized tomography in relation to the neurobehavioral sequelae of mild and moderate head injuries, *J. Neurosurg.*, 66:706, 1987.

319. Godersky, JC, Gentry, LR, Tranel, D, et al., Magnetic resonance imaging and neurobehavioral outcome in traumatic brain injury, *Acta Neurochir. Suppl. (Wien)*, 51:311, 1990.

320. Mittl, RL, Grossman, RI, Hiehle, JF, et al., Prevalence of MR evidence of diffuse axonal injury in patients with mild head injury and normal head CT findings, *AJNR Am. J. Neuroradiol.*, 15:1583, 1994.

321. Blatter, DD, Bigler, ED, Gale, SD, et al., MR-based brain and cerebrospinal fluid measurement after traumatic brain injury: correlation with neuropsychological outcome, *AJNR Am. J. Neuroradiol.*, 18:1, 1997.

322. Lang, DA, Hadley, DM, Teasdale, GM, et al., Gadolinium DTPA enhanced magnetic resonance imaging in acute head injury, *Acta Neurochir. (Wien)*, 109:5, 1991.

323. Thatcher, RW, Biver, C, McAlaster, R, et al., Biophysical linkage between MRI and EEG amplitude in closed head injury, *Neuroimage*, 7:352, 1998.

324. Milton, WJ, Hal O'Dell, R, Warner, EG, MRI of lightening injury: Early white matter changes associated with cerebral dysfunction, *J. Okla. State Med. Assoc.*, 89:93, 1996.

325. Fischer, H, Wik, G, Fredrikson, M, Functional neuroanatomy of robbery re-experience: affective memories studied with PET, *Neuroreport*, 7:2081, 1996.

326. Roberts, MA, Manshadi, FF, Bushnell, DL, Hines, ME, Neurobehavioral dysfunction following mild traumatic brain injury in childhood: a case report with positive findings on positron emission tomography (PET), *Brain Inj.*, 9:427, 1995.

327. Bergsneider, M, Hovda, DA, Shalmon, E, et al., Cerebral hyperglycolysis following severe traumatic brain injury in humans: a positron emission tomography study, *J. Neurosurg.*, 86:241, 1997.

328. Nagamachi, S, Nishikawa, T, Ono, S, et al., A comparative study of 123I-IMP SPECT and CT in the investigation of chronic-stage head trauma patients, *Nucl. Med. Commun.*, 16:17, 1995.

329. Gray, BG, Ichise, M, Chung, DG, et al., Technetium-99m-HMPAO SPECT in the evaluation of patients with a remote history of traumatic brain injury: a comparison with x-ray computed tomography, *J. Nucl. Med.*, 33:52, 1992.

330. Ichise, M, Chung, DG, Wang, P, et al., Technetium-99m-HMPAO SPECT, CT and MRI in the evaluation of patients with chronic traumatic brain injury: A correlation with neuropsychological performance, *J. Nucl. Med.*, 35: 217, 1994.

331. Abu-Judeh, HH, Singh, M, Masdeu, JC, Abdel-Dayem, HM, Discordance between FDG uptake and technetium-99m-HMPAO brain perfusion in acute traumatic brain injury, *J. Nucl. Med.*, 39:1357, 1998.

332. Yamakami, I, Yamaura, A, Isobe, K, Types of traumatic brain injury and regional cerebral blood flow assessed by 99mTc-HMPAO SPECT, *Neurol. Med. Chir. (Tokyo)*, 33:7, 1993.

333. Choksey, MS, Costa, DC, Iannotti, F, et al., 99TCm-HMPAO SPECT studies in traumatic intracerebral haematoma, *J. Neurol. Neurosurg. Psychiatry*, 54:6, 1991.

334. Umile, EM, Plotkin, RC, Sandel, ME, Functional assessment of mild traumatic brain injury using SPECT and neuropsychological testing, *Brain Inj.*, 12:577, 1998.

335. Oder, W, Goldenberg, G, Spatt, J, et al., Behavioural and psychosocial sequelae of severe closed head injury and regional cerebral blood flow: a SPECT study, *J. Neurol. Neurosurg. Psychiatry*, 55:475, 1992.

336. Abdel-Dayem, HM, Abu-Judeh, H, Kumer M, et al., SPECT brain perfusion abnormalities in mild or moderate traumatic brain injury, *Clin. Nucl. Med.*, 23:309, 1998.

337. Della Corte, F, Giordano, A, Pennisi, MA, et al., Quantitative cerebral blood flow and metabolism determination in the first 48 hours after severe head injury with a new dynamic SPECT device, *Acta Neurochir. (Wien)*, 139:636, 1997.

338. Nedd, K, Sfakianakis, G, Ganz, W, et al., 99mTc-HMPAO SPECT of the brain in mild to moderate traumatic brain injury patients: compared with CT — a prospective study, *Brain Inj.*, 7:469, 1993.

339. Jacobs, A, Put, E, Ingels, M: et al., One-year follow-up of technetium-99m-HMPAO SPECT in mild head injury, *J. Nucl. Med.*, 37:1605, 1996.

340. Jacobs, A, Put, E, Ingels, M, Bossuyt, A, Prospective evaluation of technitium-99m-HMPAO SPECT in mild and moderate traumatic brain injury, *J. Nucl. Med.*, 35: 942, 1994.

341. Rappaport, M, Hemmerle, AV, Rappaport, ML, Short and long latency auditory evoked potentials in traumatic brain injury patients, *Clin. Electroencephalogr.*, 22:199, 1991.

342. Rappaport, M, Hemmerle, AV, Rappaport, ML, Intermediate and long latency SEPs in relation to clinical disability in traumatic brain injury patients, *Clin. Electroencephalogr.*, 21:188, 1990.

343. Wang, WP, Qiu, MD, Ren, HJ, Zhang, XH, Relations of intracranial pressure, creatine kinase and brainstem auditory evoked potential in patients with traumatic brain edema, *Chin. Med. J. (Engl.)*, 107:205, 1994.

344. Kugler, CF, Petter, J, Platt, D, Age-related dynamics of cognitive brain functions in humans: an electrophysiological approach, *J. Gerontol. A Biol. Sci. Med. Sci.*, 51:B3, 1996.

345. Wirsen, A, Stenberg, G, Rosen, I, Ingvar, DH, Quantified EEG and cortical evoked responses in patients with chronic traumatic frontal lesions, *Electroencephalogr. Clin. Neurophysiol.*, 84:127, 1992.

346. Sangal RB, Sangal JM, Closed head injury patients with mild cognitive complaints without neurological or psychiatric findings have abnormal visual P300 latencies, *Biol. Psychiatry*, 39:305, 1996.

347. Von Bierbrauer, A, Weissenborn, K, P300 after minor head injury (a follow-up examination), *Acta Neurol. Belg.*, 98:21, 1998.

348. Rappaport, M, Leonard, J, Ruiz Portillo, S, Somatosensory evoked potential peak latencies and amplitudes in contralateral and ipsilateral hemispheres in normal and severely traumatized brain-injured subjects, *Brain Inj.*, 7:3, 1993.

349. Rappaport, M, Clifford, JO, Jr., Winterfield, KM, P300 response under active and passive attentional states and uni- and bimodality stimulus presentation conditions, *J. Neuropsychiatry Clin. Neurosci.*, 2:399, 1990.

350. Unsal, A, Segalowitz, SJ, Sources of P300 attenuation after head injury: single-trial amplitude, latency jitter and EEG power, *Psychophysiology*, 32:249, 1995.

351. Sangal, RB, Sangal, JM, Belisle, C, P300 latency and age: a quadratic regression explains their relationship from age 5 to 85, *Clin. Electroencephalogr.*, 29:1, 1998.

352. Werner, RA, Vanderzant, CW, Multimodality evoked potential testing in acute mild closed head injury, *Arch. Phys. Med. Rehabil.*, 72:31, 1991.

353. Soustiel, JF, Hafner, H, Chistyakov, AV, et al., Trigeminal and auditory evoked responses in minor head injuries and post-concussion syndrome, *Brain Inj.*, 9:805, 1995.

354. Montgomery, EA, Fenton, GW, McClelland, RJ, et al., The psychobiology of minor head injury, *Psychol. Med.*, 21:375, 1991.

355. Baguley, IJ, Felmingham, KL, Lahz, S, et al., Alcohol abuse and traumatic brain injury: Effect on event-related potentials, *Arch. Phys. Med. Rehabil.*, 78:1248, 1997.

356. Padula, WV, Argyris, S, Ray, J, Visual evoked potentials (VEP) evaluating treatment for post-trauma vision syndrome (PTVS) in patients with traumatic brain injuries (TBI), *Brain Inj.*, 8:125, 1994.

357. Thatcher, RW, Walker, RA, Gerson, I, Geisler, FH, EEG Discriminant analyses of mild head trauma, *Elecroencephologr. Clin. Neurophysiol.*, 73:94, 1989.

358. Karabudak, R, Ciger, A, Erturk, I, Zileli, T, EEG and the linear skull fractures, *J. Neurosurg. Sci.*, 36:47, 1992.

359. Matousek, M, Takeuchi, E, Starmark, JE, Stalhammar, D, Quantitative EEG analysis as a supplement to the clinical coma scale RLS85, *Acta Anesthesiol. Scand.*, 40:824, 1996.

360. Evans, BM, Bartlett, JR, Prediction of outcome in severe head injury, based on recognition of sleep related activity in the polygraphic electroencephalogram, *J. Neurol. Neurosurg. Psychiatry*, 59:17, 1995.

361. Doyon, J, Owen, AM, Petride, M, et al., Functional anatomy of visuomotor skill learning in human subjects examined with positron emission tomography, *Eur. J. Neurosci.*, 8:637, 1996.

362. Gomez Beldarrain, M, Garcia-Monco, JC, Quintana, JM, et al., Diaschisis and neuropsychological performance after cerebellar stroke, *Eur. Neurol.*, 37:82, 1997.

363. Desmond, JE, Gabrieli, JD, Wagner, AD, et al., Lobular patterns of cerebellar activation in verbal working-memory and finger-tapping tasks as revealed by functional MRI, *J. Neurosci.*, 17:9675, 1997.

364. Dronkers, NF, A new brain region for coordinating speech articulation, *Nature*, 384: 159, 1996.

365. Hotz, G, Helm-Estabrooks, N, Perseveration, Part II: a study of perseveration in closed-head injury, *Brain Inj.*, 9:161, 1995.

366. Lane, RD, Reiman, EM, Bradley, MM, et al., Neuroanatomical correlates of pleasant and unpleasant emotion, *Neuropsychologia*, 35:1437, 1997.

367. Levy, LM, Henkin, RI, Hutter A, et al., Mapping brain activation to odorants in patients with smell loss by functional MRI, *J. Comput. Assist. Tomogr.*, 22:96, 1998.

368. Deiber, MP, Wise, SP, Honda, M, et al., Frontal and parietal networks for conditional motor learning: a positron emission tomography study, *J. Neurophysiol.*, 78:977, 1997.

369. Fischer, RP, Carlson, J, Perry, JF, Postconcussive hospital observation of alert patients in a primary trauma center, *J. Trauma*, 21:920, 1981.

370. Mendelow, AD, Teasdale, G, Jennett, B, et al., Risks of intracranial hematoma in head injured adults, *Br. Med. J.*, 287:1173, 1983.

371. Dacey, RG, Alves, WM, Rimel, RW, et al., Neurosurgical complications after apparently minor head injury. Assessment of risk in a series of 610 patients, *J. Neurosurg.*, 65:203, 1986.

372. Miller, JD, Murray, LS, Teasdale, GM, Development of a traumatic intracranial hematoma after a "minor" head injury, *Neurosurg.*, 27:699, 1990.

373. Bailey, BN, Gudeman, SK, Minor head injury, in Becker, DP, Gudeman, SK, (Eds.), *Textbook of Head injury*, WB Saunders, Philadelphia, 303, 1989.

374. Young, HA, Gleave, RW, Schmidek, HH, Gregory, S, Delayed traumatic intracerebral hematoma: report of 15 cases operatively treated. *Neurosurgery*, 14:22, 1984.

375. Marion, DW, Head and spinal cord injury. *Neurol. Clin.*, 16:485, 1998.

376. Stratton, MC, Gregory, RJ, What happens after a traumatic brain injury?: Four case studies, *Rehabil. Nurs.*, 20:323, 1995.

377. Coburn, K, Traumatic brain injury: the silent epidemic, *AACN Clin. Issues Crit. Care Nurs.*, 3:9, 1992.

378. Katz, RT, DeLuca, J, Sequelae of minor traumatic brain injury, *Am. Fam. Physician*, 46:1491, 1992.

379. Levin, HS, Head trauma, *Curr. Opin. Neurol.*, 6:841, 1993.

380. Kushner, D, Mild traumatic brain injury: toward understanding manifestations and treatment, *Arch. Intern. Med.*, 158:1617, 1998.

381. Rosenthal, M, Mild traumatic brain injury system, *Ann. Emerg. Med.*, 22:1048, 1993.

382. Chambers, J, Cohen, SS, Hemminge, L, et al., Mild traumatic brain injuries in low-risk trauma patients, *J. Trauma*, 41:976, 1996.

383. Rawlinson, JN: The early management of head injury, *Curr. Opin. Neurol. Neurosurg.*, 5:3, 1992.

384. Esselman, PC, Uomoto, JM, Classification of the spectrum of mild traumatic brain injury, *Brain Inj.*, 9:417, 1995.

385. Harrington, DE, Malec, J, Cicerone, K, Katz, HT, Current perceptions of rehabilitation professionals towards mild traumatic brain injury, *Arch. Phys. Med. Rehabil.*, 74:579:86, 1993.

386. Parkerson, JB, Taylo, Z, Flynn, JP, Brain injured patients: comorbidities and ancillary medical requirements, *Md. Med. J.*, 39:259, 1990.

387. Raskin, SA,The relationship between sexual abuse and mild traumatic brain injury, *Brain Inj.*, 11:587, 1997.

388. Klein, M, Houx, PJ, Jolles, J, Long-term persisting cognitive sequelae of traumatic brain injury and the effect of age, *J. Nerv. Ment. Dis.*, 184:459, 1996.

389. Brown, DS, Nell, V, Recovery from diffuse traumatic brain injury in Johannesburg: a concurrent prospective study, *Arch. Phys. Med. Rehabil.*, 73:758, 1992.

390. Arienta, C, Caroli, M, Balbi, S, Management of head-injured patients in the emergency department: a practical protocol, *Surg. Neurol.*, 48:213, 1997.

391. Sakata, R, Ostby, S, Leung, P, Functional status, referral and cost of treatment for persons with traumatic head injury, *Brain Inj.*, 5:411, 1991.

392. Wrigley, JM, Yoels, WC, Webb, CR, Fine, PR, Social and physical factors in the referral of people with traumatic brain injuries to rehabilitation. *Arch. Phys. Med. Rehabil.*, 75:149, 1994.

393. Lestina, DC, Miller, TR, Smith, GS, Creating injury episodes using medical claims data, *J. Trauma*, 45:565, 1998.

394. Borromei, A, Cavrini, G, Guerra, L, et al., Elective neurotraumatology and therapeutic strategies in early post-trauma, *Funct. Neurol.*, 12:89, 1997.

395. Englander, J, Hall, K, Stimpson, T, Chaffin, S, Mild traumatic brain injury in an insured population: subjective complaints and return to employment, *Brain Inj.*, 6:161, 1992.

396. Hsiang, JN, Yeung, T, Yu, AL, Poon, WS, High-risk mild head injury, *J. Neurosurg.*, 87:234, 1997.

397. Lee, ST, Liu, TN, Wong, CW, et al., Relative risk of deterioration after mild closed head injury, *Acta Neurochir. (Wien)*, 135:136, 1995.

398. Klufas, RA, Hsu, L, Patel, MR, Schwartz, RB, Unusual manifestations of head trauma, *A.J.R. Am. J. Roentgenol.*, 166:675, 1996.

399. Cheatham, ML, Block, EF, Nelson, LD, Evaluation of acute mental status change in non-head-injured trauma patient, *Am. Surg.*, 64:900, 1998.

400. Borczuk, P, Predictors of intracranial injury in patients with mild head trauma, *Ann. Emerg. Med.*, 25:731, 1995.

401. Stiell, IG, Wells, GA, Vandemheen, K, et al., Variation in ER use of computed tomography for patients with minor head injury, *Ann. Emerg. Med.*, 30:14, 1997.

402. Servadei, F, Nasi, MT, Cremonini, AM, et al., Importance of a reliable admission Glasgow Coma Scale score for determining the need for evacuation of posttraumatic subdural hematomas: a prospective study of 65 patients, *J. Trauma*, 44:868, 1998.

403. Nagurney, JT, Borczuk, P, Thomas, SH, Elder patients with closed head injury: a comparison with nonelder patients, *Acad. Emerg. Med.*, 5:678, 1998.

404. Dunham, CM, Coates, S, Cooper, C, Compelling evidence for discretionary brain computed tomographic imaging in those patients with mild cognitive impairment after blunt trauma, *J. Trauma*, 41:679, 1996.

405. Ingebrigtsen, T, Romner, B, Routine early CT-scan is cost saving after minor head injury, *Acta Neurol. Scand.*, 93:207, 1996.

406. Murshid, WR, Management of minor head injuries: admission criteria, radiological evaluation and treatment of complications, *Acta Neurochir. (Wien)*, 140:56, 1998.

407. Holmes, JF, Baier, ME, Derlet, RW, Failure of the Miller criteria to predict significant intracranial injury in patients with a Glasgow Coma Scale score of 14 after minor head trauma, *Acad. Emerg. Med.*, 4:788, 1997.

408. Persinger, MA, Clinical neurological indicators are only moderately correlated with quantitative neuropsychological test scores in patients who display mild-moderate brain impairment following closed head injuries, *Percept. Mot. Skills*, 81:1283, 1995.

409. Landy, PJ, Neurological sequelae of minor head and neck injuries, *Injury*, 29:199, 1998.

410. Sabhesan, S, Natarajan, M, Biomechanics and head injury outcome, *J. Indian Med. Assoc.*, 93:448, 1995.

411. Stambrook, M, Moore, AD, Kowalchuk, S, et al., Early metabolic and neurologic predictors of long-term quality of life after closed head injury, *Can. J. Surg.*, 33:115, 1990.

412. Hetherington, CR, Stuss, DT, Finlayson, MA, Reaction time and variability 5 and 10 years after traumatic brain injury, *Brain Inj.*, 10:473, 1996.

413. Luber, SD, Brady, WJ, Brand, A, et al., Acute hypoglycemia masquerading as head trauma: a report of four cases, *Am. J. Emerg. Med.*, 14:543, 1996.

414. Lee, ST, Lue, TN, Early seizures after mild closed head injury, *J. Neurosurg.*, 76:435, 1992.

415. Neidermeyer, F, Immediate transition from a petit mal absence to a grand mal seizure, Case Report, *Eur. Neurol.*, 14:11, 1976.

416. Verduyn, WH, Hilt, J, Roberts, MA, Roberts, RJ, Multiple partial seizure-like symptoms following minor closed head injury, *Brain Inj.*, 6:245, 1992.

417. Haas, DC, Lourie, H: Trauma-triggered migraine: an explanation for common neurological attacks after mild head trauma. Review of the literature, *J. Neurosurg.*, 68:181, 1988.

418. Haan, J, Ferrari, MD, Brouwer, OF, Acute confusional migraine. Case report and review of the literature, *Clin. Neurol. Neurosurg.*, 68:275, 1988.

419. Haas, DC, Ross, GS, Transient global amnesia triggered by mild head trauma, *Brain*, 109:251, 1986.

420. Kennedy, MP, Trauma-precipitated migrainous hemiparesis, *Ann. Emerg. Med.*, 20:1023, 1991.

421. Salber, PR, Byington, D, Trauma-induced migraine: a case of altered mental status after mild head injury. *Am. J. Emerg. Med.*, 9:296, 1991.

422. Jay, GW, Posttraumatic headache and the posttraumatic syndrome, *J. Disability*, 1:153, 1990.

423. Berman, JM, Fredrickson, JM, Vertigo after head injury- a five-year follow-up, *J. Otolaryngol.*, 7:237, 1978.

424. Shutty, MS, Dawdy, L, McMahon, M, Buckelew, SP, Behavioral treatment of dizziness secondary to benign positional vertigo following head trauma, *Arch. Phys. Med. Rehabil.*, 72:473, 1991.

425. Hinoki, M, Otoneurological observations on whiplash injuries to neck with special reference to the formation of equilibrial disorder, *Clin. Surg. (Tokyo)*, 22:1683, 1967.

426. Hinoki, M, Vertigo due to whiplash injury: a neuro-otological approach, *Acta Otolaryngol. (Stockh.)*, 419 Suppl:9, 1985.

427. Sandstrom, J, Cervical syndrome with vestibular symptoms, *Acta Otolaryngol. (Stockh.)*, 54:207, 1962.

428. Boquet, J, Moore, N, Boismare, F, Monnier, JC, Vertigo in post-concussional and migrainous patients: implication of the autonomic nervous system, *Agressologie*, 24:235, 1983.

429. Levin, HS, High, WM, Eisenberg, HM, Impairment of olfactory recognition after closed head injury, *Brain*, 108:579, 1985.

430. Rouit, RL, Murali, R, Injuries of the cranial nerves, in Cooper, PR, (Ed.), *Head Injury*, 2nd Ed., Williams and Wilkins, Baltimore, 141, 1987.
431. Parsons, LC, Ver Beek, D, Sleep-awake patterns following cerebral concussion, *Nurs. Res.*, 31:260, 1982.
432. Ron, S, Algm, D, Hary, D, Cohen, M, Time-related changes in the distribution of sleep stages in brain injured patients, *Electroencephalogr. Clin. Neurophysiol.*, 48:432, 1980.
433. Prigatono, GP, Stahl, ML, Orr, WC, Zeiner, HK, Sleep and dreaming disturbances in closed head injury patients, *J. Neurol. Neurosurg. Psychiatry*, 45:78, 1982.
434. Kowatch, RA, Sleep and head injury, *Psychiatr. Med.*, 7:37, 1989.
435. Bohnen, N, Twijnstra, A, Kroeze, J, Jolles, J, A psychophysiological method for assessing visual and acoustic hyperaesthesia in patients with mild head injury, *Br. J. Psychiatry*, 159:860, 1991.
436. Bohnen, N, Twijnstra, A, Wijnen, G, Jolles, J, Tolerance for light and sound of patients with persistent post-concussional symptoms six months after mild head injury, *J. Neurol.*, 238:443, 1991.
437. Bohnen, N, Twijnstra, A, Wijnen, G, Jolles, J, Recovery from visual and acoustic hyperaesthesia after mild head injury in relation to patterns of behavioral dysfunction, *J. Neurol. Neurosurg. Psychiatry*, 55:222, 1992.
438. Waddell, PA, Gronwell, DM, Sensitivity to light and sound following minor head injury, *Acta Neurol. Scand.*, 69:270, 1984.
439. Biary, N, Cleeves, L, Findley, L, Koller, W, Post traumatic tremor, *Neurology*, 39:103, 1989.
440. Doczi, T, Tarjanyi, J, Huszka, E, Kiss, J, Syndrome of inappropriate secretion of antidiuretic hormone (SIADH) after head injury, *Neurosurgery*, 10:685, 1982.
441. Hadani, M, Findler, G, Shaked, I, Sahar, A, Unusual delayed onset of diabetes insipidus following closed head trauma, *J. Neurosurg.*, 63:456, 1985.
442. Kern, KB, Meislin, HW, Diabetes insipidus: Occurrence after minor head trauma, *J. Trauma*, 24:69, 1984.
443. Yoshida Shiroozu, A, Zaitsu, A, et al., Diabetes insipidus after trauma of two extremes in severity, *Yonsei. Med. J.*, 31:71, 1990.
444. Marion, MS, Cevette, MJ, Tinnitus, *Mayo Clin. Proc.*, 66:614, 1991.
445. Emmett, JR, Shea, JJ, Treatment of tinnitus with tocainide hydrocloride, *Otolaryngol Head Neck Surg.*, 88:442, 1980.
446. Ram, Z, Hadani, M, Spiegelman, R, et al., Delayed nonhemorrhagic encephalopathy following mild head trauma, *J. Neurosurg.*, 71:608, 1989.
447. Annegers, JF, Hauser, WA, Lee, JR, Rocca, WA, Incidence of acute symptomatic seizures in Rochester Minnesota, 1935–1984, *Epilepsia*, 36:327, 1995.
448. Annegers, JF, Hauser, WA, Coan, SP, Rocca, WA, A population based study of seizures after traumatic brain injuries, *N. Engl. J. Med.*, 338:20, 1998.
449. Verduyn, WH, Hilt, J, Roberts, MA, Roberts, RJ, Multiple partial seizure-like symptoms following minor closed head injury, *Brain Inj.*, 6:245, 1992.
450. Varney, NR, Hines, ME, Bailey, C, Roberts, RJ, Neuropsychiatric correlates of theta bursts in patients with closed head injury, *Brain Inj.*, 6:499, 1992.
451. Roberts, MA, Verduyn, WH, Manshadi, FF, Hines, ME, Episodic symptoms in dysfunctioning children and adolescents following mild and severe traumatic brain injury, *Brain Inj.*, 10:739, 1996.
452. Lee, ST, Lui, TN, Wong, CW, et al., Early seizures after moderate closed head injury, *Acta Neurochir. (Wien)*, 137:151, 1995.

453. Lee, ST, Lui, TN, Wong, CW, et al., Early seizures after severe closed head injury, *Can. J. Neurol. Sci.*, 24:40, 1997.

454. De Santis, A, Sganzerla, E, Spagnoli, D, et al., Risk factors for late posttraumatic epilepsy, *Acta Neurochir. Suppl. (Wien)*, 55:64, 1992.

455. Pohlmann-Eden, B, Bruckmeir, J, Predictors and dynamics of posttraumatic epilepsy, *Acta Neurol. Scand.*, 95:257, 1997.

456. Da Silva, AM, Vaz, AR, Ribeiro, I, et al., Controversies in posttraumatic epilepsy, *Acta Neurochir. Suppl. (Wien)* 50:48, 1990.

457. Heikkinen, ER, Ronty, HS, Tolonen, U, Pyhtinen, J, Development of posttraumatic epilepsy, *Stereotact Funct. Neurosurg.*, 54-55:25-33, 1990.

458. Temkin, NR, Dikmen, SS, Winn, HR, Management of head injury posttraumatic seizures, *Neurosurg. Clin. N. Am.*, 2:425, 1991.

459. Deahl, M, Trimble, M, Serotonin reuptake inhibitors, epilepsy and myoclonus, *Br. J. Psychiatry*, 159:433, 1991.

460. Rabinowicz, AL, Correale, J, Boutros, RB, et al., Neuron-specific enolase is increased after single seizures during inpatients video/EEG monitoring, *Epilepsia*, 37:122, 1996.

461. Correale, J, Rabinowicz, AL, Heck, CN, et al., Status epilepticus increases CSF levels of neuron-specific enolase and alters the blood-brain barrier, *Neurology*, 50:1388, 1998.

462. Rao, TH, Libman, RB, Patel, M, Seizures and 'disappearing' brain lesions, *Seizure*, 4:61, 1995.

463. Arnold, LM, Privitera, MD, Psychopathology and trauma in epileptic and psychogenic seizure patients, *Psychosomatics*, 37:438, 1996.

464. Barry, E, Krumholz, A, Berge, GK, et al., Non-epileptic posttraumatic seizures, *Epilepsia*, 39:427, 1998.

465. Tisher, PW, Holzer, JC, Greenberg, M, et al., Psychiatric presentations of epilepsy, *Harv. Rev. Psychiatry*, 1:219, 1993.

466. Shaumann, BA, Annegers, JF, Johnson, SB, et al., Family history of seizures in posttraumatic and alcohol-related seizure disorders, *Epilepsia*, 35:48, 1994.

467. Armstrong, KK, Sahgal, V, Bloch, R, et al., Rehabilitation outcomes in patients with posttraumatic epilepsy, *Arch. Phys. Med. Rehabil.*, 71:156, 1990.

468. Haltiner, AM, Temkin, NR, Winn, HR, Dikmen, SS, The impact of posttraumatic seizures on 1-year neuropsychological and psychosocial outcome of head injury, *J. Int. Neuropsychol. Soc.*, 2:494, 1996.

469. Zafonte, RD, Mann, NR, Millis, SR, et al., Posttraumatic amnesia: Its relation to functional outcome, *Arch. Phys. Med. Rehabil.*, 78:1103, 1997.

470. McMillan, TM, Jongen, EL, Greenwood, RJ, Assessment of post-traumatic amnesia after severe closed head injury: retrospective or prospective? *J. Neurol. Neurosurg. Psychiatry*, 60:422, 1996.

471. Wilson, JT, Teasdale, GM, Hadley, DM, et al., Post-traumatic amnesia: Still a valuable yardstick, *J. Neurol. Neurosurg. Psychiatry*, 57:198, 1994.

472. Corrigan, JD, Mysiw, WJ, Gribble, MW, Chock, SK, Agitation, cognition and attention during post-traumatic amnesia, *Brain Inj.*, 6:155, 1992.

473. Morris, MK, Bowers, D, Chatterjee, A, Heilman, KM, Amnesia following a discrete basal forebrain lesion, *Brain*, 15(Pt 6):1827, 1992.

474. Mattioli, F, Grassi, F, Peerani, D, et al., Persistent post-traumatic retrograde: A neuropsychological and (18F) FDG PET study, *Cortex*, 32:121, 1996.

475. Schwartz, ML, Carruth, F, Binns, MA, et al., The course of post-traumatic amnesia: three little words, *Can. J. Neurol. Sci.*, 25:108, 1998.

476. King, NS, Crawford, S, Wenden, FJ, et al., Measurement of post-traumatic amnesia: How reliable is it, *J. Neurol. Neurosurg. Psychiatry*, 62:38, 1997.

477. Saneda, DL, Corrigan, JD, Predicting clearing of post-traumatic amnesia following closed head injury, *Brain Inj.*, 6:167, 1992.

478. Mutyala, S, Holmes, JM, Hodge, DO, Young, BR, Spontaneous recovery rate in traumatic sixth-nerve palsy, *Am. J. Ophthalmol.*, 122:898, 1996.

479. Doty, RL, Yousem, DM, Pham, LT, et al., Olfactory dysfunction in patients with head trauma, *Arch. Neurol.*, 54:1131, 1997.

480. Yousem, DM, Geckle, RJ, Bilker, WB, et al., Posttraumatic olfactory dysfunction: MR and clinical evaluation, *AJNR Am. J. Neuroradiol.*, 17:1171, 1996.

481. Sartoretti-Schefer, S, Scherler, M, Wichmann, W, Valavanis, A, Contrast-enhanced MR of the facial nerve in patients with posttraumatic peripheral facial nerve palsy, *AJNR Am. J. Neuroradiol.*, 18:1115, 1997.

482. Haig, AJ, Ho, KC, Ludwig, G, Clinical, physiologic, and pathologic evidence for vagus dysfunction in a case of traumatic brain injury, *J. Trauma*, 40:441, 1996.

483. Mariak, Z, Mariak, Z, Stankiewicz, A, Cranial nerve II-VII injuries in fatal closed head trauma, *Eur. J. Ophthalmol.*, 7:68, 1997.

484. Lellerstein, LF, Freed, S, Maples, WC, Vision profile of patients with mild brain injury, *J. Am. Optom. Assoc.*, 66:634, 1995.

485. Lepore, FE, Disorders of ocular motility following head trauma, *Arch. Neurol.*, 52:924, 1995.

486. Schenk, T, Zihl, J, Visual motion perception after brain damage: I. Deficits in global motion perception, *Neuropsychologia*, 35:1289, 1997.

487. Whyte, J, Fleming, M, Polansky, M, et al., The effects of visual distraction following traumatic brain injury, *J. Int. Neuropsychol. Soc.*, 4:127, 1998.

488. Miller, LA, Tippett, LJ, Effects of focal brain lesions on visual problem-solving, *Neuropsychologia*, 34:387, 1996.

489. Hills, EC, Geldmacher, DS, The effect of character and array type on visual spatial search quality following traumatic brain injury, *Brain Inj.*, 12:69, 1998.

490. Freed, S, Hellerstein, LF, Visual electrodiagnostic findings in mild traumatic brain injury, *Brain Inj.*, 11:25, 1997.

491. Heinze, HJ, Muntge, TF, Gobiet, W, et al., Parallel and serial visual search after closed head injury: electrophysiological evidence for perceptual dysfunctions, *Neuropsychologia*, 30:495,1992.

492. Breslau, J, Dalley, RW, Tsuruda, JS, et al., Phased-array surface coil MR of the orbits and optic nerves, *AJNR Am. J. Neuroradiol.*, 16:1247, 1995.

493. Silverman, IE, Galetta, SL, Gray, LG, et al., SPECT in patients with cortical visual loss, *J. Nucl. Med.*, 34:1447, 1993.

494. Krantz, JL, Psychosocial aspects of vision loss associated with head trauma, *J. Am. Optom. Assoc.*, 63:589, 1992.

495. Tjell, C, Rosenhall, U, Smooth pursuit neck torsion test: a specific test for cervical dizziness, *Am. J. Otol.*, 19:76, 1998.

496. Rubin, AM, Wooley, SM, Dailey, VM, Goebel, JA, Postural stability following mild head or whiplash injuries, *Am. J. Otol.*, 16:216, 1995.

497. Davies, RA, Luxon, LM, Dizziness following head injury: a neuro-otological study, *J. Neurol.*, 242:222, 1995.

498. Deguine, O, Latil d'Albertas, D, Fraysse, B, Comparison of postoperative results in suspected and confirmed cases of perilymphatic fistula, *Rev. Laryngol. Otol. Rhinol. (Bord.)*, 116:95, 1995.

499. Fitzgerald, DC, Persistent dizziness following head trauma and perilymphatic fistula, *Arch. Phys. Med. Rehabil.*, 76: 1017, 1995.

500. Shutty, MS, Dawdy, L, McMahon, M, Buckelew, SP, behavioral treatment of dizziness secondary to benign positional vertigo following head injury, *Arch. Phys. Med. Rehabil.*, 72:473, 1991.

501. Hu, CJ, Chan, KY, Lin, TJ, et al., Traumatic brainstem deafness with normal brainstem auditory evoked potentials, *Neurology*, 48:1448, 1997.

502. Grossman, AR, Tempereau, CE, Brones, MF, et al., Auditory and neuropsychiatric behavior patterns after electrical injury, *J. Burn Care Rehabil.*, 14:169, 1993.

503. Krauss, JK, Trankle, R, Kopp, KH, Post-traumatic movement disorders in survivors of severe head injury, *Neurology*, 47:1488, 1996.

504. Kant, R, Zeiler, D, Hemiballismus following closed head injury, *Brain Inj.*, 10:155, 1996.

505. Silver, JK, Lux, WE, Early onset dystonia following traumatic brain injury, *Arch. Phys. Med. Rehabil.*, 75:885, 1994.

506. Krauss, JK, Jankovic, J, Tics secondary to craniocerebral trauma, *Mov. Disord.*, 12:776, 1997.

507. Mysiw, WJ, Corrigan, JD, Gribble, MW, The ataxic subgroup: a discrete outcome after traumatic brain injury, *Brain Inj.*, 4:247, 1990.

508. Jankovic, J, Post-traumatic movement disorders: Central and peripheral mechanisms, *Neurology*, 44:2006, 1994.

509. Krauss, JK, Treankle, R, Kopp, KH, Posttraumatic movement disorders after moderate or mild head injury, *Mov. Disord.*, 12:428, 1997.

510. Scott, BL, Jankovic, J, Delayed-onset progressive movement disorders after static brain lesions, *Neurology*, 46:68, 1996.

511. Scarano, VR, Jankovic, J, Post-traumatic movement disorders: Effect of the legal system on outcome, *J. Forensic Sci.*, 43:334, 1998.

512. Childers, MK, Rupright, J, Jones, PS, Merveille, O, Assessment of neuroendocrine dysfunction following traumatic brain injury, *Brain Inj.*, 12:517, 1998.

513. Hackl, JM, Gottardis, M, Wieser, C, et al., Endocrine abnormalities in severe traumatic brain injury: a cue to prognosis in severe craniocerebral trauma? *Intensive Care Med.*, 17:25, 1991.

514. Kishikawa, H, Diabetes insipidus after trauma of two extremes in severity, *Yonsei. Med. J.*, 31:71, 1990.

515. Webster, JB, Bell, KR, Primary adrenal insufficiency following traumatic brain injury: a case report and review of the literature, *Arch. Phys. Med. Rehabil.*, 78:314, 1997.

516. Lee, SC, Zasler, ND, Kreutzer, JS, Male pituitary gonadal dysfunction following severe traumatic brain injury, *Brain Injury*, 8:571, 1994.

517. Lezak, ML, Living with the characterologically altered brain injured patient, *J. Clin. Psychiatry*, 39:592, 1978.

518. Lilly, R, The human Kluver-Bucy syndrome, *Neurology*, 33:1141, 1983.

519. Herzog, A, Russell, V, Vaitokaitis, JL, et al., Neuroendocrine dysfunction in temporal lobe epilepsy, *Arch. Neurol.*, 39:133, 1982.

520. Herzog, A, Seibel, M, Schomer, D, et al., Reproductive endocrine disorders in men with partial seizures of temporal lobe origin, *Arch. Neurol.*, 43:347, 1986.

521. Herzog, A, Seibel, M, Schomer, D, et al., Reproductive endocrine disorders in women with partial seizures of temporal lobe origin, *Arch. Neurol.*, 43:341, 1986.

522. Sandel, ME, Williams, KS, Dellapietra, L, Derogatis, LR, Sexual functioning following traumatic brain injury, *Brain Inj.*, 10:719, 1996.

523. Kreuter, M, Dahllof, AG, Gudjonsson, G, et al., Sexual adjustment and its predictors after traumatic brain injury, *Brain Inj.*, 12:349, 1998.

524. Choi, D, Spann, R, Traumatic cerebrospinal fluid leakage: risk factors and the use of prophylactic antibiotics, *Br. J. Neurosurg.*, 10:571, 1996.

525. Eljamel, MS, Foy, PM, Post-traumatic CSF fistulae, the case for surgical repair, *Br. J. Neurosurg.*, 4:479, 1990.

526. Childers, MK, Rupright, J, Smith, DW, Post-traumatic hyperthermia in acute brain injury rehabilitation. *Brain Inj.*, 8:335, 1994.

527. Jackson, RD, Mysiw, WJ, Fever of unknown origin following traumatic brain injury, *Brain Inj.*, 5:93, 1991.

528. Clinchot, DM, Otis, S, Colachis, SC, 3rd, Incidence of fever in the rehabilitation phase following brain injury, *Am. J. Phys. Med. Rehabil.*, 76:323, 1997.

529. Wildburger, R, Zarkovic, N, Egger, G, et al., Basic fibroblast growth factor (BFGF) immunoreactivity as a possible link between head injury and impaired bone fracture healing, *Bone Miner*, 27:183, 1994.

530. Goodman, TA, Merkel, PA, Perlmutter, G, et al., Heterotopic ossification in the setting of neuromuscular blockade, *Arthritis Rheum.*, 40:1619, 1997.

531. Oostra, K, Everaert, K, Van Laere, M, Urinary incontinence in brain injury, *Brain Inj.*, 10:459, 1996.

532. Burney, TL, Senapati, M, Desai S, et al., Acute cerebrovascular accident and lower urinary tract dysfunction: a prospective correlation of the site of brain injury with urodynamic findings, *J. Urol.*, 156:1748, 1996.

533. Helm-Estabrooks, N, Hotz, G, Sudden onset of "stuttering" in an adult: neurogenic or psychogenic? *Semin Speech Lang*, 19:23, 1998.

534. King, ML, Lichtman, SW, Seliger, G, et al., Heart-rate variability in chronic traumatic brain injury, *Brain Inj.*, 11:445, 1997.

535. Allison, SC, Abraham, LD, Peterson, CL, Reliability of the Modified Ashworth Scale in the assessment of plantarflexor muscle spasticity in patients with traumatic brain injury, *Int. J. Rehabil. Res.*, 19:67, 1996.

536. Allison, SC, Abraham, LD, Correlation of quantitative measures with the Modified Ashworth scale in the assessment of plantar flexor spasticity in patients with traumatic brain injury, *J. Neurol.*, 242:699, 1995.

537. Rasmusson, DX, Brandt, J, Martin, DB, Folstein, MF, Head injury as a risk factor in Alzheimer's disease, *Brain Inj.*, 9:213, 1995.

538. Di Trapani, G, Carnevale, A, Scerrati, M, et al., Post-traumatic malignant glioma. Report of a case, *Ital. J. Neurol. Sci.*, 17:283, 1996.

539. Prall, JA, Lloyd, GL, Breeze, RE, Traumatic brain injury associated with an intradiploic epidermoid cyst: case report, *Neurosurgery*, 37:523, 1995.

540. Goldberg, MB, Mock, D, Ichise M, et al., Neuropsychologic deficits and clinical features of posttraumatic temporomandibular disorders, *J. Orofac. Pain*, 10:126, 1996.

541. Middleboe, T, Anderson, HS, Birket-Smith, M, Friis, ML, Minor head injury: impact on general health after 1 year, *Acta Neurol. Scand.*, 85:5, 1992.

542. Woischneck, D, Firsching, R, Ruckert, N, et al., Clinical predictors of the psychosocial long-term outcome after brain injury, *Neurol. Res.*, 19:305, 1997.

543. Hibbard, MR, Uysal, S, Sliwinski, M, Gordon, WA, Undiagnosed health issues in individuals with traumatic brain injury living in the community, *J. Head Trauma Rehabil.*, 13:47, 1998.

544. Keidel, M, Diener, HC, Post-traumatic headache, *Nervenarzt.*, 68:769, 1997.

545. Uomoto, JM, Esselman, PC, Traumatic brain injury and chronic pain: differential types and rates by head injury severity, *Arch. Phys. Med. Rehabil.*, 74:61, 1993.

546. Kojadinovic, Z, Momcilovic, A, Popovic, L, et al., Brain concussion — a minor craniocerebral injury, *Med. Pregl.*, 51:165–8, 1998.
547. Muller, GE, Atypical early posttraumatic syndromes, *Acta Neurol. Belg.*, 74:163, 1974.
548. Goldstein, J, Posttraumatic headache and the postconcussion syndrome, *Med. Clin. North Am.*, 75:641, 1991.
549. Bring, G, Westman, G, Chronic posttraumatic syndrome after whiplash injury. A pilot study of 22 patients, *Scand. J. Prim. Health Care*, 9:135, 1991.
550. Denny-Brown, D, Russell, WR, Experimental cerebral concussion, *Brain*, 64:93, 1941.
551. Jay, GW, *Headache Handbook: Diagnosis and Treatment*, CRC Press, Boca Raton, 17, 1999.
552. Packard, RC, Ham, LP, Pathogenesis of posttraumatic headache and migraine: a common headache pathway? *Headache*, 37:42, 1997.
553. Buchholz, DW, Reich, SG, The menagerie of migraine, *Semin. Neurol.*, 16:83, 1996.
554. Leisman, G, Lateralized effects of migraine and ANS seizures after closed head injury. *Int. J. Neurosci.*, 54:63, 1990.
555. Sakas, DE, Whittaker, KW, Whitwell, HL, Singounas, EG, Syndromes of posttraumatic neurological deterioration in children with no focal lesions revealed by cerebral imaging: evidence of a trigeminovascular pathophysiology, *Neurosurgery*, 41:661, 1997.
556. Schmidtke, K, Ehmsen, L, Transient global amnesia and migraine. A case control study, *Eur. Neurol.*, 40:9, 1998.
557. Vohanka, S, Zouhar, A, Transient global amnesia after mild head injury in childhood, *Act. Nerv. Super. (Praha)*, 30:68, 1988.
558. Harrison, DW, Walls, RM, Blindness following minor head trauma in children: a report of two cases with a review of the literature, *J. Emerg. Med.*, 8:21, 1990.
559. Harker, LA, Rassekh, C, Migraine equivalent as a cause of episodic vertigo, *Laryngoscope*, 98:160, 1988.
560. Baloh, RW, Neurotology of migraine, *Headache*, 37:615, 1997.
561. Vohanka, S, Zouhar, A, Benign posttraumatic encephalopathy, *Act. Nerv. Super. (Praha)*, 32:179, 1990.
562. Jay, GW, *Headache Handbook: Diagnosis and Treatment*, CRC Press, Boca Raton, 45, 1999.
563. Dorpat, TL, Holmes, TH, Mechanisms of skeletal muscle pain and fatigue, *Arch. Neurol. Psychiatry*, 74:628, 1955.
564. Perl, S, Markle, P, Katz, LN, Factors involved in the production of skeletal muscle pain, *Arch. Intern. Med.*, 53:814, 1934.
565. Langemark, M, Olesen, J, Pericranial tenderness in tension headache. A blind controlled study, *Cephalalgia*, 7:249, 1987.
566. Langemark, M, Jensen, K, Myofascial mechanisms of pain, in *Basic Mechanisms of Headache*, Olesen, J, Edvinsson, L, (Eds.), Elsevier Science, Amsterdam, 321, 1988.
567. Cailliet, R, *Pain: Mechanisms and Management*, F.A. Davis, Philadelphia, 83, 1993.
568. Jay, GW, The autonomic nervous system: Anatomy and pharmacology, in *Pain Medicine-A Comprehensive Review*, Raj, P, (Ed.), C. V. Mosby, St. Louis, 461, 1996.
569. Travell, J, Rinzler, SH, The myofascial genesis of pain, *Postgrad. Med.*, 11:425,1952.
570. Jay, GW, Chronic daily headache and myofascial pain syndromes: Pathophysiology and treatment, in: *Treating the Headache Patient*, Cady, RK, Fox, AW, (Eds.), Marcel Dekker, New York, 211, 1995.

571. Fricton, JR, Myofascial Pain Syndrome, in: *Advances in Pain Research and Therapy*. Vol. 17, Fricton, JR, Awad, E, (Eds.), Raven Press, New York, 107, 1990.

572. Basbaum, AI, Fields, HL, Endogenous pain control systems: Brainstem spinal pathways and endorphin circuitry, *Ann. Rev. Neurosci.*, 7:309, 1984.

573. Andersen, E, Dafny, N, An ascending serotonergic pain modulation pathway from the dorsal raphe nucleus to the parafascicularis nucleus of the thalamus, *Brain Res.*, 269:57, 1983.

574. Raskin, NH, On the origin of head pain, *Headache*, 28:254, 1988.

575. Raskin, NH, *Headache*, 2nd Ed. Churchill Livingstone, New York, 1988.

576. Fields, HL, Sources of variability in the sensation of pain, *Pain*, 33:195, 1988.

577. Wall, PD, Stability and instability of central pain mechanisms, in: *Proceedings of the Fifth World Conference on Pain*, Dubner, R, Bond, MR, (Eds.), Elsevier Science, Amsterdam, 13, 1988.

578. Sicuteri, F, Natural opiods in migraine, in: *Advances in Neurology*, Vol. 33, Critchley, M, Friedman, AP, Gorini, S, et al, (Eds.), Raven Press, New York, 65, 1982.

579. Sicuteri, F, Spillantini, MG, Fanciullacci, M, "Enkephalinase" in migraine and opiate addiction, in: *Migraine: Proceedings of the Fifth International Migraine Symposium*, Rose, C, (Ed.), S. Karger, Basel, 86, 1985.

580. Mosnaim, AD, Diamond, S, Wolf, ME, et al., Endogenous opiod-like peptides in headache: An overview, *Headache*, 29:368, 1989.

581. Genazzani, AR, Nappi, G, Gacchinetti, F, et al., Progressive impairment of CSF B-EP levels in migraine sufferers, *Pain*, 18:127, 1984.

582. Facchinetti, F, Genazzani, AR, Opiods in cerebrospinal fluid and blood of headache sufferers, in: *Basic Mechanisms of Headache*, Olesen, J, Edvinsson, L, (Eds.), Elsevier Science, Amsterdam, 261, 1988.

583. Nappi, G, Gacchinetti, G, Legnante, G, et al., *Impairment of the central and peripheral opiod system in headache*. Paper presented at the Fourth International Migraine Trust Symposium, London, 1982.

584. Rolf, LH, Wiele, G, Brune, GG, 5-Hydroxytryptamine in platelets of patients with muscle contraction headache, *Headache*, 21:10, 1981.

585. Giacovazzo, M, Bernoni, RM, Di Sabato, F, Martelletti, P, Impairment of 5HT binding to lymphocytes and monocytes from tension-type headache patients, *Headache*, 30:20, 1990.

586. Shimomura, T, Takahashi, K, Alteration of platelet serotonin in patients with chronic tension-type headache during cold pressor test, *Headache*, 30:581, 1990.

587. Pernow, B, Substance, P, *Pharmacol. Rev.*, 35:85, 1983.

588. Almay, BGL, Johansson, F, von Knorring, L, et al., Substance P in CSF of patients with chronic pain syndromes, *Pain*, 33:3, 1988.

589. Takeshima, T, Takao, YU, Urakami, K, et al., Muscle contraction headache and migraine. Platelet activation and plasma norepinephrine during the cold pressor test, *Cephalalgia*, 9:7, 1989.

590. Kowa, H, Shimomura, T, Takahashi, K, Platelet gamma-amino butyric acid levels in migraine and tension-type headache, *Headache*, 32:229, 1992.

591. Sicuteri, F, Nicolodi, M, Fusco, BM, Abnormal sensitivity to neurotransmitter agonists, antagonists and neurotransmitter releasers, in: *Basic Mechanisms of Headache*, Olesen, J, Edvinsson, L, (Eds.), Elsevier Science, Amsterdam, 275, 1988.

592. Langemark, M, Jensen, K, Jensen, TS, Olesen, J, Pressure pain thresholds and thermal nociceptive thresholds in chronic tension-type headache, *Pain*, 38:203, 1989.

593. Dwyer, A, Aprill, C, Bogduk, N, Cervical zygapophyseal joint pain patterns I: a study in normal volunteers, *Spine*, 15:453, 1990.

594. Bogduk, N, Corrigan, B, Kelly, et al., Cervical headache, *Med. J. Austr.*, 143:202, 1985.

595. Sjaastad, O, Fredriksen, TA, Pfaffenrath, V, Cervicogenic headache diagnostic criterion, *Headache*, 30:725, 1990.

596. Bogduk, N, The anatomical basis for cervicogenic headache, *J. Manipulative Physiol. Ther.*, 15:67, 1992.

597. Blume, HG, Diagnosis and treatment modalities of cervicogenic headaches, *Head and Neck Pain*, newsletter of the Cervicogenic Headache International Study Group, 4:1, 1997.

598. Poletti, CE, Proposed operation for occipital neuralgia: C2 and C3 root decompression, *Neurosurgery*, 12:221, 1983.

599. Pikus, H, Phillips, J, Characteristics of patients successfully treated for cervicogenic headache by surgical decompression of the second cervical nerve root, *Headache*, 35:621, 1995.

600. Blume, HG, Kakolewski, JW, Richardson, RR, Rojas, CH, Radiofrequency denaturation in occipital pain: results in 450 cases, *Appl. Neurophysiol.*, 45:543, 1982.

601. Rogal, OJ, Rhizotomy procedures about the face and neck for headaches. Paper presented at the North American Cervicogenic Headache Conference, Toronto, Canada, September 1995.

602. Sluijter, ME, Radiofrequency lesions in the treatment of cervical pain syndromes, *Procedure Technique Series*, Holland: Radionics, 2, 1990.

603. Blume, HG, Radiofrequency denaturation in occipital pain: a new approach in 114 cases, *Adv. Rain Res. Ther.*, 1:691, 1976.

604. Blume, HG, Kakolewski, JW, Richardson, RR, Rojas, CH, Selective percutaneous radiofrequency thermodenervation of pain fibers in the treatment of occipital neuralgia: results in 450 cases, *J. Neurol. Orth. Surg.*, 2:261, 1981.

605. Blume, HG, Ungar-Sargon, J, Neurosurgical treatment of persistent occipital myalgia-neuralgia syndrome, *J. Craniomandibular Practice*, 4:65, 1986.

606. Rogal OJ, Successful treatment for head, facial and neck pain. The TMJ Dental Trauma Center, 1:3, 1986.

607. Jansen, J, Spoerri, O, Atypical retro-orbital pain and headache due to compression of upper cervical roots, in: Pfaffenrath, V, Lundberg, PO, Sjaastad, O, (Eds.), *Updating in Headache*, Springer-Verlag, Berlin, 14, 1985.

608. Zwart, JA, Neck mobility in different headache disorders, *Headache*, 37:6, 1997.

609. Sjaastad, O, Bovim, G, Stovner, LJ, Laterality of pain and other migraine criteria in common migraine. A comparison with cervicogenic headache, *Funct. Neurol.*, 7:289, 1992.

610. Leone, M, D'Amico, D, Grazzi, L, et al., Cervicogenic headache: a critical review of the current diagnostic criteria, *Pain*, 78:1, 1998.

611. Pfaffenrath, V, Kaube, H, Diagnostics of cervicogenic headache, *Funct. Neurol.*, 5:159, 1990.

612. Treleaven, J, Jull, G, Atkinson, L, Cervical musculoskeletal dysfunction in post-concussional headache, *Cephalalgia*, 14:273, 1994.

613. Obelieniene, D, Bovim, G, Schrader, H, et al., Headache after whiplash: a historical cohort study outside the medico-legal context, *Cephalalgia*, 18:559, 1998.

614. Evans, RW, The postconcussion syndrome and the sequelae of mild head injury, *Neurol. Clin.*, 10:815, 1992.

615. Cicerone, KD, Psychological management of post-concussive disorders, *Phys. Med. Rehabil. State Art. Rev.*, 6:129, 1992.

616. Elkind, AH, Headache and facial pain associated with head injury, *Otolaryngol. Clin. North Am.*, 22:1251, 1989.

617. Merskey, H, Woodford, JM, Psychiatric sequelae after minor head injury, *Brain*, 95:521, 1972.

618. Ruff, RM, Camenzuli, L, Muelle, J, Miserable minority: Emotional risk factors that influence the outcome of a mild traumatic brain injury, *Brain Inj.*, 10:551, 1996.

619. Arcia, E, Gualtieri, CT, Association between patient report of symptoms after mild head injury and neurobehavioral performance, *Brain Inj.*, 7:481, 1993.

620. Hibbard, MR, Uysal, S, Kepler, K, et al., Axis 1 psychopathology in individuals with traumatic brain injury, *J. Head Trauma Rehabil.*, 13:24, 1998.

621. Van Reekum, R, Bolago, I, Finlayson, et al., Psychiatric disorders after traumatic brain injury, *Brain Inj.*, 10:319, 1996.

622. Fann, JR, Katon, WJ, Uomoto, JM, Esselman, PC, Psychiatric disorders and functional disability in outpatients with traumatic brain injuries, *Am. J. Psychiatry*, 152:1493, 1995.

623. Wright, JC, Telford, R, Psychological problems following minor head injury: a prospective study, *Br. J. Clin. Psychol.*, 35:399, 1996.

624. Nochi, M, "Loss of self" in the narratives of people with traumatic brain injuries: a qualitative analysis, *Soc. Sci. Med.*, 46:869, 1998.

625. Morton, MV, Wehman, P, Psychosocial and emotional sequelae of individuals with traumatic brain injury: a literature review and recommendations, *Brain Inj.*, 9:81, 1995.

626. Bowen, A, Neumann, V, Conner, M, et al., Mood disorders following traumatic brain injury: identifying the extent of the problem and the people at risk, *Brain Inj.*, 12:177, 1998.

627. Busch, CR, Alpern, HP, Depression after mild traumatic brain injury: a review of current research, *Neuropsycho. Rev.*, 8:95, 1998.

628. Burke, JM, Imhoff, CL, Kerrigan, JM, MMPI correlates among post-acute TBI patients, *Brain Inj.*, 4:223, 1990.

629. Persinger, MA: Depression following brain trauma is enhanced in patients with mild discrepancies between intelligence and impairment on neuropsychological scores, *Percept. Mot. Skills*, 84:1284, 1997.

630. Welch, M, Clients' experiences of depression during recovery from traumatic injury, *Clin. Nurse Spec.*, 9:92, 1995.

631. Parker, RS, Rosenblum, A, IQ loss and emotional dysfunctions after mild traumatic head injury incurred in a motor vehicle accident, *J. Clin. Psychol.*, 52:32, 1996.

632. Malia, K, Powell, G, Torode, S, Personality and psychosocial function after brain injury, *Brain Inj.*, 9:697, 1995.

633. Prigatano, GP, Personality disturbances associated with traumatic brain injury, *J. Consult. Clin. Psychol.*, 60:360, 1992.

634. Kurtz, JE, Putnam, SH, Stone, C, Stability of normal personality traits after traumatic brain injury, *J. Head Trauma Rehabil.*, 13:1, 1998.

635. Lannoo, E, de Deyne, C, Colardyn, F, et al., Personality change following head injury: assessment with the NEO Five-Factor Inventory, *J. Psychosom. Res.*, 43:505, 1997.

636. Raskin, SA, The relationship between sexual abuse and mild traumatic brain injury, *Brain Inj.*, 11:587, 1997.

637. Malia, KM, Powell, G, Torode, S, Coping and psychosocial function after brain injury, *Brain Inj.*, 9:607, 1995.

638. Malt, UF, Coping with accidental injury, *Psychiatr. Med.*, 10:135, 1992.

639. Streeter, CC, Van Reekum, R, Shorr, RI, Bachman, DL, Prior head injury in male veterans with borderline personality disorder, *J. Nerv. Ment. Dis.*, 183:577, 1995.

640. Van Reekum. R, Links. PS, Finlayson. MA, et al., Repeat neurobehavioral study of borderline personality disorder, *J. Psychiatry Neurosci.*, 21:13, 1996.

641. Fugate. LP, Spacek. LA, Kresty. LA, et al., Definition of agitation following traumatic brain injury: I. A survey of the brain injury Special Interest Group of the American Academy of Physical Medicine and Rehabilitation, *Arch. Phys. Med. Rehabil.*, 78:917,1997.

642. Harvey, AG, Bryant, RA, Predictors of acute stress following mild traumatic brain injury, *Brain Inj.*, 12:147,1998.

643. Harvey, AG, Bryant, RA, Acute stress disorder after mild traumatic brain injury, *J. Nerv. Ment. Dis.*, 186:333, 1998.

644. Bryant, RA, Harvey, AG, Acute stress response: a comparison of head injured and non-head injured patients, *Psychol. Med.*, 25:869, 1995.

645. Bryant, RA, Harvey, AG, Relationship between acute stress disorder and posttraumatic stress disorder following mild traumatic brain injury, *Am. J. Psychiatry*, 155:625, 1998.

646. Hickling, EJ, Gillen, R, Blanchard, EB, et al., Traumatic brain injury and posttraumatic stress disorder: a preliminary investigation of neuropsychological test results in PTSD secondary to motor vehicle accidents, *Brain Inj.*, 12: 265, 1998.

647. Ohry, A, Rattok, J, Solomon, Z, Post-traumatic stress disorder in brain injury patients, *Brain Inj.*, 10:687, 1996.

648. Warden, DL, Labbate, LA, Salazar, AM, et al., Posttraumatic stress disorder in patients with traumatic brain injury and amnesia for the event? *J. Neuropsychiatry Clin. Neurosci.*, 9:18, 1997.

649. Sbordone, RJ, Liter, JC, Mild traumatic brain injury does not produce post-traumatic stress disorder, *Brain Inj.*, 9:405, 1995.

650. Shalev, AY, Freedman, S, Peri, T, et al., Prospective study of posttraumatic stress disorder and depression following trauma, *Am. J. Psychiatry*, 155:630, 1998.

651. McMillan, TM, Post-traumatic stress disorder following minor and severe closed head injury: 10 single cases, *Brain Inj.*, 10:749, 1996.

652. Fuller, MG, Fishman, E, Taylor, CA, Wood, RB, Screening patients with traumatic brain injuries for substance abuse, *J. Neuropsychiatry Clin. Neurosci.*, 6:143, 1994.

653. Sander, AM, Witol, AD, Kreutzer, JS: Alcohol use after traumatic brain injury: concordance of patient's and relatives' reports, *Arch. Phys. Med. Rehabil.*, 78:138, 1997.

654. Wood, RL, Yurdakul, LK, Change in relationship status following traumatic brain injury, *Brain Inj.*, 11:491, 1997.

655. Hallett, JD, Zasler, ND, Maurer, P, Cash, S,, Role change after traumatic brain injury in adults, *Am. J. Occup. Ther.*, 48:241, 1994.

656. Fleming, JM, Strong, J, Ashton, R, Self-awareness of deficits in adults with traumatic brain injury: How best to measure? *Brain Inj.*, 10:1, 1996.

657. Linn, RT, Allen, K, Willer, BS, Affective symptoms in the chronic stage of traumatic brain injury: a study of married couples, *Brain Inj.*, 8:135, 1994.

658. Klinczak, NJ, Donovick, PJ, Burright, R, The malingering of multiple sclerosis and mild traumatic brain injury, *Brain Inj.*, 11:343, 1997.

659. Lees-Haley, PR, Dunn, JT, The ability of naïve subjects to report symptoms of mild brain injury, post-traumatic stress disorder, major depression and generalized anxiety disorder, *J. Clin. Psychol.*, 50:252, 1994.

660. Frederick, RI, Carter, M, Powel, J, Adapting symptom validity testing to evaluate suspicious complaints of amnesia in medicolegal evaluations, *Bull. Am. Acad. Psychiatry Law*, 23:231, 1995.

661. Zwil, AS, McAllister, TW, Cohen, I, Halpern, LR, Ultra-rapid cycling bipolar affective disorder following a closed head injury, *Brain Inj.*, 7:147, 1993.

662. Formisano, R, Saltuari, L, Gerstenbrand, F, Presence of Kluver-Bucy syndrome as a positive prognostic feature for the remission of traumatic prolonged disturbances of consciousness, *Acta Neurol. Scand.*, 91:54, 1995.

663. Kant, R, Smith-Seemiller, L, Duffy, JD, Obsessive-compulsive disorder after closed head injury: review of literature and report of four cases, *Brain Inj.*, 10:55, 1996.

664. Zeilig, G, Drubach, DA, Katz-Zielig, M, Karatinos, J, Pathological laughter and crying in patients with closed traumatic brain injury, *Brain Inj.*, 10:591, 1996.

665. Fornazzari, L, Farcnik, K, Smith, I, et al., Violent visual hallucinations and aggression in frontal lobe dysfunction: clinical manifestations of deep orbitofrontal foci, *J. Neuropsychiatry Clin. Neurosci.*, 4:42, 1992.

666. Grigsby, J, Kaye, K, Incidence and correlates of depersonalization following head trauma, *Brain Inj.*, 7:507, 1993.

667. Vaughan, N, Agner, D, Clinchot, DM, Perseveration and wandering as a predictor variable after brain injury, *Brain Inj.*, 11:815, 1997.

668. Whyte, J, Polansky, M, Fleming, M, et al., Sustained arousal and attention after traumatic brain injury, *Neuropsychologia*, 33:797, 1995.

669. Whyte, J, Polansky, M, Cavallucci, C, et al., Inattentive behavior after traumatic brain injury, *J. Int. Neuropsychol. Soc.*, 2:274, 1996.

670. Giubilei, F, Formisano, R, Fiorini, M, et al., Sleep abnormalities in traumatic apallic syndrome, *J. Neurol. Neurosurg. Psychiatry*, 58:484, 1995.

671. Blostein, PA, Jones, SJ, Buechler, CM, Vandongen, S, Cognitive screening in mild traumatic brain injuries: analysis of the neurobehavioral cognitive status examination when utilized during initial trauma hospitalization, *J. Neurotrauma.*, 14:171, 1997.

672. Cicerone, KD, Smith, LC, Ellmo, W, et al., Neuropsychological rehabilitation of mild traumatic brain injury, *Brain Inj.*, 10:277, 1996.

673. Veltman, RH, VanDongen, S, Jones, S, et al., Cognitive screening in mild brain injury, *J. Neurosci. Nurs.*, 25:367, 1993.

674. Parasuraman, R, Mutter, SA, Molloy, R, Sustained attention following mild closed-head injury, *J. Clin. Exp. Neuropsychol.*, 13:789, 1991.

675. Capruso, DX, Levin, HS, Cognitive impairment following closed head injury, *Neurol. Clin.*, 10:879, 1992.

676. Barth, JT, Macciocchi, SN, Giordani, B, et al., Neuropsychological sequelae of minor head injury, *Neurosurgery*, 13:529, 1983.

677. Bohnen, N, Jolles, J, Twijnstra, A, Neuropsychological deficits in patients with persistent symptoms six months after mild head injury, *Neurosurgery*, 30:692, 1992.

678. Lishman, WA, Pathogenesis and psychogenesis in the post-concussional syndrome, *Br. J. Psychiatry*, 153:460, 1988.

679. Jane, JA, Rimel, RW, Prognosis in head injury, *Clin. Neurosurg.*, 29:346, 1982.

680. Hugenholtz, HK, Stuss, DT, Stethem, LL, et al., How long does it take to recover from a mild concussion? *Neurosurgery*, 22:853, 1988.

681. Gentilini, M, Nichelli, P, Schoenhuber, H, et al., Assessment of attention in mild head injury, in: Levin, HS, Eisenberg, HM, Benton, AL, (Eds.), *Mild Head injury*, Oxford University Press, New York, 163, 1989.

682. Kay, T, Neuropsychological diagnosis: Disentangling the multiple determinants of functional disability after mild traumatic brain injury, *Phy. Med. Rehabil. State of the Art Rev.*, 6:109, 1992.

683. Gronwall. D. Cumulative and persisting effects of concussion on attention and cognition, in: Levin, HS, Eisenberg, HM, Benton, AL, (Eds.), *Mild Head Injury*, Oxford University Press, New York, 153, 1989.

684. Gronwal, D, Wrightson, P, Delayed recovery of intellectual function after minor head injury, *Lancet,* 1:605, 1974.

685. Kay, T, Neuropsychological treatment of mild traumatic brain injury, *J. Head Trauma Rehabil.*, 8:153, 1993.

686. Schapiro, SR, Sacchetti, TS, Neuropsychological sequelae of minor head trauma, in: Mandel, S, Sataloff, RT, Schapiro, SR, (Eds.), *Minor Head Trauma, Assessment, Management and Rehabilitation*, Springer-Verlag, New York, 86, 1993.

687. Lezak, MD, *Neuropsychological Assessment.* 3d Ed, Oxford University Press, New York, 97, 1985.

688. Sherer, M, Boake, C, Levin, E, et al., Characteristics of impaired awareness after traumatic brain injury, *J. Int. Neuropsychol. Soc.*, 4:380, 1998.

689. Fleming, JM, Strong, J, Ashton, R, Self-awareness of deficits in adults with traumatic brain injury: How best to measure? *Brain Inj.*, 10:1, 1996.

690. Cicerone, DK, Attention deficits and dual task demands after mild traumatic brain injury, *Brain Inj.*, 10:79, 1996.

691. Ferraro, FR, Cognitive slowing in closed-head injury. *Brain Cogn.*, 32:429, 1996.

692. McDowell, S, Whyte, J, D'Esposito, M, Working memory impairments in traumatic brain injury: Evidence from a dual-task paradigm, *Neuropsychologia*, 35:1341, 1997.

693. Robertson, IH, Manly, T, Andrade, J, et al., 'Oops': Performance correlates of everyday attentional failures in traumatic brain injured and normal subjects, *Neuropsychologia*, 35:747, 1997.

694. Ichise, M, Chung, DG, Wang, P, et al., Technetium-99m-HMPAO SPECT, CT and MRI in the evaluation of patients with chronic traumatic brain injury: A correlation with neuropsychological performance, *J. Nucl. Med.*, 35:217, 1994.

695. Webb, C, Rose, FD, Johnson, DA, Attree, EA, Age and recovery from brain injury: Clinical opinions and experimental evidence, *Brain Inj.*, 10:303, 1996.

696. Mazzucchi, A, Cattelani, R, Missale G, et al., Head-injured subjects aged over 50 years: Correlations between variables of trauma and neuropsychological follow-up, *J. Neurol.*, 239:256, 1992.

697. Rothweiler, B, Temkin, NR, Dikman, SS, Aging effect on psychosocial outcome in traumatic brain injury, *Arch. Phys. Med. Rehabil.*, 79: 881, 1998.

698. Johnstone, B, Childers, MK, Hoerner, J, The effects of normal aging on neuropsychological functioning following traumatic brain injury, *Brain Inj.*, 12:569, 1998.

699. American Speech Language and Hearing Association: Position Statement: The role of Speech-Language Pathologists in the Identification, Diagnosis and Treatment of Individuals with Cognitive-Communication Impairments. March, 1988.

700. Paul-Cohen, R, The role of the speech-language pathologist in the treatment of mild brain injury: A community based approach, in: Mandel, S, Sataloff, RT, Schapiro, SR, (Eds.), *Minor Head Trauma, Assessment, Management and Rehabilitation*, Springer-Verlag, New York, 261, 1993.

701. Sohlberg, MM, Mateer, CA, The assessment of cognitive-communicative functions in head injury*, Topics Lang Dis.*, 9:15, 1989.

702. Jay, GW, Goka, RS, Arakaki, A, Minor traumatic brain injury: Review of clinical data and appropriate evaluation and treatment, *J. Ins. Med.*, 27:262, 1997.

703. Katz, N, Hefner, D, Reuben, R, Measuring clinical change in cognitive rehabilitation of patients with brain damage: two cases, traumatic brain injury and cerebral vascular accident, in: Johnson, JA, Krefting, LH, (Eds.), *Occupational Therapy Approaches to Traumatic Brain Injury*, Haworth Press, New York, 23, 1990.

704. Zweber, B, Malec, J, Goal attainment scaling in post-acute brain injury rehabilitation, in: Johnson, JA, Krefting, LH, (Eds.), *Occupational Therapy Approaches to Traumatic Brain Injury*, Haworth Press, New York, 45, 1990.

705. Chen, SH, Thomas, JD, Glueckauf, RL, Bracy, OL, The effectiveness of computer-assisted cognitive rehabilitation for persons with traumatic brain injury, *Brain Inj.*, 11:197, 1997.

706. Neimann, H, Ruff, RM, Baser, CA, Computer-assisted retraining in head-injured individuals: a controlled efficacy study of an outpatient program, *J. Consult. Clin. Psychol.*, 58:811, 1990.

707. Christiansen, C, Abreu, B, Ottenbacher, K, et al., Task performance in virtual environments used for cognitive rehabilitation after traumatic brain injury, *Arch. Phys. Med. Rehabil.*, 79:888, 1998.

708. Cope, DN, An integration of psychopharmacological and rehabilitation approaches to traumatic brain injury rehabilitation, *J. Head Trauma Rehabil.*, 9:1, 1994.

709. Christensen, AL, Outpatient management and outcome in relation to work in traumatic brain injury patients, *Scand. J. Rehabil. Med. Suppl.*, 26:34, 1992.

710. Wade, DT, King, NS, Wenden, FJ, et al., Routine follow up after head injury: a second randomized controlled trial, *J. Neurol. Neurosurg. Psychiatry*, 65:177, 1998.

711. McLaughlin, AM, Peters, S, Evaluation of an innovative cost-effective programme for brain injury patients: response to a need for flexible treatment planning, *Brain Inj.*, 7:71, 1995.

712. King, NS, Crawford, S, Wenden, FJ, et al., Interventions and service need following mild and moderate head injury: The Oxford Head Injury Service, *Clin. Rehabil.*, 11:13, 1997.

713. Chittum, WR, Johnson, K, Chittum, JM, et al., Road to awareness: An individualized training package for increasing knowledge and comprehension of personal deficits in persons with acquired brain injury, *Brain Inj.*, 10:763, 1996.

714. Hetherington, CR, Stuss, DT, Finlayson, MA, Reaction time and variability 5 and 10 years after traumatic brain injury, *Brain Inj.*, 10:473, 1996.

715. Darragh, AR, Sample, PL, Fisher, AG, Environment effect of functional task performance in adults with acquired brain injuries: use of the assessment of motor and process skills, *Arch. Phys. Med. Rehabil.*, 79:418, 1998.

716. Davis, PK, Chittum, R, A group-oriented contingency to increase leisure activities of adults with traumatic brain injury, *J. Appl. Behav. Anal.*, 27:553, 1994.

717. Haaland, KY, Temkin, N, Randahl, G, Dikmen, S, Recovery of simple motor skills after head injury, *J. Clin. Exp. Neuropsychol.*, 16:448, 1994.

718. Wong, AM, Lee, MY, Kuo, JK, Tang, FT, The development and clinical evaluation of a standing biofeedback trainer, *J. Rehabil. Res. Dev.*, 34:322, 1997.

719. Swaine, BR, Sullivan, SJ, Relation between clinical and instrumental measures of motor coordination in traumatically brain injured persons, *Arch. Phys. Med. Rehabil.*, 73:55, 1992.

720. Sullivan, SJ, Richer, E, Laurent, F, The role of and possibilities for physical conditioning programmes in the rehabilitation of traumatically brain-injured persons, *Brain Inj.*, 4:407, 1990.

721. Gordon, WA, Sliwinski, M, Echo J, et al., The benefits of exercise in individuals with traumatic brain injury: a retrospective study, *J. Head Trauma Rehabil.*, 13:58, 1998.

722. Jankowski, LW, Sullivan, SJ, Aerobic and neuromuscular training: Effect on the capacity, efficiency, and fatigability of patients with traumatic brain injuries, *Arch. Phys. Med. Rehabil.*, 71:500, 1990.

723. Vitale, AE, Sullivan, SJ, Jankowski, LW, et al., Screening of health risk factors prior to exercise or a fitness evaluation of adults with traumatic brain injury: a consensus by rehabilitation professionals, *Brain Inj.*, 10:367, 1996.

724. Greenman, PE, McPartland, JM, Cranial findings and iatrogenesis from craniosacral manipulation in patients with traumatic brain syndrome, *J. Am. Osteopath. Assoc.*, 95:182, 1995.

725. Baker-Price, LA, Persinger, MA, Weak, but complex pulsed magnetic fields may reduce depression following traumatic brain injury, *Percept. Mot. Skills*, 83:491, 1996.

726. Smith, RB, Tiberi, A, Marshall, J, The use of cranial electrotherapy stimulation in the treatment of closed head injured patients, *Brain Inj.*, 8:357, 1994.

727. Brooke, MM, Questad, KA, Patterson, DR, Valois, TA, Driving evaluation after traumatic brain injury, *Am. J. Phys. Med. Rehabil.*, 71:177, 1992.

728. Galski, T, Ehle, HT, Williams, JB, Off-road driving evaluations for persons with cerebral injury: a factor analytic study of predriver and simulator testing, *Am. J. Occup. Ther.*, 51:352, 1997.

729. Korteling, JE, Kaptein, NA, Neuropsychological driving fitness tests for brain-damaged subjects, *Arch. Phys. Med. Rehabil.*, 77:138, 1996.

730. Haselkorn, JK, Mueller, BA, Rivara, FA, Characteristics of drivers and driving record after traumatic and nontraumatic brain injury, *Arch. Phys. Med. Rehabil.*, 79:738, 1998.

731. Millis, SR, Rosenthal, M, Lourie, IF, Predicting community integration after traumatic brain injury with neuropsychological measures, *Int. J. Neurosci.*, 79:165, 1994.

732. McColl, MA, Carlson, F, Johnston, J, et al., The definition of community integration: perspectives of people with brain injuries, *Brain Inj.*, 12:15, 1998.

733. Webb, CR, Wrigley, M, Yoel, W, Fine, PR, Explaining quality of life for persons with traumatic brain injuries 2 years after injury, *Arch. Phys. Med. Rehabil.*, 76:1113, 1995.

734. Finset, A, Dyrnes, S, Krogstad, JM, Bernstad, J, Self-reported social networks and interpersonal support 2 years after severe traumatic brain injury, *Brain Inj.*, 9:141, 1995.

735. Burleigh, SA, Farber, RS, Gillard, M, Community integration and life satisfaction after traumatic brain injury, *Am. J. Occup. Ther.*, 52:45, 1998.

736. Asikainen, I, Kaste, M, Sarna, S, Patients with traumatic brain injury referred to a rehabilitation and re-employment programme: social and professional outcome for 508 Finnish patients 5 or more years after injury. *Brain Inj.*, 10:883, 1996.

737. Wood, RL, Yurdakul, LK, Change in relationship status following traumatic brain injury, *Brain Inj.*, 11:491, 1997.

738. Leathem, J, Heath, E, Woolley, C, Relatives' perceptions of role change, social support and stress after traumatic brain injury, *Brain Inj.*, 10:27, 1996.

739. Kreutzer, JS, Gervasio, AH, Camplair, PS, Primary caregivers' psychological status and family functioning after traumatic brain injury, *Brain Inj.*, 8:197, 1994.

740. Kreutzer, JS, Gervasio, AH, Camplair, PS, Patient correlates of caregivers' distress and family functioning after traumatic brain injury, *Brain Inj.*, 8:211, 1994.

741. Gillen, R, Tennen, H, Affleck, G, Steinpreis, R, Distress, depressive symptoms, and depressive disorder among caregivers of patients with brain injury, *J. Head Trauma Rehabil.*, 13:31, 1998.

742. Knight, RG, Devereux, R, Godfrey, HP, Caring for a family member with a traumatic brain injury, *Brain Inj.*, 12:467, 1998.

743. Leach, LR, Frank, RG, Bouman, DE, Farmer, J, Family functioning, social support and depression after traumatic brain injury, *Brain Inj.*, 8:599, 1994.

744. Hall, KM, Karzmark, P, Stevens, M, et al., Family stressors in traumatic brain injury: a two-year follow-up, *Arch. Phys. Med. Rehabil.*, 75:876, 1994.

745. Peters, LC, Stambrook, M, Moore, AD, Esses, L, Psychosocial sequelae of closed head injury: Effects on the marital relationship, *Brain Inj.*, 4:39, 1990.

746. Douglas, JM, Spellacy, FJ, Indicators of long-term family functioning following severe traumatic brain injury in adults, *Brain Inj.*, 10:819, 1996.

747. Wallace, CA, Bogner, J, Corrigan, JD, et al., Primary caregivers of persons with brain injury: life changes 1 year after injury, *Brain Inj.*, 12:483, 1998.

748. Seel, RT, Kreutzer, JS, Sander, AM: Concordance of patients' and family members' ratings of neurobehavioral functioning after traumatic brain injury, *Arch. Phys. Med. Rehabil.*, 78:1254, 1997.

749. Sander, AM, Seel, RT, Kreutzer, JS, et al., Agreement between persons with traumatic brain injury and their relatives regarding psychosocial outcome using the Community Integration Questionnaire, *Arch. Phys. Med. Rehabil.*, 78:353, 1997.

750. Hayden, ME, Mild traumatic Brain injury, A primer for understanding its impact on employee return to work, *AAOHN J.*, 45:635, 1997.

751. Englander, J, Hall, K, Stimpson, T, Chaffin, S, Mild traumatic brain injury in an insured population: Subjective complaints and return to employment, *Brain Inj.*, 6:161, 1992.

752. Greenspan, AI, Wrigley, JM, Kresnow, M, et al., Factors influencing failure to return to work due to traumatic brain injury, *Brain Inj.*, 10:207, 1996.

753. Wehman, P, Kregel, J, West, M, Cifu, D, Return to work for patients with traumatic brain injury, Analysis of costs, *Am. J. Phys. Med. Rehabil.*, 73:289, 1994.

754. West, M, Wehman, P, Kregel, J, et al., Costs of operating a supported work program for traumatically brain-injured individuals, *Arch. Phys. Med. Rehabil.*, 72:127, 1991.

755. Ip, RY, Dornan, J, Schentag, C, Traumatic brain injury: Factors predicting return to work or school, *Brain Inj.*, 9:517, 1995.

756. Wehman, P, Kregel, J, Sherron, P, et al., Critical factors associated with the successful supported employment placement of patients with severe traumatic brain injury, *Brain Inj.*, 7:31, 1993.

757. Stambrook, M, Moore, AD, Peters, LC, et al., Effects of mild, moderate and severe closed head injury on long-term vocational status, *Brain Inj.*, 4:183, 1990.

758. O'Neill, J, Hibbard, MR, Brown, M, et al., The effect of employment on quality of life and community integration after traumatic brain injury, *J. Head Trauma Rehabil.*, 13:68, 1998.

759. Rappaport, M, Hall, KM, Hopkins, K, et al., Disability rating scale for severe head trauma: coma to community, *Arch. Phys. Med. Rehabil.*, 63:118, 1982.

760. Hamilton, BB, Granger, CV, Sherwin, FS, et al., A uniform national data system for medical rehabilitation, in: Fuhrer, MJ, (Ed.), *Analysis and Measurement*, Brookes Publishing Co., Baltimore, MD, 1987.

761. Mahoney, FI, Barthel, DW, Functional evaluation: Barthel Index, *M. State Med. J.*, 14:61, 1965.

762. Linacre, JM, Heinemann, AW, Wright, BD, et al., The structure and stability of the Functional Independence Measure, *Arch. Phys. Med. Rehabil.*, 2:57, 1987.

763. American Medical Association: *Guide to the Evaluation of Permanent Impairment*, 3rd ed. (revised), American Medical Association, Milwaukee, WI, 1990.

764. DiScalas, C, Grant, CC, Brooke, MM, Gans, BM, Functional outcome in children with traumatic brain injury: Agreement between clinical judgement and the Functional Independence Measure, *Am. J. Phys. Med. Rehabil.*, 71:145, 1992.

765. Whitlock, JA, Jr, Hamilton, BB, Functional outcome after rehabilitation for severe traumatic brain injury, *Arch. Phys. Med. Rehabil.*, 76:1103,1995.

766. Stineman, MG, Goin, JE, Granger, CV, et al., Discharge motor FIM-function related groups, *Arch. Phys. Med. Rehabil.*, 78:980, 1997.

767. Kaplan, CP, Corrigan, JD, The relationship between cognition and functional independence in adults with traumatic brain injury, *Arch. Phys. Med. Rehabil.*, 75:643, 1994.

768. Grimby, G, Gudjonsson, G, Rodhe, M, et al., The functional independence measure in Sweden: experience for outcome measurement in rehabilitation medicine, *Scand. J. Rehab. Med.*, 28:51, 1996.

769. Dombovy, ML, Olek, AC, Recovery and rehabilitation following traumatic brain injury, *Brain Inj.*, 11:305, 1997.

770. Corrigan, JD, Smith-Knapp, K, Granger, CV, Validity of the functional independence measure for persons with traumatic brain injury, *Arch. Phys. Med. Rehabil.*, 78:828, 1997.

771. Tesio, L, Cantagallo, A, The functional assessment measure (FAM) in closed traumatic brain injury outpatients: a Rasch-based psychometric study, *J. Outcome Meas.*, 2:79, 1998.

772. Gomez, PA, Lobato, RD, Ortega, JM, De La Cruz, J, Mild head injury: differences in prognosis among patients with a Glasgow Coma Scale score of 13 to 15 and analysis of factors associated with abnormal CT findings, *Br. J. Neurosurg.*, 10:453, 1996.

773. Lajtman, Z, Gasparovic, S, Prognostic value of Glasgow Coma Scale for tracheotomy in head injured patients, *Acta Med. Croatica*, 50:133, 1996.

774. Zafonte, RD, Hammond, FM, Mann, NR, et al., Relationship between Glasgow coma scale and functional outcome, *Am. J. Phys. Med. Rehabil.*, 75:364, 1996.

775. Born, JD, The Glasgow-Liege Scale, *Acta Neurochir.*, 91:1, 1988.

776. Whitlock, JA, Jr, Functional outcome of low-level traumatically brain-injured admitted to an acute rehabilitation programme, *Brain Inj.*, 6:447, 1992.

777. Dikmen, SS, Ross, BL, Machamer, JE, Temkin, NR, One year psychosocial outcome in head injury. *J. Int. Neuropsychol. Soc.*, 1:67, 1995.

778. Gordon, E, von Holst, H, Rudehill, A, Outcome of head injury in 2298 patients treated in a single clinic during a 21-year period, *J. Neurosurg. Anesthesiol.*, 7:235, 1995.

779. Masson, F, Maurette, P, Salmi, LR, et al., Prevalence of impairments 5 years after a head injury and their relationship with disabilities and outcome, *Brain Inj.*, 10:487, 1996.

780. Ditunno, JF, Functional assessment measures in CNS Trauma, *J. Neurotrauma.*, (Suppl 1):S301, 1992.

781. Conzen, M, Ebel, H, Swart, E, et al., Long-term neuropsychological outcome after severe head injury with good recovery, *Brain Inj.*, 6:45, 1992.

782. Jennet, B, Teasdale, G, *Management of Head Injuries*, F.A. Davis, Philadelphia, 1981.

783. Katz, DI, Alexander, MP, Traumatic brain injury, predicting course of recovery and outcome for patients admitted to rehabilitation, *Arch. Neurol.*, 51:661, 1994.

784. Semlyen, JK, Barnes, MP, The further validation and precision of the NIAF-R, *Brain Inj.*, 12:155, 1998.

785. Torenbeek, M, van der Heijden, GJ, de Witte, LP, Bakx, WG, Construct validation of the Hoensbroeck Disability Scale for brain injury in acquired brain injury rehabilitation, *Brain Inj.*, 12:307, 1998.

786. Michaels, AJ, Michaels, CE, Moon, CH, et al., Psychosocial factors limit outcomes after trauma, *J. Trauma*, 44:644, 1998.

787. McPherson, KM, Pentland, B, Disability in patients following traumatic brain injury — which measure? *Int. J. Rehabil. Res.*, 20:1, 1997.

788. Horton, AM, Jr, Cross-validation of the alternative impairment index, *Percept. Mot. Skills*, 81:1153, 1995.

789. Diringer, MN, Edwards, DF, Does modification of the Innsbruck and the Glasgow Coma Scales improve their ability to predict functional outcome? *Arch. Neurol.*, 54:606, 1997.

790. Crawford, S, Wenden, FJ, Wade, DT, The Rivermead head injury follow up questionnaire: a study of a new rating scale and other measures to evaluate outcome after head injury, *J. Neurol. Neurosurg. Psychiatry*, 60:510, 1996.

791. Davis, CH, Fardanesh, L, Rubner, D, et al., Profiles of functional recovery in fifty traumatically brain-injured patients after acute rehabilitation, *Am. J. Phys. Med. Rehabil.*, 76:213, 1997.

792. Ommaya, AK, Salazar, AM, Dannenberg, AL, et al., Outcome after traumatic brain injury in the U.S. military medical system, *J. Trauma*, 41:972, 1996.

793. Mendelson, G, "Compensation neurosis" revisited: Outcome studies of the effects of litigation, *J. Psychosom. Res.*, 39:695, 1995.

794. Mills, VM, Nesbeda, T, Katz, DI, Alexander, MP, Outcomes for traumatically brain-injured patients following post-acute rehabilitation programs, *Brain Inj.*, 6:219, 1992.

795. Mattson, JD, Case management in mild traumatic brain injury and post-concussive rehabilitation, *Phys. Med. Rehabil.: State of the Art Reviews*, 6:183, 1992.

796. Van den Broek, MD, Lye, R, Staff stress in head injury rehabilitation, *Brain Inj.*, 10:133, 1996.

797. Costello, M, Pedersen, C, Tan, M, et al., Acquired brain injuries — demanding nursing excellence, *Aust. Nurs. J.*, 5:24, 1997.

798. Macciocchi, SN, Eaton, B, Decision and attribution bias in neurorehabilitation, *Arch. Phys. Med. Rehabil.*, 76:521, 1995.

799. Markowsky, SJ, Skaar, DJ, Christie, JM, et al., Phenytoin protein binding and dosage requirements during acute and convalescent phases following brain injury, *Ann. Pharmacother.*, 30:443, 1996.

800. McKindley, DS, Boucher, BA, Hess, MM, Effect of acute phase response on phenytoin metabolism in neurotrauma patients, *J. Clin. Pharmacol.*, 37:129, 1997.

801. Murri, L, Arrigo, A, Bonuccelli, U, et al., Phenobarbital in the prophylaxis of late posttraumatic seizures, *Ital. J. Neurol. Sci.*, 13:755, 1992.

802. Rivey, MP, Allington, DR, Stone, JD, Serfoss, ML, Alteration of carbamazepine pharmacokinetics in patients with traumatic brain injury, *Brain Inj.*, 9:41, 1995.

803. Anderson, GD, Gidal, BE, Hendryx, RJ, et al., Decreased protein binding of valproate in patients with acute head trauma, *B. J. Clin. Pharmacol.*, 37:559, 1994.

804. Anderson, GD, Awan, AB, Adams, CA, et al., Increases in metabolism of valproate and excretion of 6-beta-hydroxycortisol in patients with traumatic brain injury, *Br. J. Clin. Pharmacol.*, 45:101, 1998.

805. Wroblewski, BA, Joseph, AB, Intramuscular midazolam for treatment of acute seizures or behavioral episodes in patients with brain injury, *J. Neurol. Neurosurg. Psychiatry*, 55:328, 1992.

806. Stanislav, SW, Cognitive effects of antipsychotic agents in persons with traumatic brain injury, *Brain Inj.*, 11:335, 1997.

807. Lott, RS, Kerrick, JM, Cohen, SA, Clinical and economic aspects of risperidone treatment in adults with mental retardation and behavioral disturbances, *Psychopharmacol. Bull.*, 32:721, 1996.

808. Rommel, O, Tegenthoff, M, Widdig, W, et al., Organic catatonia following frontal lobe injury: response to clozapine, *J. Neuropsychiatry Clin. Neurosci.*, 10:237, 1998.

809. Patterson, DE, Braverman, SE, Belandres, PV, Speech dysfunction due to trazodone — fluoxetine combination in traumatic brain injury, *Brain Inj.*, 11:287, 1997.

810. Mashiko, H, Yokoyama, H, Matsumoto, H, Niwa, S, Trazodone for aggression in an adolescent with hydrocephalus, *Psychiatry Clin. Neurosci.*, 50:133, 1996.

811. Sloan, RL, Brown, KW, Pentland, B, Fluoxetine as a treatment for emotional lability after brain injury, *Brain Inj.*, 6:315, 1992.

812. Khouzam, HR, Donnelly, NJ, Remission of traumatic brain injury: induced compulsions during venlafaxine treatment, *Gen. Hosp. Psychiatry*, 20:62, 1998.

813. Whyte, J, Hart, T, Schuster, K, et al., Effects of methylphenidate on attentional function after traumatic brain injury, a randomized, placebo-controlled trial, *Am. J. Phys. Med. Rehabil.*, 76:440, 1997.

814. Plengerf, PM, Dixon, CE, Castillo, RM, et al., Subacute methylphenidate treatment for moderate to moderately severe traumatic brain injury: A preliminary double-blind placebo-controlled study, *Arch. Phys. Med. Rehabil.*, 77:536, 1996.

815. Kaelin, DL, Cifu, DX, Matthies, B, Methylphenidate effect on attention deficit in the acutely brain-injured adult, *Arch. Phys. Med. Rehabil.*, 77:6, 1996.

816. Hornyak, JE, Nelson, VS, Hurvitz, EA, The use of methylphenidate in paediatric traumatic brain injury, *Pediatr. Rehabil.*, 1:15, 1997.

817. Wroblewski, BA, Leary, JM, Phelan, AM, et al., Methylphenidate and seizure frequency in brain injured patients with seizure disorders, *J. Clin. Psychiatry*, 53:86, 1992.

818. Hornstein, A, Lennihan, L, Seliger, G, et al., Amphetamine in recovery from brain injury, *Brain Inj.*, 10:145, 1996.

819. Wroblewski, BA, Joseph, AB, Kupfer, J, Kalliel, K, Effectiveness of valproic acid on destructive and aggressive behaviors in patients with acquired brain injury, *Brain Inj.*, 11:37, 1997.

820. Stanislav, SW, Fabre, T, Crismon, ML, Childs, A, Buspirone's efficacy in organic-induced aggression, *J. Clin. Psychopharmacol.*, 14:126, 1994.

821. Nichels, JL, Schneider, WN, Dombovy, ML, Wong, TM, Clinical use of amantadine in brain injury rehabilitation, *Brain Inj.*, 8:709, 1994.

822. Kraus, MF, Maki, PM, Effect of amantadine hydrochloride on symptoms of frontal lobe dysfunction in brain injury case studies and review, *J. Neuropsychiatry Clin. Neurosci.*, 9:222, 1997.

823. Kraus, MF, Maki, P, The combined use of amantadine and l-dopa/carbidopa in the treatment of chronic brain injury, *Brain Inj.*, 11:455, 1997.

824. Van Reekum, R, Bayley, M, Garner, S, et al., N of 1 study: amantadine for the amotivational syndrome in a patient with traumatic brain injury, *Brain Inj.*, 9:49, 1995.

825. McDowell, S, Whyte, J, D'Esposito, M, Differential effect of a dopaminergic agonist on prefrontal function in traumatic brain injury, *Brain*, 121(Pt. 6):1155, 1998.

826. Powell, JH, al-Adawi, S, Morgan, J, Greenwood, RJ, Motivational deficits after brain injury: Effects of bromocriptine in 11 patients, *J. Neurol. Neurosurg. Psychiatry*, 60:416, 1996.

827. Taverni, JP, Seliger, G, Lichtman, SW, Donepezil medicated memory improvement in traumatic brain injury during post acute rehabilitation, *Brain Inj.*, 12:77, 1998.

828. Eams, P, Sutton, A, Protracted post-traumatic confusional state treated with physostigmine, *Brain Inj.*, 9:729, 1995.

Part Two

Introduction to Part Two

As a wonderful English comedy group has said, "And now for something completely different." Many readers have complemented me on my writing style in my *Headache Handbook*. I tried to use the same style in Part One of this book. One comment I have heard frequently is that I wrote the way I lectured.

I wanted to have Part Two of this book reflect the individual styles of some of the superb clinicians and professionals with whom I was lucky enough to work. So, I asked the authors of the following chapters to each do it "their way." I wanted each author to write the way they lectured, the way they thought, the way they taught, in the style most complementary to each of them, and not to me.

I hope the reader will experience each chapter as the written voice of an expert clinician and professional. The stylistic differences are similar to those found in the lectures at a symposium.

As I asked, they did it their way.

Foreword

Specialists in a number of different fields wrote the second part of this book. Here you will be able to read the specialists' opinion regarding the various evaluations and treatments for MTBI. You will also have the ability to read a legal perspective, as well as that of several medical specialties.

It has been my privilege to have worked with most of the authors represented here. They are truly experts in their fields, and they are a powerful force in the appropriate treatment of MTBI patients. The authors I have not worked with directly are experts I wish had been close enough for me to have done so.

I feel this will round out the textbook.

11 Mild Traumatic Brain Injury: Treatment Paradigms

Richard S. Goka, M.D.

INTRODUCTION

Mild Traumatic Brain Injury (MTBI) presents in many ways with numerous concurrent symptoms. It has been said that no two patients are alike. The literature is very limited in defining the actual treatment. The variation is strictly due to the level of dysfunction. Alves (1992) said the problems experienced by mildly injured persons are not likely to be qualitatively different from the problems experienced by patients surviving severe injuries: they may simply reflect the degree of intracranial pathologic changes. This author, from his own experience, agrees that mild and moderately injured patients present with similar complaints. However, the degree of complaints might be less in the milder cases.

One will find throughout the literature different ways to treat specific deficits in brain injury without a focus on MTBI. Gronwald suggested, beyond traditional rehabilitation, that reassurance, education, support, and regular monitoring of progress are needed. Specific modalities of treatment of brain-injured patients will be similar, yet the intensity and complexity of treatment will vary depending on the degree of the injury. Furthermore, the National Institutes of Health (NIH) consensus statement in 1998 noted that MTBI is significantly underdiagnosed, and early intervention is often neglected.

Determining what is organic and what is nonorganic (psychological) in the various symptomatologies is very difficult. Factors of emotion, psychosocial dynamics, and true organic lesions can be so intertwined that the clinician cannot make specific determinations as to organic and nonorganic lesions. Alves (1992) noted that there is no answer to how socioeconomic morbidity, social factors and psychosocial processes interacted with physical recovery. Ruffolo (1999) looked at return to work. Her findings of deficits were similar for those who did or did not return to work. She raised the questions of social support intervention, discharge disposition, and type of job as factors that need to be considered. It is best to treat the symptoms knowing that some might not have an organic etiology.

The Mild Brain Injury Committee of the Brain Injury Special Interest Group, American Congress of Rehabilitation Medicine has six areas that are felt to be important in the treatment of MTBI:

0-8493-1955-2/00/$0.00+$.50
© 2000 by CRC Press LLC

1. Etiology/Pathology
2. Preinjury Status
3. Injury/Illness-related
4. Impairments
5. Disability
6. Handicap

The impairments are the actual deficits. The disability and handicap will vary among individuals. A disability is how the impairment affects the individual, i.e., the effect of loss of a digit affects individuals in different ways. For example, the loss of the index finger on the right hand has a different effect if it is the dominant index finger of a laborer versus the nondominant finger of an executive. The handicap is what society makes of the impairment and disability, i.e., the cosmetic consequence will be of greater significance to an executive than to a laborer. The impairments, disability, and handicap must be part of the treatment plan.

As the patient lingers after injury without a diagnosis, symptoms may worsen and frustration, anxiety, and depression can elevate. These psychological factors can and do increase the cognitive impairment. The treatment process needs to minimize the potential exacerbation of those symptoms.

The National Institutes of Health in 1998 presented a consensus statement on Rehabilitation of Traumatic Brain Injury (TBI). Essentially, it stated that there was not enough information, and it encouraged more research. Alternative treatment sites were advocated.

The treatment format and setting with mild traumatic brain injury (MTBI) are strictly dependent on the deficits and how these deficits relate to functional activities at home, work, or school. A majority of patients are not diagnosed in an acute care setting. Most individuals are seen in a physician's or psychologist's office. The key is how the deficits are related to the ability to function.

Once the presumptive diagnosis of MTBI has been confirmed by appropriate measures, a treatment plan can be developed. The symptom complex can be very broad and include other entities such as pain, headaches, dizziness, etc., which should be treated both earlier and simultaneously, if possible. Some of the symptoms, e.g., pain, and the pharmacological management, can impair cognition. The practitioner must keep a close eye on the medications, their interactions, and the potential to alter cognition. On the flip side, if the pain is not adequately controlled, then the individual's ability to concentrate can impair cognitive retraining.

Therefore, it is prudent to develop a close working team, either interdisciplinary or multi-disciplinary, to manage a case of MTBI. Close communication is essential. Generally, it is not prudent to do mono-treatment in the beginning. One discipline usually cannot develop a plan that will be effective. The "bare bones" would be a physician and either a speech-language pathologist or psychologist to work on developing cognitive strategies to overcome the functional problems.

The participation in group therapy sessions with other MTBI patients is helpful to gain an understanding of the disease and limit the frustration of the unknown. However, it can also make a person more disabled. The group leader must keep the individuals on track and minimize potential symptom magnification. Group therapy can also help the caregivers or significant others to gain an understanding of the disease complex.

The treatment of Mild Traumatic Brain Injury can become very complex and needs the expertise of individuals who are knowledgeable and understand how to maximize function in the shortest time. The team members and their roles will be outlined below and in other portions of this text. There is no set formula, number of visits, or duration of treatment that will work for all. The degree of impairment in MTBI is variable, and each patient's treatment must be individualized. Guidelines should be used as guidelines and not viewed as a formula for success.

Concurrent related or unrelated medical problems need to be addressed. Horn and Zasler's "Rehabilitation of Post-Concussive Disorders" outlines the diagnosis and management of many of the related concurrent medical presentations. It is very comprehensive and is a suggested reading.

Periodic reassessment is a must. It has been shown that during treatment or immediately after treatment, no significant change occurs on the neuropsychological testing, however, function has improved. How can this be? One reason could be that the testing was not specific enough for the deficits. This is true especially when testing the nondominant frontal lobe. Another example is a patient who can do specific tasks in an artificially structured environment (clinic), but is unable to perform when presented with the task in the "real world." During treatment, compensatory strategies may have been developed to compensate for an area of a specific deficit. The treatment of these functional deficits must be honed in a real-world situation.

With functional recovery, it is assumed that the altered neuropathway was "reestablished" or a new one was "developed." Therefore, the reassessment should not only include the neuropsychological-cognitive effects, but also how the individual is able to function in the real world.

The goals of treatment are to maximize functional independence and minimize any disability or handicap. A major difficulty in managing these cases is the wide variation of deficits one may encounter in MTBI. Therefore, an overview of the potential impairments, suggestions that have been useful in the past, and the team members are presented.

RECOVERY PATTERN

It is generally accepted that most individuals with a brain insult will undergo a period of spontaneous recovery within the first six months after injury. It is felt that after the period of spontaneous recovery, the residual deficits are permanent. The severity of the deficits will vary in each case. Spontaneous recovery does not indicate that a treatment plan must wait until the residual deficits become permanent. Early intervention can prevent development of dysfunctional scenarios (Kay, 1993). The recovery pattern can be enhanced with specific cognitive treatment.

During the acute phase, the patient gradually becomes aware of a problem(s), e.g., memory or higher processing deficits, and becomes frustrated. This, in turn, can lead to anxiety, depression, frustration, etc. Participation in individual and group therapies helps to minimize the frustration. Sometime the use of antidepressant medication is beneficial. Furthermore, the family is an important part of the team. The family must understand that the problems are real and need to be addressed and provided with assistance. However, the family must further realize that to take over a task is not always the best answer. Careful individual and family counseling will assist in the recovery pattern. Specific therapy should be geared to the functional deficits.

Chronic patients, those with residuals after the period of spontaneous recovery, who have not received treatment, can benefit from a structured multi-, interdisciplinary treatment approach. Since their deficits are felt to be permanent, the approach would be to develop compensatory strategies. Generally, the psychological, psychosocial, and pain behaviors are much more difficult to treat and require a longer time if early intervention has not occurred. Again, compensatory strategies to overcome the functional loss is the best approach.

DEFICITS AND TREATMENT

The literature has many surveys of symptoms. Alves et al., between 1981 and 1984, studied 1151 patients. The most frequent symptoms were headaches (45.8%), dizziness (14.2%), memory problems (13.0%), weakness (10.4%), etc. The major cognitive problems were short-term memory, concentration, and easy distractibility.

The treatment is to reestablish neuropathways or develop compensatory strategies. In essence, it is a type of learning. A simple, yet complex example is learning to ride a bicycle. Riding a bicycle is a complex sensory, motor, and cognitive process. The motor function of pedaling, the sensory function of balance and vision, and the cognitive function of direction in which one goes and avoids obstacles or unsafe areas are all involved. To master the use of a bicycle one must practice. Practice or repetitive stimulation of a specific nature will establish or reestablish learning or memorization within the brain. Repetitive stimulation is how rehabilitation reestablishes function. This is the basic learning process of the brain. Daily repetition of a task will develop the pathway and permanently program or reprogram the brain.

PAIN

Pain must be minimized. The most common pain complaints include cervical strain/sprain or headaches. Horn and Zasler outlined the mechanism of pain and headaches. The headaches are usually myofascial or cervical in origin. Essentially, the brain cannot feel.

The first approach, once a definitive diagnosis is obtained, would be to have a physical therapist work on range of motion and strengthening. A massage to the tight muscles will decrease some of the pain symptoms.

Strengthening the neck muscle will protect the neck and decrease the pain. The physician might opt to perform trigger point injections or more specific facet or epidural blocks, if indicated. Medications are variable. Muscle relaxants and analgesics can help the symptoms, but may also cause some alteration in cognition. Careful titration of any medications is important. The treatment of pain goes far beyond the scope to this article. The reader is referred to the suggested reading and more specific articles and texts that are readily available.

COGNITION

Kay (1993) defined cognitive deficits as objective and subjective. Differentiating the two is very useful in the development of a treatment plan. He noted that objective cognitive deficits are those primary cognitive changes determined directly by damage to the brain, while subjective cognitive deficits are the breakdowns in mental processing that are experienced by the person and manifested on neuropsychological testing. The processing deficits can be caused by both objective deficits due to brain injury or psychological and physical factors.

Treatment of specific cognitive deficits must be individualized. The reader is again referred to the specific literature for said treatment. As noted earlier, the emphasis of treatment is on how the deficits affect function.

PSYCHOLOGICAL

Minimizing subjective cognitive deficits and controlling the anxiety and frustration are simplistic ways of presenting psychological treatment. Counseling is usually best. However, pharmacological intervention might be indicated. Decreasing the depression, anxiety, and frustration will help decrease the subjective intensity of the deficits and pain. Individual and group therapy with the patient and significant other is a must. The significant other plays an important role in the day-to-day dynamic. Gaining an understanding of the problems is usually half the treatment.

SHORT-TERM MEMORY

Short-term memory appears as a major cognitive dysfunction with MTBI and most TBI patients. Calendars, journals, etc. have been useful tools. The use of such allows the patient to have a visual record to refer to. With technology, the use of pocket computers or data-based watches might be alternatives or adjuncts to pencil and notebook. The key is to have the patient prioritize journal events and appointments. The system must be used on a daily basis to become second nature.

DISTRACTIBILITY

Distractibility is more difficult to treat. The best method is to attempt to desensitize the individual as much as possible. Sometimes doing specific treatment in a noisy environment such as a coffee shop or bowling alley is helpful. If the noise level cannot be filtered out, earplugs might help. Either a simple over-the-counter earplug or one made specifically for the patient may be utilized. The custom-made earplugs work better in industry where there is noisy machinery.

If the patient works at an office job and has specific tasks that require extended time or focused concentration, any interruption may be distracting enough to require twice the time to complete the task. A suggestion is to have the patient budget the time and advise his co-workers that he/she is not to be disturbed at specific times. Another suggestion would be to close their door or hang a "Do Not Disturb" sign. Try to determine what the disruptive factors are and either desensitize or alter the specific task or behavior.

FATIGUE

Many patients have complained of fatigue, especially in the early afternoon. During the recovery process this is more than likely the brain saying that it needs to rest. Patients would do best to perform most mental tasks in the morning, when they are fresh. This will minimize the stress of not being able to complete a task in the afternoon. Educating the patient on the simple mechanism of fatigue will greatly improve the patient's ability to adapt.

If patients cannot rearrange their schedules to accommodate morning tasks, then they must understand that it will take them twice as long to complete them when the fatigue begins. They should try to take a break before attempting the mental tasks in the afternoon.

OTHER COMPENSATORY STRATEGIES

The hand-held computer has become a very useful tool. It can be adapted so the information can be downloaded into a personal computer. There are even watches today that can communicate with personal computers.

It amazes this author how much therapists do not know about currently available technology. There are many inexpensive software programs that can assist an individual with an MTBI, let alone the general population. Occupational therapists for years have been dealing with money management and balancing the checkbook. Many noninjured individuals could never balance a checkbook. Today, there is inexpensive checkbook software that does all the work and then some. Therefore, it is useful to have one team member who is familiar with the current computer software and affordable technology.

When possible, samples of actual work that will be required are imperative. The employer knows what is required of the individual to return to the job. Rarely do clinicians have the exact details of what skills are required to return to work. Asking the employer to provide some specific tasks and reviewing these samples enables the patient to work specifically on what will be required to return to the job. If the deficits cannot be overcome, can accommodations or strategies be made? Clinical staff creativity in dealing with redevelopment of skills will enable a patient to return to work.

TEAM MEMBERS AND ROLES

All members of the team need to have an expertise in the treatment of brain injury. MTBI is a subset of brain injury in a milder form. All team members must work together to maximize functional goals in the shortest amount of time.

PHYSICIAN

The primary treating physician should be a specialist who has a good foundation in the treatment of mild traumatic brain injury. This is generally a physiatrist or neurologist. Understanding the complexities and potential sequelae, complications, and psychosocial dynamics are very important to minimize morbidity. Other specialty consultants can be used. Sometimes a psychiatrist with an understanding of the psychopharmacology and traumatic brain injury might be indicated. The primary treating physician should furthermore have an understanding of chronic pain management. He/she might wish to engage the assistance of a pain specialist to perform specific injections if indicated.

The primary treating physician should have a working knowledge of all the medications being prescribed. Drug interaction can delay or compromise recovery. Close communications with all the physicians are essential.

PSYCHOLOGIST

Psychology has become more and more specialized over the past few decades. There are neuropsychologists, behavioral-psychologists, etc., whose doctorate degrees are usually as clinical or educational psychologists.

The neuropsychologist is someone who has some knowledge of functional neuro-anatomy, has had specialty training in psychometric testing, and understands what specific testing may be used to evaluate the various functions of the brain. After an evaluation, the neuro-psychologist should be able to provide the team with more concrete evidence of any cognitive dysfunctions. He/she should be able to assist the team in determining the subjective and objective degree of impairment. However, sometimes clear delineation between subjective and objective impairment is impossible. Again, function and restoration of function is of ultimate importance.

The behavioral psychologist is generally someone trained in behavioral management of patients. Nonproductive behavior can affect treatment and outcome. Generally, nonproductive behavior is less of a problem in MTBI than in more severely impaired TBI survivors.

Psychological counseling should be provided to give patients both some understanding of their impairment(s) and an outlet for frustration. The patient and their significant other need to understand the pathology and use compensatory strategies to overcome or minimize the functional losses. Depending on the particular treatment environment, cognitive retraining can be performed by a psychologist or speech-language pathologist.

SPEECH-LANGUAGE PATHOLOGIST

The speech-language pathologist generally works on areas of speech and language. In MTBI, aphasia is not the rule. However, integrating complex, multistep thinking is generally a problem. The speech-language pathologist will work with the patient in developing compensatory strategies in specific applications. Therapy may need to be daily at first, and then gradually tapered off. Carryover of the tasks is essential, and the patient must continue the work at home.

OCCUPATIONAL THERAPIST

The occupational therapist has great skills with activities of daily living. This goes beyond basic hygiene. There are many activities, especially with community reentry, money management, etc., that can be affected by MTBI. There are occupational therapists who are trained in driving evaluations. Some patients with MTBI should not be driving due to their impairment, and this will need to be assessed.

RECREATIONAL THERAPIST

The recreational therapist has learned how games can enhance physical mobility, strength, and endurance. Furthermore, some of these games can enhance eye-hand coordination, memory, and mental processing. Just think how complex some simple games are and you will realize the amount of physical and mental work needed. Often, in close conjunction with the occupational therapist, the recreational therapist will perform community reentry tasks, e.g., shopping, transportation, etc.

PHYSICAL THERAPIST

The physical therapist has an understanding of the mobility, muscle functions, and treatment of soft tissue pain problems. Headaches and neck pain are common with MTBI. Concurrent treatment to decrease the pain and increase mobility and strength, as well as lessen balance problems, is usually needed with MTBI.

FAMILY AND EMPLOYER

One must include the family and employer. The family spends greater than 50% of the day with the patient. The family needs to be the coach and mentor of their loved one. Family dynamics must be productive. A family member should be chosen who will assist the patient and encourage the patient to continue the compensatory strategies.

The employer is needed to get the person back to their usual and customary work. A sympathetic employer will provide work samples and gradually reintegrate the patient into his/her job. Some accommodations might need to be made on the job, therefore, a close relationship with the employer is very productive.

The treatment team needs to be made up of experts. Training and experience lead to better outcomes. Working closely in a multi- or interdisciplinary fashion enhances communication and program planning. Regular team meetings help to foster good communication.

TREATMENT SETTING

The rehabilitation hospital has been the "cornerstone" of treatment for individuals with brain injury. However, post acute rehabilitation clinics are well recognized as alternative settings. The community offers many good alternatives and must be utilized to simulate the real world. The therapist should have the ability to perform the therapy wherever it can help the patient.

If one can actually recreate the environment in which the patient must function, this maximizes the therapy. An example would be noise as a distraction on one's job. If a patient works in a factory that is noisy, and the patient is unable to cognitively filter out the noise to perform tasks of the job, then the patient cannot return to his/her regular employment. Once the ability to concentrate with some distraction is overcome, the next step would be to gradually simulate the noise as a distraction. First, by using public places such as a restaurant with many conversations; then try a bowling alley with the noise of the machines. The ultimate place is the factory itself.

FUNCTIONAL GOALS

Once each team member has had the opportunity to assess the patient, it is best to have a discussion to determine what deficits are apparent and how best to approach each area. The objective should be to return the patient to his premorbid level of function, or at least as close as possible. This is generally possible with MTBI. The goals need to be realistic and practical. Obtaining preinjury information on function is very important. An example would be budget and check writing. Some patients never mastered this task; someone else always did it. In that case, it may not be practical to work on budgeting and check writing.

OUTCOME MEASUREMENT

Justification of rehabilitation has been accountable for many years. The Commission on Accreditation of Rehabilitation Facilities (CARF) established program evaluation as an accreditation criterion. More recently, payers have requested outcome measurements to justify or deny payment. It is imperative that some systems are developed with the treatment of MTBI. Unfortunately, when treatment is not performed at a facility, this usually does not occur. The author would suggest that the Disability Rating Scale by Rappaport and the Glasgow Outcome Scale by Jennett and Teasdale be looked at. The author further encourages that the Model System data bank develop some tracking system for outcome with the MTBI patients.

SUMMARY

The review of the literature is limited in specific articles for the treatment of MTBI. As Alves indicated, the symptoms are similar in most brain injuries, only the magnitude is different. Therefore, a reading list has been attached to this chapter to provide resources. One of the most comprehensive reference lists is on the National Institute of Health's website. There, one can access the consensus statement and find the reference list.

The treatment of mild traumatic brain injury is an extension of brain injury rehabilitation. The outcome is dependent on many variables. Concurrent problems, such as pain and headache, are common in this patient population. The clinicians must have expertise in the treatment to achieve reasonable outcomes in a minimal time frame. Expertise is gained by experience. The treatment plan must be realistic with the ultimate goal of enhancing function.

REFERENCES

Alves, WM, et al., Understanding posttraumatic symptoms are minor head injury, *J. Head Trauma Rehab.*, 1:2, 1986.

Alves, WM, Natural History of Post-Concussive Signs and Symptoms, *Phys. Med. Rehabil., State of the Art Reviews*, 6(1):21-32, 1992.

Gronwald, DMA, Rehabilitation programs for patients with mild head injury: components, problems, and evaluation, *J. Head Trauma Rehab.*, 1:53, 1986.

Horn, LJ, Zasler, ND, Eds., *Rehabilitation of Post-Concussive Disorders: State of the Art Reviews, Physical Medicine and Rehabilitation*, Vol. 6:1, Hanley and Belfus, Philadelphia, 1992.

Horn, LJ, Post-Concussive Headache, Horn, LJ, Zasler, ND, Eds., *Rehabilitation of Post-Concussive Disorders: State of the Art Reviews, Physical Medicine and Rehabilitation*, Vol. 6:1, Hanley and Belfus, Philadelphia, 1992.

Jennet, B, Teasdale, G, Glasgow Outcome Scale, *Management of Head Injuries*, Contemporary Neurology Series, F.A. Davis, Philadelphia, 1981.

Kay, T, Neuropsychological treatment of mild traumatic brain injury, *J. Head Trauma Rehab.*, 8:3, 1993.

Rappaport, M, et al., Disability rating scale for severe head trauma: coma to community, *Arch. Phys. Med. Rehabil.*, 63:118, 1982.

Rappaport, M, et al., Head injury outcome up to ten years later, *Arch. Phys. Med. Rehab.*, 70:885, 1989.

Ruffolo, CF, et al., Mild traumatic brain injury from motor vehicle accidents: factors associated with return to work, *Arch. Phys. Med. Rehab.*, 80:392, 1999.

Traumatic Brain Injury, Model Systems, Grants by the U.S. Dept of Education, National Institute of Rehabilitation Research (NIDRR), Washington, D.C.

Trudel, PH, Ed., Moving Ahead, Interdisciplinary Special Interest Group, *Am. Congress of Rehabilitation Medicine*, 12:3, 1998.

Zasler, ND, Neuromedical Diagnosis and Management of Post-concussive Disorders. Horn, LJ, Zasler, ND, Eds., *Rehabilitation of Post-Concussive Disorders: State of the Art Reviews, Physical Medicine and Rehabilitation*, Vol. 6:1, Hanley and Belfus, Philadelphia, 1992.

SUGGESTED READING

Journal: *Brain Injury*; Taylor and Francis.

Journal: *Rehabilitation of Traumatic Brain Injury*; Aspen Publishers

Minor Head Injury; Vol. 1:2, 1986

Mild Traumatic Brain Injury; Vol. 8:3, 1993

Posttraumatic Headaches; Vol. 14:1, 1999.

Goka, RS, Arakaki, AH, Centers of Excellence, Choosing the Appropriate Rehabilitation Center, *Journal of Insurance Medicine*, Vol. 23:1, 1991.

Hoff, JT, Anderson, TE, Cole, TM, Eds., *Mild to Moderate Head Trauma*, Blackwell Scientific, Boston, 1989.

Horn, LJ, Cope, DN, Eds., Traumatic Brain Injury, *State of the Art Review: Physical Medicine and Rehab.*, Vol. 3:1, Feb. 1989.

Horn, LJ, Cope, DN, Eds., Rehab. of Post-Concussive Disorders, *State of the Art Review: Physical Medicine and Rehab.*, Vol. 6:1, Feb. 1992.

Levin, HS, et al., *Neurobehavioral Consequences of Closed Head Injury*, Oxford University Press, New York, 1982.

Levin, HS, et al., *Mild Head Injury*, Oxford University Press, New York, 1989.

National Institute on Health; Consensus Statement on the Traumatic Brain Injury, NIH, 1998. (Website: consensus.NIH.Gov.).

Rosenthal, et.al., *Rehabilitation of the Adult and Child with Traumatic Brain Injury*, 3rd ed., FA Davis, Philadelphia, 1999.

12 The Physical Therapy Evaluation

Denise Baugh, PT

A patient seen in physical therapy with a minor acquired traumatic brain injury can be a challenge for even the seasoned physical therapist. Very often patients are referred to physical therapy by the physician after a motor vehicle accident or an injury on the job. Depending on the type of physician, the patient may only have a diagnosis of cervical sprain/strain and/or headache. Physicians treat patients based on their specialty and/or background.[1] This often poses a challenge for those patients who have minor traumatic head injuries that are undiagnosed.

These patients may present with treatable physical therapy issues; however, they have additional underlying difficulties that effect the outcome of physical therapy. Much has been written about posttraumatic headache following brain injury, but consistent treatment has not been found.[2-5] This chapter will look at the common findings of patients who have been sent to physical therapy with possible minor traumatic brain injury, and recommendations for treatment. The overall treatment must be based on the findings in physical therapy and identified needs for referral. It is also important that the physical therapist know how to identify possible signs of a brain injury and how to work appropriately with these patients. It is the responsibility of the physical therapist to complete an appropriate evaluation and treatment plan as well as to identify the need for additional referrals. The physical therapist identifies not only the physical limitations but also any complicating factors, and in the case of brain injury, any referrals to additional health care providers.

INITIAL EVALUATION

As with any patient seen in physical therapy, treatment cannot commence without the proper evaluation to address areas of dysfunction; this sets the groundwork for the treatment that will follow. Physical therapy evaluation and treatment should follow the guidelines published by the APTA in the *Guide to Physical Therapist Practice*.[6-8] For simplicity, this will follow the medical directed approach using a SOAP format.[9]

SUBJECTIVE

The initial interaction with the patient allows the therapist to acquire pertinent information from the patient and, if needed, from family members or other caretakers. As with other areas of medicine, patient confidentiality is important and the

0-8493-1955-2/00/$0.00+$.50
© 2000 by CRC Press LLC

patient must give permission for the therapist to talk to caregivers. When dealing with MTBI caregivers, you should have important information about how the patient is functioning at home. Very often, patients with brain injury underreport their difficulties.[10,11] It is therefore important, if the therapist suspects the patient's report is not complete, that caregivers be contacted. It is also very important to address pain and the patient's perception of difficulties with home, work, and leisure activities, as well as difficulties with positional tolerance, sleeping, or driving. The therapist needs to direct the questions toward a patient's ability to complete tasks such as cooking, cleaning, bathing, self-feeding, and shopping. In addition, it is of great importance for the therapist to address issues of interaction with other people such as conversation, memory, communication skills, money management, and interaction with family and coworkers. This information will help the therapist to not only have an idea about possible brain injury, but to also address the need for immediate referral.

Many therapists choose to use the mini-mental status test.[12] It should be noted at this time that patients who have a minor TBI might demonstrate or report impairment in one of the following areas: money management, memory, or interaction with others. In addition, what is often seen clinically is that these patients will perservate on pain or one area of their life in dysfunction. This subjective evaluation can be divided in to the following categories:

1. History of accident. This includes the date of injury, a brief summary of what happened, and any current or previous treatment for this injury. Also important are whether the symptoms are changing, and if any previous treatment has helped.

2. Previous medical history. This should include any previous injuries to the same area or with similar pain, as well as any preexisting medical conditions.

3. Diagnostic tests. These will include any information the patient knows about results of diagnostic tests, or results forwarded to the therapist from a physician or radiologist.

4. Medications. These include any current medications, either from this injury or for other medical problems.

5. Location and severity of pain. This includes description, severity, and location of pain, and anything that makes the pain better or worse. Pain levels should be recorded using a measurable scale: a 0-10 scale, or a 0-100 scale and/or a visual analogue scale. It may often be helpful for a therapist to use the McGill Pain Questionnaire.[13]

6. Positional tolerance. This should include positions that make pain better or worse, and the length of time the patient is able to maintain one position, sitting, standing, or walking, especially those needed for work. In addition, this should include sleeping position and ability to sleep, as many patients with brain injury report insomnia.[14] Also included in this area should be driving, including positions of comfort or discomfort.

7. Functional difficulty. This includes activities of daily living, leisure activities, working outside the home, and interaction with family, friends, and coworkers.
8. Additional complaints of patient or areas the therapist feels are important for this evaluation.

OBJECTIVE

This is the part of the evaluation where the therapist uses specific measures to address the above concerns and any treatable physical therapy diagnosis, following physical therapy guidelines.[6-8]

Inspection

Look at posture sitting and standing, looking for any significant abnormality. Also look at how the patient holds his/her arms and neck, and weight bearing. It is also important to look for any scars or open wounds.

Medical Function

Look at vital signs including respiration, pulse, and blood pressure to establish baseline measurements. These may also present information needed for additional referrals.

Range of Motion

Active and passive range measured with goniometer or inclinometer. Range of motion should address all locations where the patient complains of pain or difficulties. If a head injury is suspected, it is important to look at cervical range of motion, even if the patient is not complaining of cervical pain. When measuring range of motion it is important to attempt to get the patient to start in a neutral position.[15] Movement must also be noted for not only range, but also for quality of movement. One additional area that should be addressed is the temporal mandibular joint, especially if the patient was involved in a motor vehicle accident. Temporal mandibular joint dysfunction has been noted as a contributor to posttraumatic headache.[16]

Specific Joint Function

This will address all joints at which a patient complains of pain, as well as those proximal to the pain. This may be included with active and passive range of motion, with the addition of resistive pressure, compression/distraction, and mobility testing. There are various techniques to address joint mobility; these are dependent on the joint and the training of the therapist, but all look at the mobility of the joint.[17-19]

Neurological

Testing includes reflexes/tone, upper motor neuron signs, motor function (looking at key muscles), sensation, and balance testing. Most important for these patients are motor function, sensation, and balance.

Motor

Function is assessed with the use of manual muscle testing.[20, 21] In addition to looking at overall strength you must also look for nerve root involvement with the use of key muscle and break-way testing.[22]

Sensory

This testing should include addressing any complaints that the patient has, specifically complaints of numbness and tingling or lack of control of the hands. Sensory testing can include pinprick, sharp/dull, light touch, hot/cold, and proprioception. In addressing sensory dysfunction, it is necessary to look at dematomal and myotomal patterns in the appropriate extremities. However, impaired sensation may not follow a set pattern. It is also important to look at cranial nerve function. In addition, it may also be necessary to complete the upper limb tension tests.

Balance

Testing includes, but is not limited to, single limb and double limb stance with eyes open and closed, "Foam and Dome" testing, Rhomberg, and heel/toe gait.[17,23] For facilities that have advanced moving platforms, balance assessment on these apparati is appropriate.

Palpation

It is very important to address areas of pain as well as muscular tightness to reveal myofascial dysfunction and abnormal bony alignment. This will address hypertonic muscle versus muscle spasm. Palpation can also help identify areas of joint dysfunction based on the noted muscles. It is important during palpation to request feedback from the patient as to areas of pain or discomfort.

Gait

Address the patient's ambulatory status with and without appropriate assistive devices. Based on the patient's level of pain, assistive devices may be necessary early in treatment.

Special Tests

Depending on the facility, this may include the use of isokinetic machines and work assessment skills.

ASSESSMENT

As with every initial evaluation, the findings must be assessed to set goals. It is in this part of the evaluation that the therapist can take what is reported by the patient in the subjective, compare it with objective findings, and develop an appropriate list of problems and goals. The therapist must set appropriate functional goals using the objective findings along with the patient goals, and these need to be measurable. One of the most important goals to address in physical therapy is pain control. This is very important in the presence of brain injury as has been previously mentioned. If a patient has high levels of pain, testing for brain injury will not be accurate.[2,3,25,26]

PLAN

This is the area of the initial evaluation to address what will be accomplished in physical therapy, how this will be completed, and in what time frame. It is also important to address any possible referrals that the patient may need during physical therapy or after including specialist medical doctors; temporal mandibular joint specialists; ear, nose, and throat physicians; occupational therapists; speech therapists; and psychologists.

COMMON FINDINGS

Some of the most common physical therapy findings include pain, decreased range of motion and joint function, impaired sensation, decreased strength, abnormal balance, difficulties completing activities of daily living at home and work, myofascial dysfunction, and decreased endurance.

Pain is generally the reason why patients are referred to physical therapy. Headache pain is the most common, especially after a motor vehicle accident and with previous head injuries.[27] These are often described as continuous and can vary from a pounding throbbing to a constant ache. Many times these patients report that nothing will change the pain. It can get worse, especially if they are reminded of the initial injury. However, if the patient is distracted and is not thinking about the pain, there may be an increase in function. Pain is often what patients monitor to determine if they are getting better. It is very common for patients to be referred to physical therapy for chronic pain. The physical therapist must remember that just because the patient has chronic pain, typically of unknown or questionable etiology, that does not mean that their pain is not real.[2,5,11,25,27,32] It is important that these patients are seen by the appropriate caregivers, and treatment by a multidisciplinary team is important.[1] There is often significant muscular tightness resulting in myofascial pain.

Decreased range of motion is most often seen cervically, but may also be present in the upper extremity, the thoracic and lumbar regions, and the TMJ. In addition, abnormal movement at facet joints primarily presents as a hypomobility limited by pain. Joint limitation may be hyper- or hypomobile, and very often is in the presence of pain. After a motor vehicle accident, dysfunction at the carpometacarpal joint of the first digit is frequently seen.

Sensation is primarily impaired, not absent, and this may be isolated to one upper extremity. This can be proximal but is most often seen distally, and may mimic carpal tunnel or thoracic outlet syndrome. However, additional nerve involvement should not be overlooked. Rarely are nerve roots involved, but there may be some disc involvement, thus sensory testing does not generally show dermatomal or myotomal patterns.

Although some patients have a noticeable decrease in strength, this may be secondary to pain. It is generally not lack of strength that keeps a patient from completing activities of daily living (ADLs).

Balance difficulties seen in patients with a severe brain injury are more obvious or significant than those seen in patients with mild traumatic brain injury.[23] MTBI patients may report occasionally running into things or needing to support themselves by holding onto a wall or furniture. Very rarely does the patient have reports of falling or loss of balance. However, those MTBI patients who complain of dizziness have more difficulties with balance. This is due to possible damage to the inner ear, especially the vestibular system, and referral is necessary for further evaluation.

The limitations in ADLs are probably most significant to the patient. They often describe limitations in all activities, however, they may still be able to maintain their homes. Very often they do not want to rely on someone else to help, and so do not admit to problems. Some of the areas of reported difficulty are vacuuming, cleaning, and outside activities, especially with upper extremity involvement on the dominant side. Often the patient will be having more difficulties than they realize; however, they do not typically think about them until such problems are addressed in physical therapy. Not only are physical limitations affecting ADLs but cognition also plays a role. This is not addressed specifically in physical therapy except for referral to other therapies during or after discharge. It is important to be aware of these findings as these play a role in the development of home exercise programs outside of formal treatment. MTBI patients may have great success if they have support from friends and family who are aware of their difficulties.

Myofascial dysfunctions are generally consistent with areas of pain. These are evaluated with various manual tools and represent the area where physical therapy is most effective with treatment. These can include, but are not limited to, trigger points, muscle tightness, hypertonic muscle, muscle spasm, and shortened muscles.[19,23,28,34]

Most patients report a decrease in activity levels after an accident. Some of them report a decrease in activity levels at home or at work, and others just report an overall decrease in endurance. This can often be the underlying factor for the need for an additional referral to a psychologist to address such pertinent issues.

RECOMMENDED TREATMENTS

Although each patient will be different, the same general guidelines apply for treatment. Treatment must begin with controlling pain. As previously mentioned, patients often use pain as the indication of whether they are getting better with treatment. It is well documented that pain can affect results of cognitive testing.[2-4,25,26] During the course of physical therapy, many other disciplines may be involved in the patient's treatment. It is important that all caregivers work together for the patient's well-being. As noted during the initial evaluation, these patients may need referrals to additional physicians, especially a neurologist if a brain injury is suspected. In addition, the physical therapist will need to work closely with any psychologist or counselor the patient is seeing. Not only are brain-injured patients seen in psychology for cognitive difficulties, they also work through psychological difficulties including depression, anxiety, and posttraumatic stress disorder. These patients also respond very well to the use of biofeedback with electromyographic (EMG) monitoring.[16] Biofeedback and physical therapy work together very well with patients who present with myofascial difficulties. Additional treatment may include brain injury rehabilitation with neuropsychology, speech therapy, and occupational therapy. In a multidisciplinary setting, the interaction between staff allows this to be an easy and contiguous process.

As previously stated, physical therapy's main goal, initially, is pain control so that the extent of the possible brain injury can be assessed. As with any physical therapy patient, treatment is dependent on what is found in the evaluation and what is addressed as problems in the assessment. Although most of these patients present with myofascial pain and posttraumatic headache, additional difficulties are often noted. Each patient must be addressed as a unique individual and treatment must be individualized.

Patients may have significant pain. Whether it is chronic or acute, they still need to have it reduced. One of the easiest ways to decrease pain is through the use of modalities. Depending on the facility as well as the patient, different forms of electrical stimulation, ultrasound, or hot/cold may be employed.

Electrical stimulation can include, but is not limited to, interferential current, transcutaneous electrical nerve stimulation (TENS), bipolar/biphasic electrical stimulation, and Russian current.[30] Electrical stimulation may also be combined with ultrasound for its deep heat properties, or with the use of topical hot/cold packs. Ultra high frequency Cortical Electrical Stimulation(CES) has been a valuable tool for headache control. When the level of serotonin is increased, the pain from the headache decreases.[31] CES is used as an adjunct to physical therapy hands-on treatment and may also be appropriate for home use.

Ultrasound is used as a deep heat for muscle relaxation and pain control, however, if the patient demonstrates signs of inflammation, ultrasound may be used in a pulsed setting for anti-inflammatory control.[33]

In addition to modalities, therapists need to use manual techniques to control pain. These can include oscillatory techniques, massage, myofacial release, and manual traction. As the patient enters the subacute and chronic phase of rehabilitation, additional manual techniques are appropriate. There are numerous forms of manual therapy that physical therapists can be trained to use. Some of the most common types of techniques include muscle energy, myofascial release, strain-counterstrain, soft tissue mobilization, joint mobilization, and trigger point therapy.[17,19,34] It is very important that each patient be evaluated for which techniques will work best for them. This is based not only on the patient's symptoms, location of pain, muscle tightness, and decreased range of motion, but also on those techniques that the therapist is most competent in performing. Once a technique is used, the results must be evaluated for change in pain and range of motion. Again, the therapist is reminded that patients with brain injuries may not have significant decrease in reports of pain levels, even if muscle tightness has decreased and range of motion has increased.

Treatment must also address any joint dysfunction present. Studies have shown that patients with headaches, especially those with mild traumatic brain injury, have cervical dysfunction. The upper cervical spine refers directly to the cranium so the most common dysfunctions occur at the occiput and C1, and C1 and C2.[2,34,35] Lower cervical dysfunction may also be present, but is not the cause of the resultant headache. This, as well as any dysfunction in the upper extremity, must be addressed. Most commonly used techniques of joint mobilization include oscillations or prolonged stretch.

Once pain has decreased and the joints are cleared, the motor and sensory function must be reevaluated. Sensory dysfunction often continues as many of these patients also present with symptoms of thoracic outlet syndrome. In order to resolve this, the ribs as well as the scalenes must be cleared. These may be treated with the previously noted manual therapy techniques.

Important to any treatment program is the use of a home program. This must start from the first day for patient involvement in care. Initially, this may be isometric exercises which can then progress to range of motion and strengthening. The therapist must remember that if the patient is given too many exercises, they will not complete them. Also, these must be exercises that are easy to complete and the patient must have written instructions so that they can remember them at home. In addition, with brain-injured patients, the therapist will need to review the exercises often. Strengthening exercises should not be added until there has been a significant decrease in pain and/or a noticeable increase in range of motion. Exercise has been shown to improve function as well as depression.[36] Especially important in brain injury patients is the need to restore function as well as minimize any side-effects of chronic pain.

One form of manual therapy that is often overlooked is addressing trigger points. This can be accomplished with the use of massage or with spray and stretch, addressing specific muscles and trigger-point injections. Injections are only possible with close interaction with the physician, again showing the importance of a multidisciplinary team approach for treatment. Reference for appropriate injections can be found using Travell and Simmons *Myofascial Pain and Dysfunction: The Trigger Point Manual.*[37]

As with any physical therapy visit, it is important to record progress. Pain is often a key indicator if treatment techniques are effective from day to day and also after daily treatment. Whichever method of pain measurement is employed, it must be used consistently before and after every treatment.

Once a decrease in pain has been established, other areas of dysfunction noted in the initial evaluation can be addressed. This is the time in which gait and balance are addressed. If the patient is falling over initially, a cane and necessary gait training may be initiated at the start of treatment. It is after pain is decreased that more specific balance activities will be addressed. Using initial testing results will determine what is appropriate for treatment. Testing techniques including gait, heel-to-toe, single and double limb support, vision challenged and unchallenged — as well as the use of the foam and dome technique — make good treatment regimes. Patients may have a difficult time with the foam and dome as it is a significant challenge and they may become very unsteady. This makes an important aspect of a home program: to gradually increase the time of static stance. Gait strategies may include heel-to-toe gait, walking on toes, walking on heels, grapevine stepping, balance beam walking, walking outside, up and down stairs, and walking forward and backward. Patients must first realize they can accomplish easy tasks before more challenging ones are added to treatment.

If the patient is not seeing occupational therapy (OT) at this time, or if OT is focusing on cognitive rehabilitation, several additional areas of treatment are pertinent for independent patient functioning. These include tasks that the patient needs to do to return to work as well as function at home. It is notable that in some facilities only an OT will work on these skills; however, no matter who works on them, they need to be addressed during treatment. Home skills can be assessed in the clinic or with a home visit, depending on how impaired the patient presents. Specific areas that may need to be addressed may include cooking, cleaning, dressing, and bathing. Very often the patient just needs education to complete the tasks with minimal pain and the difficulty goes away. One area in the work environment that is very important is the ergonomic design of workstations. Although this can be accomplished in the clinic, brain-injured patients may have a difficult time transferring skills from the clinic to the work site. If the patient is not returning to work for a while, then a temporary setting may be established in the clinic or a nearby established workstation.

If the patient is working, it is important to address proper body mechanics and posture at work to eliminate any further pain or exacerbation of symptoms. These may be addressed with education on adjustments to current work settings, as well as by working with the employer to make additional adaptations.

In addition, sleeping and driving positions need to be explored. Patients generally do well with education for modified positions or the use of pillows or available postural supports.

FOLLOW-UP

Follow-up with these patients is very important, even if they are discharged from physical therapy without pain. Most of these patients will have a home exercise program that may need to be reviewed or modified. Once pain is decreased and appropriate cognitive function can be tested, they will continue with brain injury treatment.[16,25] Research shows that if these patients receive appropriate treatment they have a better chance to return to work.[32] Coordination with the brain injury treatment team is important. Those exercises the patients received as part of physical therapy treatment will need to be incorporated into the cognitive training, such as the use of a day planner. In addition, follow-up may be necessary to progress the patient to a health club or recreation center for furthering their exercise regime.

FINAL THOUGHTS

It is the evaluation and treatment of the physical therapy problems that improves the MTBI patient's function. It has been shown that these patients will get better; however, treatment with MTBI patients may take longer than a therapist would expect, and this should not be a reason for doubting the patient's difficulties, or doubting your (the therapist's) activities.[26]

REFERENCES

1. Zasler, ND, Posttraumatic headache: caveats and controversies, *J. Head Trauma Rehab.*, 14:1, 1999.
2. Uomoto, JM, Esselman, PC, Traumatic brain injury and chronic pain: differential types and rates by head injury severity, *Arch. Phys. Med. Rehabil.*, 74:61, 1993.
3. Lahz, S, Bryand, RA, Incidence of chronic pain following traumatic brain injury, *Arch. Phys. Med. Rehabil.*, 77:889, 1996.
4. Katz, RT, Deluca, J, Sequelae of minor traumatic brain injury, *Am. Fam. Phys.*, 46:1491, 1992.
5. Cope, DN, Effectiveness of traumatic brain injury rehabilitation: a review, *Brain Injury*, 9:649, 1995.
6. Guide to physical therapy practice, Part One: A description of patient/client management, *Physical Therapy*, 77:1177, 1997.
7. Guide to physical therapy practice, Part Two: Preferred practice patterns. *Physical Therapy*, 77:1229, 1997.
8. Magee, DJ, *Orthopedic Physical Assessment*, WB Saunders, Philadelphia, PA, 1992.
9. Lee, G, Fraser, SS, Ed nursing SOAP Notes, *J. Emerg. Nurs.*, 7:216, 1981.
10. Sbordone, RJ, Sepranian, GD, Ruf, RM, Are the subjective complaints of traumatically brain injured patients reliable? *Brain Injury*, 12:525, 1998.
11. Hillier, SL, Metzer, J, Awareness and perception of outcomes after traumatic brain injury, *Brain Injury*, 11:525, 1997.
12. Schwamm, LH, Van Dyke, C, Kiernan, RJ, et al., The neurobehavioral cognitive status examination: Comparison with the cognitive capacity screening examination and the mini-mental state examination in a neurosurgical population, *Ann. Intern. Med.*, 107:486, 1987.
13. Melzack, R, The McGill pain questionnaire: major properties and scoring methods, *Pain*, 1:277, 1975.
14. Beetar, JT, Guilmette, TJ, Sparadeo, FR, Sleep and pain complaints in symptomatic traumatic brain injury and neurological populations, *Arch. Phys. Med. Rehabil.*, 77:1298, 1996.
15. Norkin, CC, White, DJ, *Measurement of Joint Motion: Goniometry*, FA Davis, Philadelphia, PA, 1985.
16. Martelli, MF, Grayson, RL, Zasler, ND, Posttraumatic headache: neuropsychological and psychological effects and treatment implications, *J. Head Trauma Rehabil.*, 14:49, 1999.
17. Scully, RM, Barnes, MR, *Physical Therapy*, JB Lippincott, Philadelphia, PA, 1989.
18. Greenman, PE, *Principles of Manual Medicine*, Williams and Wilkins, Baltimore, MD, 1989.

19. Basmajian, JV, Nyberg, R, Eds., *Rational Manual Therapies*, Williams and Wilkins, Baltimore, MD, 1993.

20. Kendal, FP, McCreary, EK, *Muscle Testing and Function,* 3rd Ed., Williams and Wilkins, Baltimore, MD, 1983.

21. Daniels, L, Worthingham, C, *Muscle Testing Techniques of Manual Exam*, WB Saunders, Philadelphia, PA, 1980.

22. Class notes from: Level 1- Differential Diagnosis North American Institute of Orthopaedic Manual Therapy. November 1, 1995.

23. Geurts, AC, Ribbers, GM, Knoop, JA, van Linbeek, J, Identification of static and dynamic postural instability following traumatic brain injury, *Arch. Phys. Med. Rehabil.*, 77:639, 1996.

24. Davidoff, RA, Trigger points and myofascial pain: toward understanding how they affect headaches, *Cephalalgia*, 18:436, 1998.

25. Anderson, JM, Kaplan, MS, Felsenthal, G, Brain injury obscured by chronic pain: A preliminary report, *Arch. Phys. Med. Rehabil.*, 71:703, 1990.

26. Andery, MT, Creve, N, Ganzel, K, Traumatic brain injury/chronic pain syndrome: a case comparison study, *Clin. J. Pain*, 13:244, 1997.

27. Rimel, RW, Giordani, B, Barth, JT, et al., Disability caused by minor head injury, *Neurosurgery*, 9:221, 1981.

28. Packard, RC, Epidemiology and pathogenesis of posttraumatic headache, *J. Head Trauma Rehabil.*, 14:9, 1999.

29. Gordon, WA, Brown, M, Sliwinski, M, et al., The enigma of "hidden" traumatic brain injury, *J. Head Trauma Rehabil.*, 13:39, 1998.

30. Nelson, RM, Currier, DP, *Clinical Electrotherapy*, 2nd Ed., Appleton and Lange, East Norwalk, Connecticut, 1991.

31. Shealy, CN, Cady, RK, Wilkie, RG, et al., Depression: a diagnostic, neurochemical profile and therapy with cranial electrical stimulation (CES), *J. Neurological Orthopedic Med. Surg.*, 10:301, 1989.

32. Deadorff, WW, Comprehensive multidisciplinary treatment of chronic pain: a follow-up study of treated and non-treated groups, *Pain*, 45:35, 1991.

33. Gam, AN, Warming, S, Larsen, LH, Treatment of myofascial trigger points with ultrasound combined with massage and exercise: a randomized controlled trial, *Pain*, 77:73, 1998.

34. Bell, KR, Kraus, EE, Zasler, ND, Medical management of posttraumatic headaches: Pharmacological and physical treatment, *J. Head Trauma Rehabil.*, 14:34, 1999.

35. Travealen, J, Jull, G, Atkinson, L, Cervical musculoskeletal dysfunction in post-concussion headache, *Cephalalgia*, 14:273, 1994.

36. Nordin, M, Campello, M, Physical therapy: exercises and the modalities: when, what, why, *Neurologic Clinics*, 17:75, 1999.

37. Travel, JG, Simons, DG, *Myofascial Pain and Dysfunction: The Trigger Point Manual*, Williams and Wilkins, Baltimore, MD, 1983.

38. Hellerstein, LF, Freed, S, Maples, WC, Vision profile of patients with mild brain injury, *J. AM. Optometric. Assoc.*, 66:634, 1995.

13 Acquired Brain Injury and the Speech-Language Pathologist: A Primer for the SLP Entering the Brain Injury Industry

Pamela A. Law, CBIS/CI-CE, CCC-SLP

INTRODUCTION

Each year there are 2 million brain injuries (BI) in the United States as a result of motor vehicle accidents (MVA) falls, firearms, and sports and recreational injuries.

- 500,000 of these persons require hospitalization.
- 90,000 have some form of permanent disability.
- Seventy percent of these brain injuries are to persons between the ages of 17 and 28.[1]
- Many persons with brain injuries remain in rehabilitation of some form for three to five years.[2]

Survivors of severe brain injuries increased from more than 20% in the 1970s to more than 60% in the 1990s.[3] With a life expectancy near that of noninjured individuals, persons surviving severe brain injuries require individually tailored services to address the lifelong effects of BI. The challenge of the BI industry is to provide comprehensive, care-coordinated services tailored to meet the lifelong needs of persons with brain injuries and their families through high-quality, cost-effective service delivery.

Cost-effective treatment can be facilitated through the development of a coordinated continuum of care that begins with timely identification of BI and promotes progression through treatment sites. Enhancement of communication among team members and sites may facilitate successful transitions.

One group addressing the quality of BI services is the American Academy of Certification for Brain Injury Specialists (AACBIS). AACBIS convened a Consensus

Conference in 1993 to enhance the recognition of programs that demonstrate high standards in service delivery to persons with brain injuries and their families. AACBIS has developed a voluntary certification program designed to enhance quality service delivery by assisting programs in retaining specially trained staff through the promotion of competency-based training standards. AACBIS began its voluntary certification program with providers of postacute brain injury services, primarily because of dramatic growth in this segment of the industry. In 1980 there were fewer than 12 postacute brain injury programs nationwide. There are now more than 700. These programs are designed to assess the ability of persons with brain injuries to live independently in home communities, and to promote long-term living alternatives. However, BI programs remain largely unregulated in their provision of therapy in real-world settings.[4]

The lead of AACBIS is augmented by the National Institutes of Health, which, in October 1998, convened a Consensus Development Conference on Rehabilitation of Persons with Traumatic Brain Injuries (TBI) as a result of the TBI Act (1996). Practice recommendations made as a result of this consensus conference that are pertinent to this chapter's discussion of approaches to BI rehabilitation include:

- Interdisciplinary, comprehensive rehabilitation programs are recommended for the treatment of persons with moderate-to-severe brain injuries.
- Services prescribed should match identified functional strengths and limitations of the person with brain injury, and should be modified as necessary.
- Cognitive and behavioral assessments and treatment should be included in comprehensive programming for the person with brain injury.
- Rehabilitation programs should seek to include the input of the person with brain injury and his/her family in the development of interdisciplinary treatment plans, and should promote access to needed services across stages of recovery.
- Interdisciplinary programs should provide for the support and education of families and communities across stages of recovery.
- Programs should include community-based, nonmedical services as part of their continuum.[5]

TERMINOLOGY

One of the first challenges found by newcomers to the BI industry is the fact that BI terminology "remains imprecise and often unclear."[6] For purposes of this chapter, the terminology will be:

ACQUIRED BRAIN INJURY (ABI)

This refers to "an acquired injury to the brain caused by an external physical force, resulting in total or partial functional disability or psychosocial impairment or both." Prior terms include traumatic brain injury (TBI) and head injury (HI), with specification as to open head injury (OHI) or closed head injury (CHI). It is not uncommon to see the terminology of postconcussive syndrome (PCS) used for mild traumatic brain injury (MTBI).

COMMUNITIES

This refers to the place of residence prior to injury and the roles and supports found therein. Communities include primary residence (home, apartment, etc.), family, friends, church/synagogue, and other social outlets that connect the person with brain injury to meaningful life activities.

PERSONS WITH BRAIN INJURIES AND SURVIVORS

These terms will be used interchangeably to reflect that the person with a brain injury is more than his/her injury. It is the author's conviction that persons with brain injuries are survivors. Each individual who suffers a brain injury must meet great challenges and adversity to nurture a life filled with meaning and contribution. The author acknowledges these and wishes to convey respect for individuals meeting these challenges with dignity and courage.

ABI is the result of primary and secondary injuries to the brain. As effects ripple through the brain, both of these types of injuries damage the internal network of the brain beyond the site of injury.[7]

TABLE 13.1
Differentiation Between Primary and Secondary Injuries

Primary Injury	Secondary Injury
• Movement of the brain in the skull	• Seizure disorders
• Axonal shearing, cerebral edema, contusions, coup-contrecoup effects	• Hydrocephalus
	• Anoxia

Axonal shearing refers to the compression and stretching of axons, causing severe brain damage.

Cerebral edema refers to the swelling of the brain after injury, causing severe brain damage.

Contusion refers to the tearing of small blood vessels or bruising that can lead to neuronal death.

Coup-contrecoup refers to bruising at the site opposite the injury.[7,31]

ASSESSMENT MEASURES

The severity of brain injury is described in part through the use of the Glasgow Coma Scale (GCS), a three-part scale implemented in acute stages of injury where binary issues are death or survival. The GCS score ranges from 3 to 15 points based on scores for eye opening, best motor response, and best verbal response.[8] BI severity is classified by GCS as:

TABLE 13.2
Glasgow Coma Scale Scores[8,29]

Brain Injury Severity GCS Scores

Mild Traumatic Brain Injury	13–15
Moderate Traumatic Brain Injury	9–12
Severe Traumatic Brain Injury	3–8

The role of the SLP at this time is generally limited to introduction of sensory stimulation only when the person is medically stable. Ongoing assessment of swallow function may occur to determine the appropriate initiation of oral feedings.[6]

Another means of classifying brain injury is the Ranchos Los Amigos (RLA) Scale, an eight-tiered scale describing the cognitive and behavioral hallmarks of recovery from Traumatic Brain Injury (TBI).[9,10]

TABLE 13.3
Ranchos Los Amigos Scale at a Glance[9,10]

RLA I - No Responses
No response to pain, touch, sound, or sight.

RLA II – Generalized Reflex Response
Generalized reflex response with earliest response generally to pain.
Inconsistent responses may include physiological changes, gross body movements, or vocalizations.

RLA III – Localized Response
Examples of responses may include blinks to strong light, turning to or away from sound, response to physical discomfort, or inconsistent responses to commands.

RLA IV – Confused-Agitated
Alert, very active.
Aggressive or bizarre behaviors.
Performs motor activities but behavior is nonpurposeful.
Extremely short attention span.

RLA V – Confused, Nonagitated
Gross inattention to environment.
Highly distractible.
Requires continual redirection.
Difficulty learning new tasks.
Agitated by too much stimulation.
May engage in social conversations with inappropriate verbalizations present.

RLA VI – Confused-Appropriate
Inconsistent orientation to time and place.
Retention span and recent memory impaired.
Begins to recall past.

TABLE 13.3 (CONTINUED)
Ranchos Los Amigos Scale at a Glance[9,10]

Consistently follows simple directions.
Goal-directed behavior with assistance.

RLA VII – Automatic Appropriate

Performs daily routine in highly familiar environment in automatic, robot-like manner.
Skills noticeably deteriorate in unfamiliar environment.
Lacks realistic planning for own future.

RLA VIII – Purposeful-Appropriate

Alert and oriented times four.
Good recall of past events.
Memory deficits for recent events possible.
Able to learn new information, though not as quickly as preinjury.
Reduced stress tolerance.
Difficulty with abstract reasoning.
Possible problems with decision making.
May function at reduced levels in society.

Although these severity assessments are not reliable for predicting outcome at one-year post injury, they can offer a more complete diagnostic picture when combined with assessment of functional skills, abilities, and performance.[35] Prognostic indicators include:

- length of coma
- length of posttraumatic amnesia
- age at time of injury
- medical complications including anoxia, intracranial pressure (ICP), electrolyte imbalance, cerebral edema, increase or decrease in blood pressure, intracranial hemorrhages, hyperthermia, and seizures
- location, extent, and severity of cerebral damage
- premorbid (preinjury) personality, behaviors
- family support[3,32,34,35]

RECOVERY

Following severe closed head injury, persons with brain injuries typically progress through stages of recovery defined by cognitive, behavioral, and communication functions.[11] Recovery from brain injury is variable, dependent on:

- type and severity of injury
- location of injury

- medical management of brain injury
- severity of complications and other injuries
- premorbid personality, intelligence, and learning style[12]

Ylvisaker et al.[17] have proposed a treatment model based on the facts that recovery from TBI is evolutionary, and that cognitive and behavioral functioning is distinct in each stage of recovery.

TABLE 13.4
Treatment Model Based on Stage of Recovery

Stage of Recovery	Early Stage	Middle Stage	Late Stage
RLA Levels	RLA II, III	RLA IV, V, VI	RLA VII, VIII
Therapy Approaches	Sensory stimulation	Structure	Functional tasks to increase
	Sensory integration	Environmental	independence
		Management	Community Re-entry
		Compensatory	Compensatory strategies
		Strategies	Cognitive aids

EARLY STAGE OF RECOVERY FROM BRAIN INJURY

The role of the SLP in the early stage of recovery from brain injury is primarily one of sensory stimulation as this is a period when the person with brain injury begins to respond inconsistently to his or her environment. Therapy approaches are tailored to increase arousal of the person and the recognition of his or her environment.[13] Involvement of the SLP in the early stage of recovery is also valuable for family education and support regarding brain injury and its recovery process.[14]

As the person with brain injury progresses through the early stage of recovery, sensory stimulation approaches progress to sensory integration approaches. The two approaches are distinguished by their distinct purposes:

Sensory stimulation goals are designed to increase responsiveness to the environment.
Sensory integration goals are designed to enhance the brain's response to two or more sensory stimuli.[12]

There is a small percentage (10–20%) of survivors of severe brain injury who remain minimally and inconsistently responsive to environmental stimuli (RLA II, RLA III) for an extended time period, usually three to six months. Ansell[15] has proposed that these persons be referred to as the "Slow to Recover (STR)." The STR individual is distinguished from persons in coma by the presence of spontaneous eye opening and differential sleep/wake cycles. The role of the SLP in treating these persons includes approaches found in the early stage of recovery table above. Specific approaches include:

- carefully controlled sensory stimulation
- use of modality and speed specific (slowed, carefully controlled intervals between stimuli)
- quiet periods built into treatment schedule
- use of enriched environments
- use of augmentative and alternative communication (AAC) systems to facilitate the person's interaction with his or her environment.[15]

SLPs often take the lead in interdisciplinary brain injury teams in establishing stimulation schedules. Close collaboration with each member of the interdisciplinary team is essential. Treatment recommendations should include:

TABLE 13.5
Intervention for Persons in the Early Stage of Recovery from BI

Sensory Stimulation and Integration[16]

- Limit the number of visitors to two or fewer at a given time.
- Introduce self and tasks to be performed.
- Attempt to normalize the person's routine.
- Interpretation of the person's environment.
- Use of AAC systems to facilitate interactions with the environment.

Each person who interacts with the STR individual should be instructed to assume the person receiving stimulation understands all that is being said. Continual stimulation via television or radio is not recommended, as these become similar to background noise and do not yield opportunities to increase responsiveness to the environment.[16]

The Western Neurosensory Stimulation Profile (WNSSP) is the only standardized assessment tool for persons in the early stage of recovery from BI. The WNSSP is a 33-item test that assesses arousal, attention, verbal expression, and response to auditory, visual, tactile, and olfactory stimuli. It is designed to reflect change over time and is beneficial for informing third-party payers of progress for continuation of funding for rehabilitation therapies.[15]

MIDDLE STAGE OF RECOVERY FROM BRAIN INJURY

Persons in the middle stage of recovery from brain injury are alert, generally responsive, and disoriented to variable degrees. The ongoing focus of SLP treatment should be on reducing confusion, increasing orientation, and increasing information processing abilities by structuring the environment to facilitate learning and to increase safety.[13] Family education and support remain an ongoing component of treatment of the SLP and the interdisciplinary BI team.

TABLE 13.6
Intervention for Persons in the Middle Stage of Recovery from BI[14]

Neurobehavioral Intervention	Increase control, reduce chaos
Cognitive Rehabilitation	Increase comprehension, reduce confusion
Psychosocial Adjustment/Emotional Support	Increase confidence, reduce catastrophic reactions

LATE STAGE OF RECOVERY FROM BRAIN INJURY

The aims of therapy in the late stage of recovery from BI are increasing adaptability and the development of compensatory strategies designed to facilitate increased independence in the community.[13] Specific skills targeted by the SLP include adapting behavior in structured environments. Progression to the least restrictive environment is recommended when appropriate. Family education and support regarding the long-term consequences of BI remain an important focus of the SLP.[14]

Social interactions are often complicated by disinhibition, reduced initiation, and reduced pragmatic skills during this stage of recovery. Individual and group therapies may target increasing social skills and communicative adaptability through pragmatic skills training in social settings.[17] Specific pragmatic skills will be addressed later in this chapter, in the section on social cognition.

GROUP INTERVENTIONS

Group interventions may be utilized during each stage of recovery from BI, and interventions are a typical component of comprehensive BI programs. SLPs can and should take the lead in evaluation of persons with brain injuries prior to group placements. SLPs can also be instrumental in establishing group protocols, including admission and discharge criteria. Groups offer an opportunity for creative programming throughout the BI continuum of care.[18] Purposes of group therapy include:

- To increase social interaction and self-monitoring skills in a more natural environment
- To increase self-esteem and self-motivation
- To increase the ability to develop meaningful short- and long-term goals
- To share the feelings and needs of persons with brain injuries in a supportive environment
- To provide and receive peer review of behaviors

Development of goals is pertinent especially for persons in the early stage of recovery from BI. All purposes are pertinent for persons in the middle and late stages of recovery from BI.

Both group, and individually-tailored interventions provided by the interdisciplinary team in BI settings are designed to maximize remaining and recovering skills and abilities.[12] Rehabilitation refers to organized treatment tailored to maximize functional abilities through skill retraining or compensatory methods in the least

TABLE 13.7
Goals of Group Interventions for Each Stage of Recovery[18,19,35]

Early Stage of Recovery	Middle Stage of Recovery	Late Stage of Recovery
Increase responsiveness to environment via sensory stimulation using varied stimuli.	Increase orientation X4. Includes orientation to person, place, time, and circumstance. Reduce confusion by increasing routine, adaptive behaviors in increasingly complex settings.	Increase problem solving in functional living skills of home and money management, transportation, and self-advocacy skills.
Increase reality orientation.	Increase cognitive flexibility for problem solving and reduce impulsivity.	Focus on cognitive-communicative skills of self-monitoring, social comprehension, word retrieval strategies and increased social interaction opportunities.
Increase alerting and attending to distinguish between stimuli.	Develop compensatory strategies to increase recall, including external and internal aids.	Develop leisure skills. SLP works with recreation therapy in group setting to facilitate achievement of interdisciplinary goals.

restrictive environment. Compensatory strategies are beneficial, as rehabilitation may not restore functional abilities to preinjury levels.[20]

Jacobs identified the "purpose of rehabilitation is to change destiny" through the establishment of goals which facilitate recovery.[20] Principles which communicate respect to the person with brain injury and help to open and maintain communication that may be applied to rehabilitation include:[21]

1. Separation of the person with brain injuries from problems he/she has interacting with environment.
2. Focusing on the interest of the person with BI when establishing functional goals.
3. Involvement of persons with BI in the establishment of goals whenever possible.
4. Use of objective criteria to describe abilities and challenges (GCS, RLA, and Functional Rating Scales: FIM, FAM, and IADL).
5. Identifying diagnosis before determining prognosis is essential, as the clinician must understand the problems and limitations faced by a person with BI before recommending compensatory strategies. Such strategies may be successful in increasing functional independence.
6. Tailoring of interventions to be challenging, yet attainable.

Treat a man as he is, and he will remain as he is.
Treat a man as he can and should be,
And he will become as he can and should be. –Goethe

STAFF COMMUNICATION COMPETENCIES

It is interesting to note that SLPs are trained in communication disorders but often lack a complete understanding of what constitutes effective communication. Interdisciplinary teams often look to SLPs for effective communication strategies as psychosocial deficits often greatly impede successful community reentry for the person with BI. Effective communication requires empathic listening, that is, listening to understand rather than with an intent to respond. Beginning interactions with a common point of reference or interest facilitates effective communication. A key to effective communication within an interdisciplinary team is the one-on-one relationship established with team members, including the person with BI and his or her family. SLPs often take the lead in establishing effective communication (which does not always mean agreement) with each member of the interdisciplinary team.[21]

TABLE 13.8
Staff Communication Competencies

1. Give your full attention to the conversation.
2. Facilitate ability of interactors to transcend differences.
3. See from the other person's perspective.
4. Listen with your ears and your heart – when you listen, you learn.
5. Be patient and respectful.
6. Value family involvement.
7. Be open minded and genuinely interested in those served.

1-4, Covey[22], 5-7, Walker[23]

Ylvisaker, Feeney, and Urbanczyk[17] advocate good communication as essential for all who interact with persons with brain injuries. These authors identify skills specifically required when interacting with families. The SLP should:

1. Use language that works within the family's level of understanding.
2. Pace the conversation based on the receptivity of the listener.
3. Make eye contact at appropriate intervals.
4. Be sensitive through the use of appropriate empathy.
5. Make concrete observations and suggestions.

Ylvisaker, Feeney, and Urbanczyk[17] also promote the use of a positive communication culture within comprehensive BI programs based on four premises:

1. Persons who survive severe brain injuries experience substantial periods of confusion and fragmentation.
2. The most beneficial rehabilitation strategy is effective and satisfying communication with significant individuals in one's environment.
3. Frequent interactors are most responsible for the establishment of positive communication.
4. Communication and behavior are inseparable.[17,23]

SLPs who offer interdisciplinary teams strategies for effective communication also lay the foundation for building on individual member strengths to compensate for team weaknesses. Effective interdisciplinary team interactions yield rehabilitation synergy manifested in improved outcomes.[22]

The NIH Consensus Conference recommends an interdisciplinary team approach to BI rehabilitation for persons with moderate-to-severe brain injuries (1998). This author advocates an interdisciplinary team process across mild, moderate, and severe brain injuries. An interdisciplinary team process facilitates shared responsibility for therapy goals and, therefore, treatment outcomes.

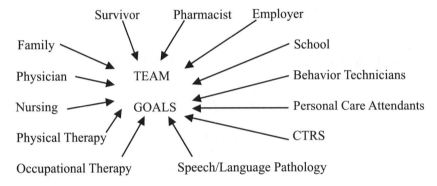

FIGURE 13.1   Schematic of Interdisciplinary Team Process.[10]

Effective interdisciplinary teams are better prepared to apply any one or a combination of different approaches to BI rehabilitation. Whatever the approach chosen by an interdisciplinary team, the ultimate aim is to see how the rehabilitation pieces (services needed) fit together in identifying available choices (resource identification), and how to access and utilize these resources to meet the lifelong needs of both survivors and families.[12] The interdisciplinary team advocates for and empowers the person with brain injury and his or her family to meet the daily challenges of life with BI.

SKILLS NEEDED IN BI REHABILITATION

BI ADVOCACY

BI advocacy manifests proactivity through coordinated case management, integrated team resources, and securing of adequate resources to meet team goals. Advocacy involves the person with brain injury as soon as possible in the decision-making process.[20] Advocacy enables team members to anticipate crises before they occur, rather than reacting to them afterwards.[12] Advocacy fosters creative partnership to ensure the needs of the person with brain injury are met through effective navigation of existing resources.[12]

BI EMPOWERMENT

Empowerment facilitates the perception of the person with BI that he or she has direct control over his or her life. Empowerment encourages the involvement of persons with brain injuries in planning and monitoring treatment so that the focus is on assets and strengths rather than limitations, and on the ongoing assessment of skills to foster increased independence for the person with BI. Families are empowered by their involvement in BI rehab programs.[24] Programs that empower survivors and families provide networking and educational opportunities. They also seek community involvement to increase opportunities for productive activities and contributions.[24] Many authors have identified personal control over one's own behavior, emotions, and life in general as essential to health — physical and psychological health.[24-27]

FUNCTIONAL APPROACHES TO BI REHABILITATION

Advocacy and empowerment lay the foundation for functional approaches to BI rehabilitation to be explored. A functional approach focuses the interdisciplinary team on the abilities of the person with BI of all levels to perform specific skills to accomplish a useful purpose.[12] A functional approach advocates improvement of skills needed for increased independence in the real world.[35] Each member of the interdisciplinary team must be trained to understand the impact of cognitive limitations on functional behaviors in order to complete functional assessments.[36] Although inconclusive, there is evidence to support the use of drills to practice skills to restore some degree of functional abilities no longer recovering spontaneously.[37] The SLP has an opportunity to lead the interdisciplinary team in applications of the functional approach and to determine when to apply drill work to augment functional gains of the interdisciplinary team.

INDEPENDENT LIVING

Application of the functional approach to BI rehabilitation lays an appropriate foundation for the implementation of the independent living model. An independent living model focuses the interdisciplinary team on the rights and responsibilities of the person with brain injury who is in control of individual treatment aims. Independent living skills training focuses on increasing the quality of life for persons with brain injuries by preparing them for fewer services in the future and increased independence.[38] Functional and independent living skills training is required as the foundation for effective community reintegration.[12] Community reintegration focuses on functional outcomes in one's community (residential facility, family home with day treatment program, other outpatient programming, or home care).[17]

Effective Home and Community-Based Services (HCBS) offer a means of providing community reintegration skills training. HCBS offers the opportunity to mobilize resources to meet the lifelong needs of persons with brain injuries in the home or community. Because of fewer indirect costs, HCBS is generally less expensive and, by its nature, more outcome oriented.[39] HCBS is comprehensive in nature and the SLP is involved in home- and community-based settings, fostering increased independence through increased safety, increased orientation, improved time and money management, and increased access to community resources.[40]

Home and Community Based Services and Community Reintegration Skills Training require the involvement and expertise of the family in meeting the lifelong needs of persons with brain injuries. The SLP, as well as other members of the interdisciplinary team, promote a family-centered approach to cognitive rehabilitation. A family-centered approach promotes the family's involvement as equal contributors to the interdisciplinary team goals of facilitating each person's rights to live in their home community with appropriate resources provided. The focus of a family-centered approach to BI rehabilitation is on functional skills required to increase independence in one's home community.[41]

FAMILY INVOLVEMENT

There are numerous benefits to family involvement in BI rehabilitation, including increased involvement (a positive prognostic indicator), improved communication among team members, promotion of the generalization of therapy gains, and opportunity to increase family support in times of emotional upheaval.[13] Building staff competence in using a family-centered approach requires competency-based education and training on family systems.[41] BI programs should readily provide training to interdisciplinary team members on family systems as many authors' experiences underscore the importance of family involvement in outcome-oriented BI rehabilitation.[10,13,42] A family-centered approach fosters a strong educational component as its core. Educated families are better prepared to "deal with the daily reality of head injury."[43] Family education and training programs promote:

- An increased understanding of BI
- Development of effective treatment regimes and compensatory strategies
- Increased resource awareness and caregiver responsibility
- Provision of an opportunity to give and receive support[43]

Family education and training programs provide an opportunity for networking with other families facing similar challenges, and an opportunity for the SLP and interdisciplinary team members to establish mentor family programs. Mentor families have faced the challenges of BI and have a willingness to share experiences with other families.[30]

Family-centered training also lays the foundation for preparing parents of persons with brain injuries to serve as educational managers facilitating successful school re-entry. Educating parents serves to reduce the feeling of being "out there on their own."[44] Lash et al.[44] propose six, two-hour workshops to train parents as educational managers. SLPs with BI and special education experience may be essential in providing specific skills training, offering suggestions for bridging gaps in communication between medical and school communities, and navigating the special education maze.

COGNITIVE-COMMUNICATIVE FUNCTIONING

Now that you, the SLP, have an understanding of approaches to BI rehabilitation, it is time for an overview of specific skills the SLP provides to an interdisciplinary team in a BI setting. This section will highlight cognitive-communication skills as they relate to persons with brain injuries. It is understood that SLPs have a comprehensive grasp of speech and language production, so these basic tenets will not be addressed. Rather, application of specific skills required by the SLP to foster interdisciplinary treatment team goals will be highlighted.

> All our mental abilities – perceiving, remembering, reasoning and many others – organized into a complex system. The overall function of which is termed cognition.[45]

The role of the SLP on an interdisciplinary BI team is to facilitate information or knowledge processing to facilitate outcome-oriented goals and objectives.[29] Prigatano has proposed a cognitive basis for communication deficits after BI.[42] Several authors and the American Speech-Language Hearing Association (ASHA) have endorsed the terminology of cognitive-communication to reflect behavioral aspects of communication not necessarily reflected in the cognitive-linguistic terminology previously used.[6,46,47] Cognitive-Communicative intervention:

1. Is directed to the reorganization of cognitive processes, NOT the modification of abnormal language.
2. Is based on working through lower-level processes to enable the emergence of higher-level activities.
3. Progresses serially to the highest level of skill.
4. Manipulates the rate, amount, duration, and complexity of stimuli consistent with abilities.[48]

Cognitive-communicative limitations after BI include impaired attention and concentration; impaired memory; slowed information (knowledge) processing; reduced initiation, planning, and organization; ineffective word retrieval; tangentiality; and talkativeness.[6] These challenges impact all areas of socialized independent living. Assessment and treatment of cognitive-communicative function by the SLP should be tailored to meet independent living concerns and needs.[49]

TABLE 13.9
Cognitive-Communicative Challenges Secondary to BI

- **Cognitive-Communicative Skill**
- **Sampling of Standardized Assessments***   **Specific Areas of Difficulty After BI**

• Attention	• Impaired attention (selective, focused, divided),
• RIPA, SCATBI	reduced concentration, heightened distractibility
• Orientation	• Disorientation to any or all: person, place, time,
• RIPA, SCATBI	and circumstance

TABLE 13.9 (CONTINUED)
Cognitive-Communicative Challenges Secondary to BI

• **Cognitive-Communicative Skill**	
• **Sampling of Standardized Assessments***	**Specific Areas of Difficulty After BI**
• Memory	• Difficulty with new learning, "forgetfulness,"
• RIPA, SCATBI, Woodcock-Johnson	Inefficient retrieval
• Reasoning and Judgment	• Difficulty reasoning through situations using
• RIPA, SCATBI	good judgment
• Thought Organization	• Reductions in ability to organize information in
• RIPA, SCATBI	logical manner, as they impact word retrieval. May see rambling, tangential conversations.
• Executive Functions	• Self-awareness, goal setting, self-monitoring,
• Ideally should involve observation, assessment tasks without structure and interviews with survivor and family. There are numerous neuropsychological batteries available.	planning, initiation, inhibition and self-evaluation, problem solving
• Social Cognition and Word Retrieval	• Pragmatic Communication Skills –
• RIPA, Boston Naming Test, Woodcock-Johnson, Western Aphasia Battery, Boston Diagnostic Aphasia Examination, Informal observation and assessment in social settings	conversational initiation, turn-taking, topic maintenance, body language, social skills, reduced cognitive flexibility and low frustration tolerance in challenging situations or interactions. Word Retrieval may be inefficient, slowed and/or full of fillers and descriptors rather than the actual word. Abstract language skills may be compromised.
• Auditory Processing	• Slowed thinking, need for frequent delay and
• RIPA, SCATBI, Woodcock-Johnson, Informal assessment in functional tasks	repetition
• Reading Comprehension and Written Expression	• May be impacted by impaired attention and
• Reading Comprehension Battery for Aphasia, Western Aphasia Battery, Boston Diagnostic Aphasia Examination, Gates-McGinitie, Functional reading tasks – newspaper, book, bank statements, etc. Functional writing tasks – paragraphs, papers, checks, shopping lists	concentration, reduced memory for information read, slowed processing, easy fatigue, or visual disturbances.

*This table is designed to give the SLP a few of the commonly used standardized assessment tools available. It is strongly recommended that these standardized assessment tools be augmented with informal assessments targeting functional skills in real-world settings. Areas for further investigation with functional measures can be determined from standardized measures.[10,13,50,51]

COGNITIVE REHABILITATION

As previously noted, the number of persons surviving severe brain injury has increased dramatically. An increase in the use of cognitive rehabilitation has resulted from an increase in professional awareness of the fact that cognitive deficits and psychosocial impairments are most likely to impede successful return to the community.[13] As with other BI terminology, there is confusion about cognitive rehabilitation definitions.[4]

Cognitive rehabilitation, cognitive remediation, and cognitive retraining are used interchangeably in the literature.[4] For the purposes of this discussion, we will use cognitive rehabilitation.

Cognitive rehabilitation refers to intervention strategies which "attempt to remediate, ameliorate, or alleviate cognitive deficits" resulting from BI.[52] This author advocates structuring cognitive rehabilitation based on stages of recovery from BI outlined at the beginning of the chapter.[13]

Regardless of the stage of recovery, development of a cognitive resource book by an SLP can be beneficial in facilitating communication between team members (including family) and promoting goal achievement.[40] Resource books (or memory notebooks) should contain pertinent, patient-specific memory aids and compensatory strategies, cueing devices, problem-solving strategies, checklists, and strategies for teachers and employers.[40]

Since no one discipline has "ownership" over cognitive domains, interdisciplinary teams should review team expertise and assign specific areas for assessment to reduce redundancy and increase quality care.[53] Specific skills of the SLP should be utilized to assess information processing, communication, orientation, memory, organization, and, of course, specific speech and language abilities. Table 13.9 outlines specific areas of assessment and treatment which may be assigned to the SLP to foster interdisciplinary collaboration.

AUDITORY PROCESSING

SLPs offer specific expertise in identifying and describing information-processing deficits. Information-processing abilities are often slowed after severe BI. The client may need additional time to get tasks done, or may have difficulty with processing new or unfamiliar information. The person with BI may receive only part of auditory instructions, and may even be unaware that they did not receive the entire message. Additionally, the person with BI may report slowed thinking or that people are talking too fast.[54]

LANGUAGE OF CONFUSION

For persons in the middle stage of recovery, a deficit worthy of further exploration as it pertains to cognitive-communicative functioning is the "language of confusion." "Language of confusion" reflects use of language that does not make sense to the listener. It is used to refer to instances where the person with BI is less able to understand his or her environment and, therefore, offers impaired responses to environmental cues. The language of confusion is characterized by bold, reckless, and impulsive production of words. Perseveration, slang, and jargon may be present. The person generally has no awareness of errors. Highly structured and frequent therapy sessions are recommended treatment by the SLP.[55,56]

ATTENTION

Attention deficits are common after BI.[8] Attention involves "admitting and holding information in consciousness."[13] Specific areas of attention addressed by the SLP include arousal, directing attention, maintaining attention, selective attention (ability to filter irrelevant information), and divided attention (ability to shift attention from among two or more competing stimuli).[13]

Identification of attention deficits begins with information-processing problems. The human brain has *limited* capacity for information processing, *the human brain can only do so much.* The ability to choose important information and ignore the rest is often impaired after BI.[45]

The SLP will describe attention in terms of:

- Attention span or the limitations on the person with BI to focus on particular stimuli
- Ability of the person to increase attention to stimuli perceived important (focused attention)
- Ability to focus on two or more things at once (divided attention)
- The ability to shift back and forth between engaging stimuli (alternating attention)[53]

The SLP will also be able to describe attention/concentration deficits through the identification of compromised ability to complete tasks, difficulty switching topics, or reports by the person with BI of feeling "unglued" or that his or her mind wanders.[54] Sohlberg and Mateer have developed a specific program for retraining attention: Attention Process Training (APT).[53] Other means the SLP may use to train attention include the following of task directions to task completion, minimizing and then increasing distractions, sequencing, and studying skills.[53]

SHORT-TERM MEMORY

Short-term memory (STM) is often compromised in persons with attention deficits after BI. This results because the person is not attending to stimuli, so he or she will be marginally successful at remembering the information at best.[54] Memory deficits are the most commonly reported deficit after severe BI.[63] Impairments in the ability to learn new information may result after brain injury involving the temporal lobes.[45] Memory involves perceiving, organizing, storing, and retrieving information at a later time when it is needed. Each of these components may be compromised after BI.

The SLP will describe three types of memory:

Immediate – repetition of information just told
Recent – events from yesterday
Remote – events from many years ago[12,13,57]

Post-traumatic amnesia (PTA) refers to the period of time after injury in which the person with BI has difficulty learning new information (period of time that *retrograde amnesia* exists).[12] The duration of PTA is used as an indicator for predicting outcome. Limitations in the validity of outcome measures were explored earlier. *Anterograde amnesia* refers to forgetting information for some time period prior to and up to the trauma.[45]

A component of STM recall that should be delineated in assessment is the presence of the recency effect. *Recency effect* refers to the effect that, even with rehearsal (practicing remembering information), the person with BI is more likely to recall later items more accurately.

In describing memory deficits after BI, the SLP should also explore the person's ability to use repetition, rehearsal, associations, or mnemonics to increase recall. These will assist in the development of compensatory strategies.[45]

EXECUTIVE FUNCTIONS

SLPs will assess executive functions in conjunction with each member of the interdisciplinary team. Executive functions are planning, prioritizing, sequencing, self-monitoring, self-correction, self-initiation, and self-inhibition. Executive function deficits are often the result of frontal lobe injury, as may be found in a person who has been thrown into the windshield in a motor vehicle accident (MVA).[12] *Executive functions* refers to the high-level cognitive processes required to formulate goals and plans to achieve goals. Skills require self-awareness of strengths and limitations.[59]

Deficits in executive functioning have been identified as the greatest impediment to returning to premorbid and competitive employment.[58] The SLP will be able to describe executive deficits through observation of disorganization, unrealistic goal setting, reduced task initiation, impulsivity, and impaired social perceptions.[54]

Ylvisaker[59] has identified eight areas in which executive system and communication deficits are evident. The SLP should address each of these areas in assessment and treatment:

- Self-Awareness
- Planning (Steps To Achieve Goals)
- Problem Solving (Recognize Alternatives And Select Most Realistic Solution)
- Goal Setting (Realistic, Attainable Goals Established)
- Self-Initiation (Begin Tasks And Conversations)
- Self-Inhibitions (Monitor Usage Of Socially Acceptable Terminology Including Profanity)
- Self-Monitoring (Assess One's Performance)
- Self-Evaluation (Perceived Versus Actual Performance Delineated Accurately)

Obviously, pre- and postinjury performances should be reflected in descriptions of performance in each of these areas.[12]

Cognitive rehabilitation evaluation of problem solving *using good judgment* involves describing specific skills to complete successful problem solving. Parente has identified nine areas for effective, successful problem solving. These areas are reflected in Table 13.10.[60]

TABLE 13.10
Components of Successful Problem Solving[60]

Evaluation and Treatment of Problem Solving Components

1. Identify the problem to be solved.
2. Classify the problem.
3. Identify the goal to be achieved.
4. Gather the necessary information to solve the problem.
5. Identify possible solutions.
6. Evaluate solutions for merit and effectiveness (inductive reasoning).
7. Determine the best solution from generated alternatives (deductive reasoning).
8. Form a plan to solve the problem (executive function).
9. Monitor the results (self-monitoring, self-evaluation).

Judgment reflects the person's ability to review available information including consequences prior to initiation of a solution. *Reasoning* reflects the drawing of conclusions after review of the information gathered.[13] *Reasoning* and problem solving are highly interrelated cognitive processes.[45]

The SLP evaluation of cognition should also describe multiple or dual tracking. *Multiple or dual tracking* is the person's ability to maintain several thoughts *simultaneously* and to switch smoothly between them.[10] Deficits in multiprocess reasoning are reflected in the ability of the person with BI to do more than one thing at a time.[54]

COMMUNICATION AND BEHAVIOR

SLPs are also responsible for describing social cognition and behavior. Communication and behavior disruption result from severe injuries, especially to the prefrontal cortex, reflected in inaccurate social perceptions and increases in frustration resulting from changes in communication ability.[17]

Social cognition refers to one's ability to interact socially with one's environment. The focus of social cognition is on dynamic interactions between the person with BI and the environment at large.[13] *Social skills* refer to the skills needed for effective participation in a social situation.[12]

Assessment of social cognition by the SLP can begin in the individual SLP evaluation. Additional data and information should be gathered from group settings where the person with BI interacts with others in a real-world setting. Groups are also effective for ameliorating social cognitive challenges.[19] The SLP should describe the presence of rambling, tangential conversations reflecting thought organization deficits.[13]

Convergent thinking refers to the ability to choose the single best answer when given specific facts or information.

Divergent thinking refers to the ability to generate numerous possible alternatives given a single fact or idea.[64]

Abstract thinking refers to theories or concepts that may be difficult to understand.[12,28]

The SLP should describe convergent and divergent naming skills. For convergent thinking, use a multiple-choice test where the idea is to identify the one best answer. A common SLP convergent thinking task is category naming. Divergent thinking is reflected in essay examinations where there are numerous alternatives, as in the common language task of category listing within a specified time frame (usually one minute). Limitations in understanding abstract language may be seen in social situations. The person may have a tendency to think literally when hearing idiomatic expressions (it is raining cats and dogs) or common social expressions.[12] Other areas where limitations in the ability to use abstract thinking occur include considering several aspects of a situation, breaking items into component parts, and using make-believe.[65]

As previously mentioned, Ylvisaker et al.[17] have described a *positive communication culture* as a means of fostering communicative effectiveness. All team members are integral to the application of this approach in social settings designed to increase functional communicative independence of persons with brain injuries. A positive communication culture can be facilitated in social skills groups through coaching and peer training in social settings.[17]

Groups are recommended for evaluation and treatment of social cognition because communication is a dynamic process where skills cannot be taught in isolation. Groups allow for an increase in social outlets for the person with BI, thus reducing social isolation. Groups enable the SLP to have an opportunity to assess pragmatic communication skills in a real-world setting. Pragmatic communication skills include:

Topic initiation – beginning a conversation without prompting
Topic maintenance – sticking with a given topic until it is finished
Turn-taking – responding when appropriate without interrupting or excusing interruptions
Appropriate body language – eye contact and postures which reflect interest
Active listening skills – attending to the conversation to get its meaning clearly[10]

Challenges for the person with BI in the area of pragmatics may be reflected in tangentiality, verbosity, topic relevance, topic transition, acknowledging, paraphrasing, and summarizing skills. Social skills training reflects an application of pragmatic communication skills in social settings. Specific tasks may include socially appropriate profanity usage, moderating loudness, use of social courtesies of "please" and "thank you," staying on task, waiting for one's turn, and excusing interruptions and derogatory comments.[40]

Peer groups for adolescents have been identified as an effective treatment regime for enhancing pragmatic skills.[19]

COMPENSATORY TECHNIQUES

An additional responsibility of the SLP is to provide compensatory techniques for cognitive challenges not ameliorated through cognitive rehabilitation. Compensatory techniques are tools or strategies designed to increase the independence of the person with brain injury.[10]

Compensatory techniques have been identified as more beneficial than restorative drill training in severe bilateral brain injury.[42] As with any technique, there are pros and cons for internal and external aids. Internal aids rely heavily on the ability of the person with BI. External aids can be costly and require extensive training; however, they may also increase independence.

TABLE 13.11
Cognitive Aids[10,18,30,42,45,53,60,61]

External Cognitive Aids	Internal Cognitive Aids
1. Behavioral Prosthetics	1. Language Based Strategies, i.e., 5 W's and H: who, what, when, where, why and how to organize information
a. Asking for reminders	
b. Putting objects in special places (put car keys near the door)	
c. Writing notes on hand	2. Reconstruction
d. Diary	3. Mnemonics
e. Putting items back where they belong	4. Chunking
	5. Association
f. Automatic bill payments	6. Assigning Attributes
2. Cognitive Prosthetics	7. Rehearsal
a. Non-Electronic Aids	8. Self-instruction
1. Checklists	9. Visualization
2. Medication organizers	10. Repetition
3. Note pads and post-it notes	11. Engage all your senses
4. Appointment calendars	
5. Lists and signs	
6. Whistling tea pots	
b. Electronic Aids	
1. Calculators	
2. Electronic checkbooks	
3. Automatic dial telephones	
4. Speaker phones	
5. Tele-memo watches	
6. Palm Pilots	
7. Neuropage or general pagers	
8. YakBak	

TABLE 13.11 (CONTINUED)
Cognitive Aids[10,18,30,42,45,53,60,61]

External Cognitive Aids	Internal Cognitive Aids

c. Cognitive Correctors
   1. Grammar Check, Spell Check
   2. Iron with Shut Off Memory
   3. Key Finders
   4. Car Finders – blinking lights, horn sounds when button pushed.
d. Cognitive Trainers
   1. Self-instruction programs
   2. Computer activities
   3. Independent Life Skills Trainers
e. Cognitive Sources
   1. Dictionary
   2. Encyclopedia
   3. Thesaurus
   4. Atlas
   5. Notes from meetings, lectures, reading
f. Cognitive Art
   1. Floor Plans
   2. Decision Trees

BEHAVIOR

The SLP is essential to an interdisciplinary team when the team's approach to neurobehavioral intervention is: "All communication is behavior. All behavior is communicative." Ylvisaker, Feeney, and Urbanczyk advocate this approach.[17] Jacobs states that thinking and doing are different.[20] An SLP can help determine the program's position on neurobehavioral intervention. The author's professional experience concurs with Ylvisaker et al.

The SLP is involved in the interdisciplinary team's data collection of measuring targeted behaviors during intervention techniques. Behavioral measures include direct observation, self-report of the person with BI, third-party report, and standardized testing. The SLP should apply skill-based behavioral intervention focused on maintaining lasting change after the conclusion of therapy. Approaches to neurobehavioral intervention should be included in job-performance competencies for each member of the interdisciplinary team. Specific skills training for interdisciplinary team members may include specific shaping strategies, reinforcement schedule, verbal mediation strategies, or crisis prevention protocols to increase environmental safety. Behavioral intervention should always be focused on the use of the least restrictive and most facilitative procedures.[20] Behavioral analysis considers the following:

TABLE 13.12
Compensatory Techniques for Persons with Brain Injuries

1. Conserve energy.
2. Write appointments in a day planner.
3. Prioritize, schedule priorities.
4. Color code files by topic.
5. Keep a pad and pencil near the bed.
6. Use checklists, timers and alarms.
7. Use phone logs to track calls.
8. Book an appointment with self to recharge battery.
9. Have a consistent routine.
10. Double-check work.
11. Allow for additional time if needed.
12. Pace self.
13. Avoid taking on too much.
14. Be on time.
15. Be orderly to increase proficiency. Clutter impedes and slows efficiency.
16. Use gestures to enhance speech.
17. Minimize distractions.
18. Ensure that necessary aids are available at all times (resource notebook, glasses, etc.)
19. Ask for repetition of instructions, repeat them aloud and seek clarification that information is correct.
20. Encourage participation in activities that nurture the soul.[10,18,44,54,62]

TABLE 13.13
Common Behavioral Sequelae After BI[6,10,17,20,53]

General Tension	Irritability	Depression
Amotivation	Restlessness	Impulsivity
Fluctuating mood	Childishness	Disinhibition
Temper outbursts	Dependency	Apathy
Frustration	Reduced self-esteem	Emotional lability
Impulsivity	Reduced self-confidence	Anxiety
Lack of insight	Denial of physical and cognitive limitations	Confabulation
Agitation	Psychiatric disturbances	Substance abuse
Hypersexuality	Confusion	Perseveration
Regulatory problems	General mental slowing	Reduced initiation

A – Antecedents – occur prior to behavior[20]
    Focus of behavior modification strategies[17]
B – Behavior – action or activity where measure change[20]
C – Consequences – follows behavior, influences the likelihood of future occurrence[20]

CONCLUSION

The SLP is an integral member of the interdisciplinary BI team. The SLP may lead the interdisciplinary team (which includes the person with brain injury and his or her family) by assessing and treating the survivor and educating all team members about social cognition and cognitive-communicative challenges faced after BI. The SLP can facilitate increased independence of people with BI of all levels by developing compensatory techniques. SLPs who want to work in the BI industry should engage in challenging practicum experiences as graduate students and continue competency-based training as Clinical Fellowship Year (CFY) employees and throughout employment in the BI industry. Competency-based education and training are essential to the satisfaction and success of the employee, program, and person with BI, regardless of the site in the continuum of care. Employment in the BI industry is not only challenging, it is intensely rewarding.

The author has been intensely rewarded by employment in the BI industry and wishes all potential interdisciplinary BI team members success and happiness.

The author wishes to thank her family, Tucker, Emilie, and Meaghan, and her parents, Peter and Brenda Griffin, for their continual love and support. The author also gratefully acknowledges the loving contributions of her friends and important teachers, Fran Lowry and Bob Fenster, toward the completion of this manuscript.

BIBLIOGRAPHY

1. Brain Injury Association: Brain Injury Facts and Figures. Washington, DC: BIA. 1996.
2. National Head Injury Foundation: Brain Injury Fact Sheet. NHIF: Washington, DC, 1989.
3. Zasler, ND, Clifton, GL, Prospects for Improving Outcome by Research. Plenary Session at Brain Injury Association Professional Symposium, 11/5/96, Dallas, Texas.
4. Seaton, JD, Niemann, GW, Creating the AACBIS: Dialogue with the AACBIS Board of Governors. Brain Injury Association Professional Symposium, 11/4/96, Dallas, Texas.
5. *ASHA Neurogenic Communication Disorders Specialty Interest Division Newsletter*, Spring, 1999. NIH Consensus Conference article.
6. Gillis, RJ, *TBI Rehabilitation for the Speech-Language Pathologist*, Butterworth-Heinemann, Boston, 1996.
7. Savage, RC, A Beginning Therapist's Guide to the Brain and Brain Injury. Niskayuna, NY: NMCD Inservice, 1992.
8. Teasdale, G, Jennett, B, Assessment of coma and impaired consciousness: a practical scale, *Lancet*, 13: 81, 1974.
9. Hagen, C., Malkmus, D, Durham, P, Levels of Cognitive Functioning. Downey, CA: RLA Hospital Communication Disorders Service, 1972.
10. Law, PA, *ABI: Introductory Course Training Manual*, Pamela Law, Westminster, CO: 1997.
11. Hagen, C, Language Disorders Secondary to CHI: Diagnosis and Treatment. *Topics in Language Disorders*, 1:73-87, 1981.
12. BIAC. *A Regional Family Guide to TBI: Together We Stand*. BIAC: Denver, CO, 1998.

13. Szekeres, SF, Ylvisaker, M, Cohen, SB, A Framework for Cognitive Rehabilitation Therapy, in Ylvisaker, M, Gobble, EMR, *Community Re-Entry for Head Injured Adults*, College-Hill, Boston, 1987.

14. Lehr, E, Counseling Students with ABI. In Glang, A., Singer, GHS, Todis, B., Eds., *Students with ABI: The School's Response*, 277, Paul H. Brookes Publishing, Baltimore, MD, 1997.

15. Ansell, BJ, Slow-to-recover BI patients: rationale for treatment, *JSHR*, 54:1017, 1991.

16. Cumberland Rehabilitation Hospital, *Do's and Don'ts for BI Patients RLA I-IV*, Cumberland, New Kent, VA, 1993.

17. Ylvisaker, M, Feeney, TJ, and Urbanczyk, B, A Social Environmental Approach to Communication Behaviors After BI. Seminars in Speech and Language: Special Issues in TBI II, 14, #1, 74, 1993.

18. Brown, C, Graduate Seminar in Neurogenic Communication Disorders. University of North Carolina at Greensboro, 1990.

19. Wiseman-Hakes, C, Stewart, ML, Wasserman R, Schuller, R, Peer group training of pragmatic skills in adolescents with ABI, *JHTR*, 13(6):23 1998.

20. Jacobs, HE, *Behavior Analysis Guidelines and BI Rehabilitation: People, Principles & Programs*, Aspen, Gaithersburg, MD, 1993.

21. Covey, SR, *Principle-Centered Leadership*, Fireside, New York, 1991.

22. Covey, SR, *The 7 Habits of Highly Effective People*, Fireside, New York, 1989.

23. Walker, BR, Creating Effective Educational Programs Through Parent-Professional Partnerships, in Glang, A, Singer, GHS, Todis, B, Eds., ABI: The School's Response, Paul H. Brookes Publishing, Baltimore, 1997.

24. Shaw, LR, Jackson, JD, The Dilemma of Empowerment in BI Rehabilitation, in McMahon BT, Evans, RW, *The Shortest Distance*, PMD Publishers Group, Inc., Winter Park, FL, 1994.

25. Rodin, J, Aging & Health: Effects of the Sense of Control, *Science*, 233:1271, 1986.

26. Shapiro, DH, Self-Control Strategies, in Corsini, R., Ed., *Encyclopedia of Psychology*, 3, 285, Wiley, New York, 1984.

27. Peterson, C, Stunkard, A, Personal control and health promotion, *Social Science and Medicine*, 28:819, 1989.

28. The American Heritage Dictionary, Second College Edition. Houghton-Mifflin, Boston.

29. Jennett, B, How severe the BI, how good the recovery? The development of the Glasgow Coma Scales, *BI Source*, 1:14, 1997.

30. Condon, MJ, Family to Family Mentoring with TBI, Course at BIAC Symposium, Vail, CO, 1998.

31. Roberts-Stoler, D, Albers-Hill, B, *Coping with Mild Traumatic Brain Injury*, Avery Publishing Group, Garden City Park, NY, 1998.

32. Ylvisaker, M, *TBI Rehabilitation: Children and Adolescents*, 2nd Ed., Butterworth-Heinemann, Boston, 1998.

33. Linehan, C, *Instructional Implications for Persons with Brain Injuries*, NMCD Inservice, Niskayuna, NY, 7/28/92.

34. Szekeres, SF, Ylvisaker, M, Holland, AL, Cognitive Rehabilitation Therapy: A Framework for Intervention, in Ylvisaker, M, Ed., *Head Injury Rehabilitation: Children & Adolescents*, College-Hill Press, San Diego, CA, 1985.

35. Giles, GM, Clark-Wilson, J, Functional Skills Training in Severe BI, in Fussey I, Giles, GM, Eds., *Rehabilitation of the Severely Brain Injured Adult: A Practical Approach*, Croom Helm, London, 1988.

36. Diller, L, Ben-Yishay, Y, Assessment in TBI, in Bach-y-Rita, P, *Comprehensive Neurologic Rehabilitation*, Volume 2, Demos, New York, 1989.

37. Ben-Yishay, Y, Rattok, J, Ross, B, Lakin, P, Ezrachi, O, Silver, S, Diller, L, Rehabilitation of Cognitive and Perceptual Deficits in People with Traumatic Brain Damage, in *Working Approaches to Remediation of Cognitive Deficits in Brain Damaged Persons*, Rehabilitation Monograph #64, NYU Medical Center: Institute of Rehabilitation Medicine, 127, 1982.

38. Williams, J, Matthews, M, Independent Living and Brain Injury: Overview, Obstacles and Opportunities, Lawrence, KS, Research & Training Center on Independent Living for Underserved Populations.

39. Kneipp, S, Community-Based Services and Support for Individual with TBI, in Ylvisaker, M, *Seminars in Speech & Language, Special Issues* in TBI II, 14, 1, 1993.

40. Cullity, LP, Jackson, JD, Shaw, LR, Community Skills Training, in McMahon, BT, Shaw, LR, Eds., *Work Worth Doing: Advances in BI Rehabilitation*, PMD Publishers Group, Inc, Orlando, FL, 1991.

41. Williams, JM, Training Staff for Family-Centered Rehabilitation: Future Directions in Program Planning, in Durgin, CJ, Schmidt, ND, Fryer, LJ, Eds., *Staff Development and Clinical Intervention in Brain Injury Rehabilitation*, Aspen Publishers, Gaithersburg, MD, 1993.

42. Prigatano, GP, et al, *Neuropsychological Rehabilitation after Brain Injury*, The Johns Hopkins University Press, Baltimore, MD, 1986.

43. Dell Orto, AE, Power, EW, *Head Injury and the Family: A Life & Living Perspective*, CRC Press, Boca Raton, FL, 1997.

44. Lash, M, Osberg, JS, Parents as educational managers for students with brain injuries, *Brain Injury Source*, 3:22, 44, 1999.

45. Glass, AL, Holyoak, KJ, *Cognition*, Second Edition. Random House, New York, 1986.

46. Ylvisaker, M, Urbanczyk, B, Assessment and Treatment of Speech, Swallowing & Communication Disorders Following TBI, in Finlayson, MAJ, Garner, SH, Eds., *Brain Injury Rehabilitation: Clinical Considerations*, Williams & Wilkins, Baltimore, 1992.

47. Hartley, LL, *Cognitive-Communicative Abilities Following Brain Injury: A Functional Approach*, Singular Publishing, San Diego, 1995.

48. Hagen, C, Language Disorders in Head Trauma, in Costello, JM, Holland, AL, Eds., *Handbook of Speech & Language Disorders*, College Hill Press, San Diego, 1982.

49. Durgin, CJ, Cullity, LP, Devine, PM, Programming for Skill Maintenance and Generalization, in McMahon, BJ, Shaw, LR, Eds., *Work Worth Doing: Advances in Brain Injury Rehabilitation*, PMD Publishing, Orlando, FL, 1991.

50. Pepping, M, The value of group psychotherapy after brain injury: a clinical perspective, in *Brain Injury Source*, 14-21, 1998.

51. Szekeres, SF, Ylvisaker, M, Cohen, SB, A Framework for Cognitive Rehabilitation Therapy, in Ylviskaer, M, Gobble, EMR, Eds., *Community Re-Entry for Head Injured Adults*, College-Hill Press, Boston, 1987.

52. Wilson, B, Models of Cognitive Rehabilitation, in Wood, RL, Eames, P, Eds., *Models of Brain Injury Rehabilitation*, Johns Hopkins University Press, Baltimore, 1989.

53. Moore-Sohlberg, M, Mateer, CA, *Introduction to Cognitive Rehabilitation: Theory and Practice*, Guilford Press, New York, 1989.

54. Haddow, J, Hyde, S, Hague, K, Rastok, B, MTBI Symposium: Awareness Levels & Their Impact on Treatment & Recovery. BIAC Symposium, Vail, CO, October 10, 1998.

55. Code, C, *The Characteristics of Aphasia*, Taylor & Francis, New York, 1989.

56. Goldfarb, R, Halper, H, Impairments of Naming and Word-Finding, in Code, C, Eds., *Characteristics of Aphasia*, Taylor & Francis, New York, 1989.
57. Crowder, R, *Principles of Learning and Memory*, Lawrence Erlbaum Associates, Hillsdale, NJ, 1976.
58. Bayless, JD, Varney, NR, Roberts, R, Tinker toy performance and vocational outcome in patients with closed head injury, *Journal of Clinical and Experimental Neuropsychology*, 11:913, 1989.
59. Ylvisaker, M, Szekeres, SF, *Metacognitive and Executive Impairments in Head-Injured Children & Adults, Topics in Language Disorders*, 9(2), Aspen Publishers, Rockville, MD, 1989.
60. Parente, R, Cognitive Aids, Short Course at Brain Injury Association Professional Symposium, Philadelphia, PA, 1997.
61. Ylvisaker, M, Szekeres, SF, Henry, K, Sullivan, DM, Wheeler, P, Topics in Cognitive Rehabilitation Therapy, in Ylvisaker, M, Gobble, EMR, *Community Re-Entry for Head Injured Adults*, College-Hill, Boston, 1987.
62. Brown, J, Dudley, D, *The Supervisor's Guide: The Everyday Guide to Coordinating People and Tasks*, Skill Path, Mission, KS, 1989.
63. Brooks, DN, Disorders of Memory, in Rosenthal, M, Griffith, E, Bond, M, Miller, JD, Eds., *Rehabilitation of the Head Injured Adult*, F.A. Davis, Philadelphia, 1983.
64. Chapey, R, Cognitive Intervention: Stimulation of Cognition, Memory, Convergent Thinking, Divergent Thinking and Evaluative Thinking, in Chapey, R, Ed., *Language Intervention Strategies in Adult Aphasia*, Second Edition. Williams & Wilkins, Baltimore, 1986.
65. AACBIS, *Training Manual for Certified Brain Injury Specialists (CBIS)*, BIA, Washington, DC, 1996.

14 Occupational Therapy Evaluation and Treatment of the Brain Injured Patient

Stacy Rogers, OT

INTRODUCTION

Occupational therapy is an essential part of the treatment team for an individual with a traumatic brain injury. The role of the occupational therapist varies according to the treatment setting and a client's level of injury. Occupational therapists assess a patient's positioning, posture, range of motion, oculomotor skills, sensation, cognition, strength, and coordination to see how the brain injury has impacted the individual in relation to functional basic living skills, complex activities of daily living, leisure skills, social skills, and vocation.

Assessment begins with gathering information about the mechanism of injury. Was the individual injured as a result of a motor vehicle accident, fall, gunshot wound, infection, a series of concussions, an anoxic event, or a whiplash type of accident? In what position was the individual found? Did the individual lose consciousness and, if so, for how long? Did the individual hit his or her head, or is the injury related to diffuse axonal shearing?

An interview with the individual's family members is an important tool in determining a patient's premorbid lifestyle and personality, in addition to work habits, interests, and behavioral changes. The individual usually cannot remember certain facts about the accident that others might be able to identify. For example, witnesses, police reports, and emergency room information may be insightful. If a magnetic resonance imaging (MRI), computed tomography scan (CT), electroencephalography (EEG), positron emission tomography (PET), single-photon emission computed tomography (SPECT), or quantitative electroencephalography (QEEG) brain mapping was performed, what were the results? An MRI assesses the integrity of the brain, spinal cord, and soft tissue. A CT scan provides emergent diagnosis of hematomas, swelling, and ischemic lesions; however, the injury may not show up on a CT scan at admission. Ischemic lesions and slowly-accumulating subdural hematomas may take days to show up on CT. An EEG is used with prolonged video monitoring to assess possible epilepsy, focal or diffuse brain damage, and sleep disturbances. PET assesses regional cerebral blood flow or metabolic activity. PET clinical application continues to be under development.[1] SPECT indicates cerebral blood profusion that may be decreased in the damaged area. A QEEG uses a digitalized signal to compare a patient's brain with a reference database that helps determine the mechanism of head injury, typically secondary to diffuse axonal injury.

Brain injuries are classified as severe, moderate, or mild. Regardless of the classification of brain injury, changes occur that affect an individual's life roles and goals. Most persons who have brain injuries are between the ages of 18 and 30 years old, a time in human development when people typically engage in activities that define identity and roles that are important throughout their lifespans.[2]

Persons with severe brain injury may require as much as five to ten years of rehabilitation services, with lifetime costs exceeding four million dollars.[3] Only about half of all persons with moderate brain injury will return to school, work, and independent living within one year of injury. At times, individuals who suffer a brain injury do not get immediate treatment and are not even identified as having a brain injury. These individuals may be treated and released only to find out they may have a brain injury later when they experience symptoms of nausea, vomiting, dizziness, headache, blurred vision, sleep disturbance, fatigue, lethargy, sensory loss, change in cognition, irritability, or other emotional outbursts. Some or all of these symptoms may indicate the presence of a brain injury.

THE OCCUPATIONAL THERAPIST AS PART OF THE ACUTE REHABILITATION TEAM

The occupational therapist should observe and document subtle changes in tone, posture, alertness, response to stimuli, and vital signs. Individuals who have suffered a brain injury and are admitted to the Intensive Care Unit (ICU) could be in a coma and have severe injuries that affect posture, tone, alertness, cognition, and behavior.

In the ICU, the patient with a brain injury may be unstable and monitored by a variety of machines to determine heart rate, blood pressure, intracranial pressure (ICP), and temperature changes. Avoid placing the patient on a flat bed; marked hip flexion and head rotation secondary to the potential of these postures tend to increase intracranial pressure. Check with the nursing staff to determine the patient's status and be aware of changes in vital signs during treatment. If the vital signs fluctuate or do not return to normal following stimulation, discontinue treatment.

There may be several secondary injuries that the therapist needs to be aware of in order to place the individual in the best possible position. Common secondary injuries include fractures and contusions. Examine the patient for edema and areas of the body in which a limitation of motion is present. Position the patient with regard for his or her secondary injuries. Proper positioning can increase functional outcome and independence when the individual becomes more alert and mobile. Make sure the head is supported with a rolled-up towel in the cervical curvature, and aligned to decrease muscular tightness and asymmetry in the neck. A flexed neck also could impinge on the jugular vein, which in turn may increase intracranial pressure. Proper positioning of the upper extremities includes the use of rolls behind the scapula for support and increased relaxation.

Perform an assessment of upper extremity range of motion as soon as the individual is stable. Note any posturing, increase in tone, or movement in response to range of motion. Never force an extremity during a posturing reaction, instead, let the pattern occur, then incorporate inhibitory techniques before the range of motion can be continued. Handling techniques such as placing the therapist's hand on the ulnar side of the patient's hand during range of motion, ranging the fifth digit first, and abducting the thumb can assist in decreasing tone. Forcing an extremity against strong resistance is found to be linked to the occurrence of heterotropic ossification (HO), which occurs in 11% to 76% of individuals with severe brain injury who posture or have high tone or spinal cord injury (SCI) with spasticity.[4] Also called "ectopic bone," heterotropic ossification is seen when abnormal calcification of bone occurs around a joint. Symptoms involve limitation of motion, redness, pain, and swelling around the joint, and should be reported to the physician.

Specialized handling techniques can assist the occupational therapist with inhibiting posturing. Decerebrate posturing is an extensor pattern of increased tone with shoulders extended, internally rotated, adducted, elbows extended, forearms pronated, wrists flexed, and fingers flexed with thumbs tucked into fingers. Posturing of this type indicates a lower-level injury to the brain and a greater possibility of significant impairment. Decorticate posturing presents as a flexor pattern of the upper extremities with increased tone in adduction, internal rotation at the shoulders, and forearm pronation. The elbows, wrists, and fingers are all in a flexed position. Handle the upper extremities by placing your hand over the triceps when the patient is in a flexor pattern, or placing your hand over the biceps when the upper extremity is in an extensor pattern. If the patient's fingers are held in a pattern of flexion, a soft roll can be placed in his or her hand to prevent tightness and shortening of the finger muscles. Prevention of finger adduction can be achieved by placing wedges between the fingers or placing the hand in a resting hand splint with individual finger troughs. Observe and note whether the patient responds to these inhibitory techniques.

Mobilize the patient as soon as they are stable. Co-treatments with the physical therapist can accomplish changing the position of the comatose patient by rolling him or her from side to side and moving him or her into a sitting position. Movement provides the individual with the feel of weight shifting, trunk movement, and weight bearing. It will also promote increased circulation and decrease the potential for skin breakdown. Input to the patient's large muscle groups through weight bearing will assist with proprioception, and movement will stimulate the individual's vestibular system. Assess head and trunk control when the patient is in a position against gravity. Each of the therapists can collaborate for a more detailed view of the changes in tone, posture, movement, attention, and responses the patient has during the treatment session.

Sensory integration enhances postural control, ocular control, motor planning, hand-eye coordination, vision, and perception.[4] Stimulation with movement assists with spatial relations and perception of body. The sensations of slow spinning and rocking may trigger vestibular reflexes. Sensory integration assists with organizing the vestibular system and providing proprioceptive input to increase body perception. Caution should be used when implementing sensory integration techniques because sensory integration can affect heart rate and blood pressure. Monitor vital signs and responses to sensory integration carefully.

Useful information is provided to the team through assessment of oculomotor skills. Check to see that no eye injury prevents opening of eyelids if the individual is unable to open eyes spontaneously. Observe if the patient has spontaneous eye opening, eye movements, is fixating on objects, and is able to track objects. If the individual has eye opening and movement, hand-eye coordination activities will assist with increased sense of visual perception. Document the patient's field of vision so other team members are aware of the useful field of vision and are able to include it in treatment activities. Educate caregivers and family to place simple familiar visual objects in the individual's field of view, for example, a picture of one of the family members or a pet.

Knowledge of cranial nerves that supply the innervation to eye muscles makes the assessment more informative and thorough. For example, injury to cranial nerve IV, the trochlear nerve, can cause diplopia. Misalignment of the eyes can cause diplopia. Shine a penlight in the patient's eyes to assess alignment: if it does not shine in the same place on each pupil, the eyes may be misaligned. Patients experiencing double vision may respond by increased agitation to visual stimuli. This can be addressed by use of a patch or tape on the glasses in the area of the double vision. Consultation with an optometrist or ophthalmologist is beneficial.

Stimulation provided to the patient can help to calm, increase alertness, and increase orientation to day, date, and place. Stimulation also can provide input to the larger muscle groups to increase proprioception, impact muscle tone, decrease flexor/extensor patterns, and affect vital signs. It is best to consult with a nurse and attend to any changes in heart rate, blood pressure, or intracranial pressure. Discontinue treatment if it drastically changes vital signs.

INDIVIDUALS AT THE STAGE OF INPATIENT BRAIN INJURY RECOVERY

Occupational therapists in the inpatient rehabilitation setting assist the team by observing the patient's orientation; static sitting balance; dynamic sitting balance; endurance/tolerance for stimulation/activity; the functional mobility of the patient; wheelchair seating; assessment of the upper extremities for flexor/extensor patterns; muscle tone; range of motion; abnormal reflexes; and response to auditory, tactile, visual, vestibular stimuli, and balance reactions.

One way of determining a patient's stage of brain injury is through the use of functional scales. Many hospitals use the Glasgow Coma Scale, Glasgow Outcome Scale, Galveston Orientation and Amnesia Test, Rancho Los Amigos Scale, Functional Independence Measures, or the Functional Assessment of Measures as a way of assessing an individual's orientation, alertness, behavior, baseline performance of activities, and interaction with team, family, and the environment. The Glasgow Coma Scale measures motor responses, verbal responses, and eye-movement responses. Glasgow Coma Scale scores of 8 or less indicate a severe injury, a score of 9 to 12 indicates moderate injury, and a score of 13 to 15 indicates a mild injury.[5] The Glasgow

Outcome Scale rates the patient by categories: death, persistent unresponsiveness, severe disability with dependence for daily support, moderate disability in which an individual can travel using public transportation and work in a sheltered environment, and good recovery with the individual resuming a normal life.[6]

The Galveston Orientation and Amnesia Test (GOAT), which consists of 12 questions covering simple biographical information; the circumstances of the patient's injury; and the patient's knowledge of current time, place, and situation, is fairly simple to use. The test yields a global index of amnesia and disorientation out of a possible maximum score of 100, with separate estimates of retrograde and anterograde amnesia (defined in terms of latest memory before head injury and earliest memory after the accident). The GOAT should be administered at least one time daily. Duration of posttraumatic amnesia is defined as a GOAT score of less than 75.[6]

The Rancho Los Amigos Scale has the following categories: no response, verbal response, localized response, confused–agitated, confused-inappropriate, confused appropriate, automatic inappropriate, and purposeful-appropriate.[5]

Individuals who are transferred from the ICU/Acute Care setting to inpatient rehabilitation are most likely emerging from a coma. At this time the occupational therapist can assess the individual's response to stimuli. Reactions to stimuli are helpful with determining if the individual is emerging from a coma. If a patient does not respond to normal auditory, tactile, or visual stimuli, then painful stimuli may need to be applied. Examples of painful stimuli are the use of ice, pressure applied to the individual's fingernail beds, or the use of a sternal rub. Note the patient's response to stimuli and if the part of the body stimulated is withdrawn, which may indicate awareness of the painful stimuli and an appropriate response to stimuli. Other reactions to stimuli that are helpful in determining if the individual is emerging from a coma include a response in the form of a groan, spontaneous movement, or other various responses.

The next level of response is arousal to stimuli with confusion, disorientation, or response to a question or a command.

Meet with the family to gain information about the patient's preinjury lifestyle, personality, education, vocation, and interests. Often, people who suffer from a brain injury respond to familiar people, sounds, pictures, and information first. Even if the person is in a coma or emerging from the coma, encourage family members to communicate with the individual. A therapist who is aware of an individual's interests is more likely to get his or her attention. Family members may be the first to notice changes in the patient. When family members are ready, educate them about providing appropriate stimuli, assisting with positioning the patient and assisting with passive range of motion and active range of motion.

Family members can better understand an injury if they are involved. Encourage family members to attend a brain injury support group. Often the family will have questions or concerns about the degree of injury, ability of the individual to progress, and how long it will take to determine an outcome. Every individual is different and every brain injury affects an individual in a unique way. There is no exact measurement for determining the amount of recovery that will occur or the effect that injury will have on an individual. Let relatives know that progress may be slow and that stages of recovery can be difficult at times, for example, there may be times when the patient may be agitated or confused. At times, patients with brain injuries will confabulate information. If the patient is confabulating, it is important to not support the false information and to redirect the patient.

Assure the family that agitation, confusion, and confabulation are common behaviors that an individual with a significant brain injury will go through, and that the staff has been trained to help the patient deal with these behaviors as they occur.

The first time the individual is stable enough to be out of bed for longer periods of time, assessment of head and trunk control against gravity will assist in determining the type of wheelchair that will benefit the client. A reclining wheelchair is useful to assist the patient in becoming accustomed to gravity after a long period of time in bed. The occupational therapist can assist with seating assessment and supplying support for different areas of weakness, such as a headrest, lumbar roll, and lateral supports.

Proper positioning of the armrests and footrests is also assessed. Functional mobility on the edge of the bed or mat as tolerated will increase muscle strength, balance, and supply input to the joint mechanoreceptors, which should increase proprioception. Mobility also stimulates the vestibular system. Be aware of any precautions regarding increased intracranial pressure when implementing functional mobility treatment. These precautions may limit the positions that can be used. For example, the patient may not be able to lie flat on a mat or bed secondary to that position increasing intracranial pressure. Use neurodevelopmental patterns, for example, rolling from side to side, lying prone on the elbows, weight-bearing in quadruped, and kneeling activities to increase proprioception, static balance, dynamic balance, and muscular strength/endurance.

The individual may fatigue easily and require frequent rest breaks. Allowing the individual to take short breaks of five minutes or so during a treatment session, or limiting treatment sessions to 15 minutes initially, may be most productive and beneficial. If the individual begins to become agitated, monitor the type and amount of stimulation the patient is receiving and the amount of extraneous distractions in the environment affecting the patient. When the patient demonstrates increased frustration and decreased tolerance for an activity, decrease stimulation by giving limited verbal information, turning the lights down, and treating the individual in a quiet room away from other people. This will eliminate distractions and assist the patient with attending to the tasks at hand.

Basic self-care activities, such as grooming, can be used to assess the individual's initiation, organization, sequencing, attention, cognition, balance, visual/perceptual skills, and ability to follow one-, two-, or three-step commands. Check a patient's initiation during performance of grooming tasks, whether no prompt is needed, or document how much structure is needed. Does the individual follow one-step commands? If the individual is stuck and does not recall the next step of the activity, cueing by stating, "Next, brush your teeth," is helpful. It is advantageous to schedule treatment time when the individual is more alert. Use a board with basic information such as day, date, year; specific times and scheduled appointments help orient the patient. Observation of self-care also gives the occupational therapist useful information about attention, safety awareness, and problem solving. For example, does the individual get distracted by people in the hallway or the TV, or does the individual try to walk without the use of an assistive device or with socks on a slippery floor? Awareness of time can be assessed by use of the clock and schedule to reinforce the amount of time that has passed during an activity. It is helpful to use cue cards and a board to assist with sequencing events. Memory notebooks with a short phrase about the treatment session will assist patients with memory. These notebooks are good ways of communicating with the family and other team members regarding techniques to implement during basic self-care activities.

Assessment of dressing can provide the occupational therapist with information about an individual's functional mobility, proprioception, vision/perception, balance, gross motor coordination, fine motor coordination, and cognitive skills. For example, can the individual sit on the edge of the bed or does he or she need to have his or her back supported? Does he or she know what step comes next? How does he or she organize a task? Does he or she have difficulty knowing where his or her body is in space, and have difficulty bumping into objects in the environment when gathering clothes? Do objects in the environment distract the individual? Is he or she able to button clothes or use zippers? Does he or she have difficulty positioning an item of clothing or knowing what part of the body to place clothing on?

Apraxia may be discovered during functional activities. There are several types of apraxia that can occur. Even though an individual has intact physical ability, sensation, and coordination, he or she may be unable to perform certain purposeful movements. Dressing apraxia occurs when the individual has a disorder of body scheme or motor planning. An individual who cannot perform a movement on command demonstrates ideomotor apraxia; however, he or she may perform the movement spontaneously. For example, when asked to demonstrate how to drink from a cup, he or she is unable; but if he or she is thirsty, he or she may drink from a cup spontaneously. Apraxia can effect an individual's limbs, speech, and even the way that an individual thinks. Constructional apraxia is demonstrated by an inability to produce designs in two or three dimensions.[7]

Route finding on the rehabilitation unit can determine the patient's visual spatial awareness and memory. Cueing the patient to signs, room numbers, and items in the environment is helpful. This also can be a way of assessing visual scanning for items in the environment. Observe a patient's attention by his or her reaction to environmental stimulation, such as another patient in the hallway.

When the individual is ready it is good to use community mobility for route finding. Goals could include a trip to the vending machine, cafeteria, newspaper stand, or gift shop, which would address attention to environment, ability to find a route with or without cues, visual scanning, spatial awareness, simple problem solving, and simple money management.

Assessment of simple activities of daily living, such as preparing instant cereal in the microwave or preparing toast, assist the therapist in determining cognitive ability. The Assessment of Motor and Process Skills (AMPS) is one way to formally assess activities of daily living. (The AMPS will be further discussed later in this chapter.) Note the individual's ability to follow directions. Does the individual need steps or directions to be broken down further? Can they initiate the activity and retrieve all the needed supplies from the cupboard? Do they remember to set a timer and, when the timer goes off, do they remember what the timer was for? Grade activities from simple to complex, and grade the amount of cueing provided to the patient. Provide structure for the activity to increase the patient's success and safety, and compensate for cognitive impairment by use of forward chaining or backward chaining. Individuals with difficulty initiating tasks may require external cues from an occupational therapist, family member, or tape recorder.

Information about vision can be gained through observation of the patient. For example, do they squint, tilt their head to the side, or overshoot when reaching for an item? Behaviors such as these indicate difficulty with acuity or diplopia. Visual acuity can be assessed with use of the Snellen Chart Near or Far. Visual tracking, saccadic eye movements, convergence, and visual fields can be assessed with use of a penlight or object to track. Use a number cancel or line dissection activity to assess the patient's visual attention, visual neglect, organization of scanning pattern, and impulsivity. Use of the Motor Free Visual Perceptual Test can give a baseline assessment of perceptual skills, such as form constancy, figure ground, visual memory, and visual closure. The River Mead Visual Perceptual Assessment thoroughly evaluates vision and perception in higher-level patients with fair sustained attention. Other visual assessments like the OPTEC 2000 are useful for gaining information about lateral phoria, verticle phoria, contrast sensitivity, fusion, stereo depth perception, and peripheral vision. Use of the Accuvision or the Wayne Saccadic Fixator can be additional ways to measure peripheral vision, visual neglect, visual reaction time, and hand-eye coordination. Functional activities such as catching and tossing a ball and reading can provide helpful information about vision. Functional mobility provides information about vision and perception; patients who demonstrate difficulty going up and down stairs may have problems with depth perception or figure ground. Another useful technique is swinging a Marsten Ball in a circular, horizontal, and diagonal pattern to initiate visual tracking. The Marsten Ball, which can be hung from the ceiling with fishing line, has a series of numbers or letters for the patient to locate. Begin gradually with this technique and instruct the patient to tell the therapist if he or she is becoming dizzy or nauseous. This activity should be used initially for five to ten minutes secondary to the potential of the patient having the previously stated symptoms.

A patient with frontal lobe damage is likely to have difficulty obtaining and sustaining fixation.[5] Some form of visual dysfunction occurs in at least 50% of patients with traumatic brain injury.[1] As stated previously, a review of the cranial nerves associated with vision will help with evaluation.

Cranial nerve II is the optic nerve, which is responsible for conducting information from the eyes to the brain. The oculomotor nerve, cranial nerve III, controls the medial, superior, and inferior rectus and inferior oblique muscles. If the patient has difficulty with eye movement toward the nose, downward, upward, and up away from the nose, the oculomotor nerve may be effected.

Impairment of the IVth cranial nerve, the trochlear, can cause diplopia. Cranial nerve VI, the abducens, controls the lateral rectus muscle, which moves the eye laterally and away from the nose. A damaged cranial nerve VII is apparent when the individual is unable to close his or her eye. Symptoms of subconjunctival hemorrhage and verticle diplopia can be the result of orbital fractures or fractures of the maxillary sinus, which may entrap the eye muscles.[4]

Use knowledge of abnormal reflex patterns during treatment to assist in guiding handling techniques in order to break up abnormal patterns. Abnormal reflexes occur because the brain is unable to inhibit reflexes that occurred normally in earlier stages of development. Examples of abnormal reflexes are the asymmetrical tonic neck reflex (ATNR), the symmetric tonic neck reflex (STNR), and the tonic labyrinthine reflex (TLR). ATNR is characterized by extension of the upper extremity that the head is turned towards with flexion of the opposite upper extremity; the head may be held in forward flexion or hyperextension. Flexion or extension of the head causes STNR. When the neck is extended, the increased extension of the upper extremities and increased flexion of the lower extremities occurs. If the individual's neck is flexed, upper extremities become flexed and lower extremities respond with increased extension. STNR and ATNR can occur together. TLR is observed in supine and prone positions. When the patient is supine, the neck extends, shoulders retract, and the arms and legs extend with rigid adduction present. TLR is demonstrated when prone by increased flexion of the head, trunk, and all other body parts. STNR and TLR occur in individuals with brain stem injuries. ATNR is present when an individual's higher level cortical control is impacted by the brain injury.[5]

The upper extremities may be in a flexor pattern or extensor pattern. The individual's trunk may present with lateral flexion, kyphotic posture, or scoliosis. This occurs secondary to abnormal reflex patterns or as a result of long periods of immobility. The pelvis often is posteriorly tilted with residual tightness in the hip flexors and adductors. In the scapula, patterns of protraction or retraction with elevation are commonly seen.

Proper positioning in bed and sitting can assist with decreasing these abnormal patterns. Use moist heat followed by positioning so the individual experiences gentle stretching of the affected area to break up abnormal patterns and return symmetry to posture. Activities such as the use of a Swiss Ball, placed behind the patient to gently stretch the patient into trunk extension with the shoulders retracted and depressed, can create a prolonged stretch for increasing symmetry to the posture of the upper back and scapular region. Placement of the individual on the side where there is greater lateral flexion can assist with elongating the muscles on that side. Strategic placement of folded-up hand towels between the patient's shoulders and behind the scapula can increase stretch to shortened muscle groups.

Attend to any changes in tone or abnormal reflex patterns while performing passive range-of-motion exercises. Should a reflex pattern be triggered, do not force the extremity during ranging; instead, let the reflex occur, provide inhibitory handling techniques to quiet the muscles, and proceed with range of motion. As stated previously, the extremity should never be forced, as forcing the extremity can cause heterotopic ossification to occur. Passive range of motion should begin with the scapular musculature to assist with relaxation. Start with elevation, depression, protraction, retraction, and rotation of the scapula. Once the scapula has been relaxed, the upper extremity will move more freely.

Muscles may be weak from long periods of inactivity. Strength can be assessed formally through manual muscle testing, or informally through observation of the individual lifting various items in the environment. Grip and pinch strength may be measured with a dynamometer and compared to average strength of an individual in his or her age category. Treatment for muscle strength can include functional activities, progressive resistive exercises, proprioceptive neuromuscular facilitation, and an individualized home exercise program. In cases where family members or friends require instruction to assist with implementing a home exercise program, consider the use of videotaped instruction. This provides the family with a resource that they can use repetitively with individuals who need assistance initiating an exercise program.

Evaluate rapid alternating movements by having the individual move quickly from pronation to supination, and by having the individual touch his or her thumb to each finger as quickly as possible. A formal evaluation of an individual's ability to perform rapid alternating movements is the Minnesota Rate of Manipulation. It is comprised of four tests that are one-handed, or two-handed tests that require both hands. Another assessment for rapid alternating movement, gross motor coordination skills, and fine motor coordination skills is the Jebsen-Taylor Test of Hand Function. It is a standardized test of coordination which is comprised of seven subtests: writing, simulated page turning, picking up small objects, simulated feeding, stacking checkers, picking up large light objects, and picking up large heavy objects. Treatment activities that can assist with increasing rapid alternating movements are throwing, catching, ball bouncing, hand clapping, and game playing.

Assess fine motor coordination by observing the individual use buttons, fasteners, zippers, and shoelaces. The patient may also be asked to touch his or her fingers to their thumb as quickly as possible.

Some more formal assessments of fine motor coordination are the Nine-Hole Peg Test and the Purdue Peg Board. In the Nine-Hole Peg Test, the individual is asked to place the pegs in each hole individually, and then to take the pegs out of the hole one at a time while the evaluator times him or her. The time is then compared to averages for people in the patient's age category. If the individual demonstrates ease with the Nine-Hole Peg Test, then an evaluator may choose to progress to the Purdue Peg Board because it involves more pieces and more fine motor movements. Treatment of fine motor coordination can involve functional self-care activities, games, fine motor coordination exercises, and crafts.

Functional activities have an increased variety of fine motor movement patterns in comparison to tabletop activities. Research involving treatment of individuals with brain injury who have fine motor coordination deficits found that patients in the functional meal preparation group showed significantly greater improvement in dominant-hand dexterity for picking up small objects than did individuals in a fine motor coordination table-top activity group.[8]

Cognition of the individual with brain injury is assessed through attention; orientation; the ability to organize, sequence, and problem-solve; safety awareness; and the ability to follow directions. Information can be gleaned from performance of functional activities, and ability to generate solutions when problems are encountered without assistance from the therapist. Cognitive rehabilitation involves retraining and the use of compensatory techniques.[1] The therapist can break down cognitive activities into manageable segments. Activities can be structured for increased ease by the therapist gathering all the materials needed for the activity. Further structure can be supplied by simple verbal or written commands provided by the therapist.

The therapist can also control distractions in the environment. As the individual demonstrates sustained attention in a nondistracting environment, the therapist can gradually add distractions to challenge the patient.

The ability of the individual to sustain attention to a task is essential before a clear picture of the individual's cognition can be formed. Sustained attention works as a filter. The person is receiving information from the environment and sustained attention provides the individual with the ability to filter out unecessary information and attend to relevant information. Evaluate the patient in a nondistracting environment. Record length of attention, add distractions if the individual is functioning well in a non-distracting environment, and note any redirection required during the assessment. Examples of distractions are the use of a radio or television, or other people in the environment. Divided attention is the ability attend to two or more tasks simultaneously. Alternating attention is the ability to shift attention from one activity to another.

Activities can progress from single, sustained attention activities, to activities that require attention to be alternated from one activity to another. An example of this type of activity setup is having the individual prepare soup and a salad. The individual must be able to shift attention from the soup on the stovetop to the salad. Eventually, more complex divided attention tasks can be addressed; for example, turning the television on while the individual is performing a task and asking them to attend to both the task and the television. Another example involves asking the patient to discuss what the news reporter was talking about while he or she was getting dressed.

Formal assessment of memory can occur once the individual is able to demonstrate reasonable sustained attention to a task in a nondistracting environment. Memory is an important component when assessing cognition. One of the most frequent complaints of patients with traumatic brain injury is an impairment of memory.[1] Immediate recall is the ability to recall information directly following receiving the information. Short-term memory is the ability to recall information after up to three to five minutes. Recent memory is recall of events that occurred within a day. Remote memory is recall of events in the past. Long-term memory involves encoding information, storage of information, and ability to retrieve information. The River Mead Behavioral Memory Test is a formal assessment of memory for orientation, date, faces, names, hidden belongings, appointments, picture recognition, prose, recall, short routes, errands, and a new skill. A few formal cognitive assessments that are useful in evaluation are the Kohlman Evaluation of Living Skills (KELS) and the Cognitive Assessment of Minnesota (CAM). The KELS appropriately ascertains if the lower-level patient has good safety awareness, time management, awareness of address, simple money management skills, and awareness of what to do in an emergency situation. Higher-level patients can be assessed with the CAM to determine short-term memory, long-term memory, simple and complex problem solving, math skills, mental manipulation, and social awareness. Functional use of community resources like telephone books, maps, and newspapers is another way to assess the cognition of an individual with a brain injury. Simple and complex money exchanges require fair cognition. Activities such as the management of a checkbook with the use of compensatory techniques can be useful for individuals with brain injury.

If an individual has problems with memory, train the patient with a particular pattern to follow for searching the environment for cues. This pattern may use typical visual scanning patterns from left to right, top to bottom. Have the individual start in the room that he or she is in and progress to other rooms in the house in a circular pattern, from left to right. For example, if the phone rings and interrupts the patient, how can he or she conduct a systematic search of the environment for cues in order to return to the previous activity? A recorded message, reminding the patient to search left to right from the room he or she is in to additional rooms, can assist family members in reinforcing the technique of systematically searching the environment when the individual is interrupted. Another method of handling interruptions is the use of a "sticky note" on which the patient writes what he or she is doing at the moment of interruption.

Persons who have brain injury report that the long-term social ramifications of their injury can be more devastating than the physical ramifications.[2] Scheduling group therapy sessions is a way to address social interaction, behavior, and the ability of the individual to use higher-level alternating and divided attention in a socially appropriate way. Role-playing is one technique that can provide the individual with opportunities to practice social interaction in a safe environment. It gives the group members an area to observe interaction and provide feedback to one another about decisions or behavior.

Examples of group activities that may be useful in providing interactions include cooking, crafts, exercise, and role-playing. The individual may have difficulty sharing feelings with family or friends and may need to practice interactions in a group to increase confidence and decrease anxiety. Groups can also create an environment where spontaneous events may occur causing the group members to interact and generate solutions. Other examples of group activities are an informative group, a current events group, or a project group for the community.

Once the patient is able to handle distractions without increased agitation or confusion, community integration can become a goal of therapy. Group community outings are an important step in community reintegration. The group may plan where the outing will occur, how to get there, what time of day would be best, and how much the activity will cost. After the activity occurs, each member can be asked to express their feelings about the outing. Have the group make an informative poster about the outing to share with the other patients on the rehabilitation unit, to generate creative ideas, and to increase interaction. Practice on public transportation could be the goal of an outing. Grading how much intervention is required by the therapist to assist each individual access transportation may be part of the outing. Family members can participate to increase their awareness of the challenges the patient is facing.

Difficulty with time management can be addressed with compensatory techniques implemented by the therapist or the family during the outing. Often, an individual with a brain injury has experienced a change in lifestyle and leisure activities. Exploring new activities on the outing can provide the individual with opportunities to increase leisure interests.

A home evaluation is an important part of the patient returning home successfully. The occupational therapist can assess the environment and make recommendations regarding safety, adaptive equipment, and strategies for setting up the home to increase the individual's success through organization and structure.

Individuals who have decreased safety awareness may require supervision from family or friends during complex tasks. Use a watch with an alarm clock or other timers within the home as compensatory strategies to assist with increased memory, initiation, and time management. Calendars with daily, weekly, and monthly reminders placed in one familiar place are ways to reinforce structure and consistency with an individual who has a brain injury. Use of color-coding is another beneficial way to reinforce structure and assist with memory. Patients with brain injuries may benefit from home-based treatment that can maximize learning, assist with educating the family, and increase functional independence in the home.[9]

Brain injury affects each individual in a unique manner; occupational therapists need to be creative in order to facilitate the most appropriate technique for the individual and the situation.

When appropriate, videotaping the patient in particular circumstances may provide the patient, family, and therapy team with useful information. In cases where the individual has decreased insight into his or her behavior, a videotape may help the patient realize his or her behavior. When family members cannot be present for training, videotape instructions to assist the family with carrying out the particular program or techniques after discharge.

A day treatment program offers treatment for the individual while he or she is transitioning from the hospital to home and community. Day treatment is a vital part of the continuum of therapy with brain injury patients. Structure provided by the therapy staff can be graded until the individual is able to become more independent through the use of compensatory techniques, and is able to proceed to an outpatient setting with less structure.

MILD TRAUMATIC BRAIN INJURY

Mild traumatic brain injury is often referred to as the "unseen injury." The individual may look fine, but may have difficulty with managing complex activities of daily living that he or she was once able to perform independently. At times, these individuals are treated and released following an accident, or several accidents over a period of time, with a "post concussive syndrome." His or her life begins to unravel without the individual being able to identify the cause. An individual who suffers from a mild traumatic brain injury may have any or all of the following symptoms which were stated at the beginning of this chapter: nausea, dizziness, disturbed sleep patterns, emotional outbursts, headaches, and difficulty with higher-level attention or memory. It is not until the patient attempts to return to his or her normal routine that the difficulty begins. Mild traumatic brain injury can have as significant an effect on individuals as a moderate or severe injury.

A cause of mild traumatic brain injury can be axonal shearing as a result of an injury that occurred causing the head to accelerate/decelerate and twist and disturb delicate neural tissue. Mild traumatic brain injury can also be caused by a direct blow to the head, or via concussion. Perhaps the individual has been involved in a series of sporting injuries. Sometimes players in contact sports experience a concussion and return to the game within a week or two, only to have another accident that causes more damage to the brain. Another cause of mild traumatic brain injury is whiplash. As stated previously, CT scans done immediately after the accident often do not show damage to the brain. However, a later CT scan may indicate problems.

An occupational therapy evaluation of individuals with mild traumatic brain injury can assess upper extremity strength, range of motion, sensation, gross motor coordination, fine motor coordination, coordination for rapid alternating movements, proprioception, cervical range of motion, ability to perform basic self-care activities, complex activities of daily living, vision, perception, cognition, sustained attention, and higher-level divided and alternating attention to tasks. Performance of a job evaluation can provide insight and strategies for the individual to increase independence and success with issues when returning to work. Return to the complex activity of driving is another issue that can be addressed by an occupational therapist as part of a driving program.

If the individual was involved in a motor vehicle accident, there is a possibility that he or she will have soft tissue injuries. Careful observation of the individual's range of motion and the gathering of information from interviewing the patient will assist with targeting pain related to soft tissue injuries. Areas where the shoulder contacted the seatbelt are susceptible to damage. Tightness in the muscles that attach to the neck and the shoulders may contribute to pain and problems with headache. Occupational therapists can address soft tissue injuries with modalities, soft tissue massage, range of motion exercises, trigger-point release, development of an individual home exercise program, education on the use of proper body mechanics, and education on the use of pain management techniques. Analyze the position of the individual during complex activities of daily living and during work to assist with determining contributing factors to pain the individual experiences.

Address sensation by formal evaluation of an individual's response to light touch, pain, touch localization, two-point discrimination, and stereognosis. Educating the individual on the use of sensory reeducation techniques for areas of hypersensitivity or decreased sensation can be an important part of the home program. If hypersensitivity is present, start with the use of various textures to desensitize the patient's skin.

An example of an activity for decreasing hypersensitivity is for the individual to place his or her hand into a container of rice or beans. Progress to identification of moving touch, starting proximally. Have the individual look at the stimulus, close their eyes and concentrate on the sensation, and then open their eyes to confirm the sensation. Eventually, use familiar objects placed in an individual's hand following the above process to achieve recovery of stereognosis. Objects should be graded from harsh to fine, large to small, and by subtle differences in texture during late-phase sensory reeducation.

Gross motor coordination may be observed during functional mobility and complex activities of daily living. Coordination for rapid alternating movements can be assessed with the use of cerebellar movements including rapid finger to nose, finger-to-knee-nose-opposite knee, and activities such as catching a ball. Rapid alternating movements may be more formally addressed with use of the Minnesota

Rate of Manipulation. The Jebsen-Taylor Test of Hand Function can also be a useful assessment of gross motor coordination and fine motor coordination. Both of these evaluations were described previously. The Bennett Hand Tool Test may also be used to assess coordination and speed of performance.

Fine motor coordination may be addressed by having the patient move his or her thumb to touch each finger as fast as possible. Use of a Nine-Hole Peg Test and the Purdue Peg Board can address formal assessment and be used as a measure of progress. The Valpar Tools Test evaluates an individual's use of a variety of tools that are common in the fields of mechanics, printing, assembly, and construction. Treatment of gross motor and fine motor coordination can be implemented through the use of everyday activities, for example, tying shoes, typing, playing games, playing a musical instrument, and participating in an individualized home program designed by the occupational therapist.

Having the individual participate in meal planning and preparation is an insightful way to assess his or her ability to plan, organize, problem solve, and attend to the task. A formal assessment, such as, the Assessment of Motor and Process Skills (AMPS), is a useful way to evaluate and reassess progress with activities of daily living. The AMPS was designed as an occupational therapy assessment tool and is a thorough way of analyzing the activity and rating the performance. Occupational therapists who use the AMPS must attend specialized training and become certified to become raters to increase their validity and reliability in rating.

Interviewing the individual with a mild traumatic brain injury is a way of determining the effect his or her injury has had on his or her vision and perception. The occupational therapist should note any report of diplopia, blurred vision, increased headaches, difficulty with maintaining their place when reading, or increased incidence of eye strain/fatigue, which are indications that the individual may have an injury to his or her visual system. Visual tracking should be checked as well as visual saccades and convergence. Any decrease in mobility, slowness of movement, or nystagmus must be noted. Further visual assessment includes the use of the Snellen chart to assess near and far acuity, in addition to assessment of lateral and vertical phorias, depth perception, and field of vision. Use organized and disorganized number and symbol patterns to provide the evaluator with useful information regarding scanning patterns, impulsivity, and visual fields. Additional information can be gained with use of a Marsten Ball in treatment for horizontal and diagonal patterns. A large dry-erase board can be used as a tool for treatment with the use of activities such as line tangles and scanning for various numbers or letters written on the board. If the occupational therapist has access to the Accuvision and The Wayne Saccadic Fixator, these machines can be used to address visual reaction time, field of vision, hand-eye coordination, and peripheral vision, and to train the individual with compensatory techniques for vision. The OPTEC 2000 is another useful evaluation tool that addresses visual acuity near and far, contrast sensitivity, color perception, phorias, stereo depth perception, fusion, and peripheral vision. Perceptual skills can be assessed with the Motor Free Vision Perception Test. This test evaluates for form constancy, figure ground, visual memory, and visual closure. The River Mead Visual Perceptual Test is another way of assessing vision and perception.

Cognition can be evaluated through use of the Cognitive Assessment of Minnesota. This test evaluates memory for recent, remote, short-term, and long-term; mental manipulation; calculations; abstract reasoning; foresight and planning; problem solving, concrete and complex; social awareness; and awareness of safety. Observe sustained attention to task during the evaluation. Assessment of alternating and divided attention to task can be evaluated through use of controlled interruptions or distractions in the environment during the testing. More formal evaluation of alternating and divided attention is done with the use of evaluations such as the Wisconsin Card Sorting Task or the Stroop Test. Performance of complex activities of daily living with controlled distractions is another way of assessing higher-level sustained, alternating, and divided attention to tasks.

Executive functions include judgment, decision making, initiation, planning, organization, intuition, and the ability to regulate behavior. Present the patient initially with simple problems and observe his or her response. Is he or she able to anticipate outcomes and generate alternative solutions to the problem? How much structure does the therapist provide? Is the task organized or disorganized? Answers to questions such as these will provide useful information regarding the use of executive functions. Monitor the individual's behavior and frustration level. If his or her behavior starts to escalate and frustration increases, discontinue the task and initiate calming techniques or a rest break. Assist with implementation of compensatory strategies to increase the potential for success. Use repetition to reinforce compensatory strategies and progress to more complex problems. Have the individual look at the goal he or she is trying to accomplish, plan how to accomplish the goal, initiate the plan, and then review the outcome. Problem solving in this manner will help the individual with a systematic way of looking at problems, and help the occupational therapist with identifying areas to reinforce compensatory strategies. Examples of compensatory techniques for memory and organization include the use of a watch with an alarm clock, calendars, day planners, a tape recorder, and sticky notes. Also, routine systematic techniques may be used for remembering numbers through chunking the information. Other routine systematic techniques may involve helping the individual recall names by restating the name shortly after being introduced and trying to remember a salient feature about an individual. The use of schedules, alarm clocks, checklists, and daily routines can assist with use of the time management and help an individual with accomplishing goals.

The individual may need education from the occupational therapist to increase his or her awareness of distracters that are present in the environment, and to generate functional alternatives to use in decreasing the distracters. Cognitive fatigue is another issue that the occupational therapist can address with the patient in order to increase the patient's awareness of the importance of rest breaks, power naps, and the use of relaxation techniques.

The area of the brain that is affected by the injury can correlate to certain cognitive deficits. Patients who have frontal lobe damage may present with decreased initiation, ability to plan and organize, mental flexibility, and abstraction. These abilities are referred to as executive functions. Executive functions assist the individual in awareness of self, goal setting, ability to plan to accomplish a goal, monitoring the progress towards the goal, and ability to revise the plan when problems arise.[1] Damage to the brain following anoxic or hypoxic injury effects the hippocampus, which is one of the most vulnerable structures in the brain. The ability to develop new memory and integrate that memory into storage relies on the hippocampus.[1] Decreased insight is common following damage to the right hemisphere. Most patients with injuries in this area underestimate the extent of their cognitive impairments.[1]

Research has indicated that individuals with traumatic brain injury benefit from intervention as long as five years post injury. Establishing routines for the individual with brain injury through the use of structured supports related primarily to executive function, cognitive function, behavior, and communication can assist with transitions. Examples of transitions are from one therapy to another, from the beginning of the day to the end of the day, and from the hospital or outpatient clinic to home. Tasks can be structured with the use of external cues or internal cues, forward or backward chaining, repetition, photo cues in the form of a flowchart, modified tasks, and anticipation of changes in stimuli from day to day. Structure can also be enforced through control of environmental distractions.[6]

An approach established by Ylvisaker involves individuals participating in real-world tasks with sufficient external supports or "scaffolding" that assists in providing strategic behavior, emphasizing components of cognitive processing, and mastery of the task.[10] As the individual demonstrates increased independence with a task, withdraw part of the support, expand the task, and vary the environment in which the task is performed.[6] In occupational therapy these variances in task and environment have been called grading of an activity.

There is a risk of employment problems following traumatic brain injury, with estimates of unemployment varying from 50% to 99%.[1] A job-site evaluation is a useful and important assessment needed to increase a patient's independence and ability to accomplish his or her goal of return to work. The occupational therapist can analyze the physical, environmental, and cognitive aspects of the work environment.

Assessing the individual performance components of the job and determining potential areas where the individual needs intervention is an important part of the job evaluation. Generating functional solutions with the individual and the employer can help increase the potential for successful return to work. Examples of solutions that may be determined at the job evaluation are to have the individual return to work for a limited time each day and to structure the environment so they are working on one task at a time with limited distractions present. Consider having the individual shadow another employee to assure that the patient is following through with all the correct job procedures. Occupational therapy treatment may involve simulation of work tasks in the clinical setting to assist the individual with implementation of compensatory techniques, and to increase the individual's cognitive endurance for the workday. Implementing functional strategies such as color-coding, cue sheets, day planners, and other memory aids can also increase the individual's success.

An individual with mild traumatic brain injury may experience variance in performance from day to day due to factors of fatigue, stress, increased distractions, and/or responsibilities. This can increase the amount of anxiety experienced by the individual. Occupational therapists can assist with implementing techniques to increase relaxation. One method of relaxation is progressively tensing and relaxing muscle groups and concentrating on the feeling of relaxation as the individual progresses through the muscle groups. Another method of relaxation is visualization or guided imagery. The patient may benefit from biofeedback. Occupational therapists can co-treat with biofeedback professionals to ensure proper relaxation of targeted muscle groups is occurring. It is important that the patient is aware that his or her abilities may change from day to day. He or she will have good days and bad days. On the bad days, use of compensatory strategies may be his or her best resource. Open communication and support from the employer may not always be present. If the patient experiences further difficulty with return to work, encourage the patient to contact his or her therapist for support and additional problem solving.

Axonal shearing injuries of the brain create diffuse damage affecting many areas of the central nervous system, including the brainstem.[1] These injuries often affect parts of the brainstem, basal forebrain, and hypothalamus, which are structures that control the sleep/wake cycle. Appropriate diagnosis of a sleep disorder will assist with treatment. Have the patient document the amount of time that he or she is sleeping and determine the amount of time he or she would like to be able to sleep. Then have the patient attempt to delay or increase the time of sleep onset by a few hours every day.[1] The physician may prescribe a variety of medications to assist with sleep/wake cycles. Individuals with residual sleep disorders as a result of traumatic brain injury can benefit from occupational therapy intervention to address the complex activity of daily living (ADL) of driving. In the U.S. alone, in 1990 it was estimated that 200,000 motor vehicle accidents were due to falling asleep at the wheel.

Occupational therapists are valuable members of a driving program. Individuals with brain injury may have difficulty with vision, perception, physical reaction time, visual reaction time, cognition, and attention, which impacts the complex ADL of driving. To locate a qualified driving program in your area, please contact the Association for Driver Rehabilitation Specialists at P. O. Box 49, Edgerton, WI 53534, or by phone at (608) 884-8833. A driving rehabilitation program should have a qualified Certified Driving Rehabilitation Specialist (CDRS) on staff and appropriate vehicle(s), as well as equipment to provide comprehensive services in the following areas: clinical evaluation, on-road evaluation, vehicle modifications/Rx, driver training/treatment, and a final fitting. Individuals with brain injury may be found to have one or several of the following characteristics when they are driving: inappropriate speed; slow to identify and avoid potentially hazardous situations; require instruction from passengers; miss or do not observe signs, signals, or speed limits; leave out important road, traffic, or warning information; have slow or poor decisions with regard to traffic or road changes; become easily frustrated or confused; may get lost even in familiar areas; experience collisions or near misses; and blame driving mistakes on the behavior of other drivers.

In much the same way that every individual is different, every individual experiences their brain injury in a different way. The information in this chapter is meant to be a guideline for treatment of individuals with brain injury. For further information, please refer to the listed references for this chapter.

REFERENCES

1. Rizzo, R, MD, Tranel, D, Eds., *Head Injury and Postconcussive Syndrome*. Churchill Livingstone, New York, 1996.
2. Gutman, SA, Napier-Klemic, J, The experience of head injury on the impairment of gender role, *The American Journal of Occupational Therapy*, 50:535, 1996.
3. Burleigh, SA, Farber, RS, Gillard, M, Community integration and life satisfaction after traumatic brain injury: long-term findings, *The American Journal of Occupational Therapy*, 52:45, 1998.
4. Mackay, LE, Chapman, PE, Morgan, AS, *Maximizing Brain Injury Recovery: Integrating Critical Care and Early Rehabilitation*, Aspen Press, Gaithersburg, MD, 1997.
5. Pedretti, LW, Zoltan, B, *Occupational Therapy Practice Skills for Physical Dysfunction*, 3rd ed., The C.V. Mosby Company, St. Louis, 1990.
6. Richardson, JTE, *Clinical and Neuropsychological Aspects of Closed Head Injury*, Taylor & Francis, New York, 1990.
7. Siev, E, Freishtat, B, Zoltan, B, *Perceptual and Cognitive Dysfunction in the Adult Stroke Patient: A Manual for Evaluation and Treatment*, SLACK, Inc., Thorofare, NJ, 1986.
8. Neistadt, ME, The effects of different treatment activities on functional fine motor coordination in adults with brain injury, *American Journal of Occupational Therapy*, 52:877, 1994.
9. Schwartz, SM, Adults with traumatic brain injury: three case studies of cognitive rehabilitation in the home setting, *The American Journal of Occupational Therapy*, 49:655, 1995.
10. Ylvisaker, M, Feeney, TJ, *Collaborative Brain Injury Intervention: Positive Everyday Routines*, Singular Publishing Group, Inc., San Diego, 1988.

ADDITIONAL READING

1. Morse, PA, Ed., *Brain Injury: Cognitive and Prevocational Approaches to Rehabilitation*, The Tiresias Press, Inc., New York, 1986.
2. Cohen, H, Vestibular rehabilitation improves daily life function, *The American Journal of Occupational Therapy*, 52(4), 919, 1994.
3. Shimelman, A, Hinojosa, J, Gross motor activity and attention in three adults with brain injury, *The American Journal of Occupational Therapy*, 49:973, 1995.
4. Price-Lackey, P, Cashman, J, Jenny's story: reinventing oneself through occupation and narrative configuration, *The American Journal of Occupational Therapy*, 50:306, 1996.
5. Abreu, BC, Seale, G, Podlesak, J, Hartley, L, Development of critical paths for postacute brain injury rehabilitation: lessons learned, *The American Journal of Occupational Therapy*, 50:417, 1996.
6. Yuen, HK, Case report-positive talk training in an adult with traumatic brain injury, *The American Journal of Occupational Therapy*, 51:780, 1997.
7. Giles, GM, Ridley, JE, Dill, A, Frye, S, A consecutive series of adults with brain injury treated with a washing and dressing retraining program, *The American Journal of Occupational Therapy*, 51:256, 1997.

15 Neuropsychology for the Non-Neuropsychologist: Special Guidance for Working with Persons with Mild TBI (MTBI)

Karen E. Lee, Psy.D.
Richard H. Cox, Ph.D., MD, ABRP, ABPP

"No head injury is too severe to despair of, nor too trivial to ignore" Hippocrates, 4th Century B.C.

Many professionals today are faced with working with individuals who have sustained a brain injury. Brain injuries vary in degree of seriousness and sequelae of symptoms. According to Segalowitz & Lawson (1995), 70% to 90% of head injuries are classified as mild. Although much research exists on moderate-to-severe injuries, there is a need to understand the complexities of brain damage in light of individuals who have been diagnosed with a "mild" injury. There are many places to find the demographics of brain injury. Unfortunately, not all head injuries are seen by professionals; hence, not all come to the attention of professionals and are therefore not accounted for. However, recognizing the limitations of documentation, it is reported that over 700,000 patients receive hospital services each year due to head injury. Of these persons, approximately 10% will suffer severe head injury resulting in life-altering disabilities. Whereas in earlier years many persons with severe brain injury would not have survived, due to the advances in medical technology, today many will survive but with permanent and life-altering disabilities. Approximately two-thirds of head injury victims will be between the ages of 15 and 25. Even prior to the advent of managed medical care, many head injury victims did not receive sufficient rehabilitation to return to educational and/or occupational endeavors. Today, most professionals believe the number of patients receiving less than adequate rehabilitation is much higher; however, it is not possible to document these data. The purpose of this chapter is to help the nonneuropsychologist professional learn more about the field of neuropsychological evaluation and treatment, and to increase the knowledge base of the reader regarding mild traumatic brain injury (MTBI). With an increased awareness of the cognitive, emotional, and social changes brought on by a not so mild brain injury, it is the hope of these authors that professionals of all disciplines will be better equipped to serve these clients. Those with MTBI often access services provided by medical professionals, mental health professionals, attorneys, educators, and vocational services.

NEUROPSYCHOLOGY DEFINED

What exactly is "neuropsychology?" Neuropsychology is a specialty within the field of clinical psychology that studies how the brain expresses itself functionally, and how certain behaviors are caused by and controlled by certain areas of the brain. The neuropsychologist is a specialist in diagnosing brain damage by utilizing non-invasive methods, especially developed tests which reveal both mild and more severe brain function disability. These instruments involve both physical and mental participation on the part of the patient. Furthermore, the neuropsychologist can indicate the level and degree of brain damage. Mild brain damage is sometimes only demonstrable by the neuropsychological method. While medical doctors who specialize in brain trauma can often demonstrate severe brain damage, mild head injury is sometimes only revealed by the neuropsychological measurement of subtle brain functions. Medical evaluation is clearly best for severe brain injury where structural and anatomical change has occurred. Function tests are often best performed by the neuropsychologist.

Differential diagnosis is often difficult in the patient with head injury. The patient may have had psychological abnormalities, intellectual deficiencies, and/or abnormal behavior prior to the brain insult. The neuropsychologist is best able to determine the concomitant, prior, or causal relationship of such thinking and behavior in the postinjury state.

Since we now have a greater understanding of the functions of the different parts of the brain, it is possible to indicate localization of the injury by determining the anatomical locus of neuropsychological malfunction. As will be pointed out later in this chapter, this is particularly important for those injuries that result in frontal lobe insult, since most of the executive functions necessary for daily living are executed in that part of the brain.

According to Lezak (1995), the dimensions of behavior studied can be classified into three major areas: cognition, emotionality, and executive functioning. Cognition is the information-handling aspect of behavior. It has been the most studied, since it is easier to conceptualize and test, and affects a person's immediate ability to communicate orally and in writing.

The second area, emotionality, can be equally devastating to an individual experiencing a brain injury, especially if a marked change has occurred since the injury. An individual's feelings and level of motivation are often affected. A subset of the area of feelings is the area of "social disability" caused by many injuries to the brain. For example, the patient may become socially withdrawn, may suffer from a lack of acceptance by his or her family regarding residual deficits, may exhibit inappropriate social behaviors, may have problems profiting from experience, may have a loss in leisure skills and interests, may have a marked reduction in sexual activity, may experience problems with the law, and may have problems coping with financial difficulties caused by the injury and the fact that they are unemployed postinjury.

The third area, executive functioning, represents how an individual will navigate their daily life in the areas of planning, problem solving, benefiting from external feedback, and in the manner in which a person will respond to their environment, either impulsively or uninhibitedly. Only rarely is one of these functions altered as a result of a brain injury. According to Lezak (1995), "The disruptive effects of most brain lesions, regardless of their size or location, usually involve all three systems."

In summary, the neuropsychological evaluation provides information which complements the customary neurological exam and data supplied by an EEG, CAT scan, or MRI, by providing information on the nature and extent of functional impairment caused by the neurological injury or disease being investigated. The neuropsychological evaluation is sometimes a foundation for arriving at a correct diagnosis, and at other times supplemental. While the EEG, MRI, and other medical evaluations are essential in the identification of malfunctioning brain structure and some types of brain function, only the neuropsychological method can fully appreciate and diagnose memory, judgment, daily planning, and other essentials of thinking necessary for independent living, employment, and the normal pursuits of life.

Neuropsychological evaluations provide documentation necessary to rehabilitate moderate and severe brain injuries, and are also useful in detecting the presence of mild brain injury that may go undetected in routine medical and psychological examinations. Mild brain injury can be caused by a moderate blow to the head, a fall, a drug overdose, or exposure to toxic substances, to name a few. Mild brain injury can affect an individual's earning potential, so it is vital to provide adequate neuropsychological documentation to identify the presence of mild head injury. This is especially important to those individuals who are suspected of malingering. Malingering is difficult for all specialties to accurately diagnose; however, malingering is confounded in the mild head injury patient. Memory loss, judgment, difficult word-finding, incorrect word association, and numerous other symptoms are frequently present in a wide variety of disorders, including malingering. Neuropsychological tests are not totally accurate but offer the best available differential diagnostic documentation. There are specialty examinations, developed with a good degree of reliability, that assist the evaluation team in presenting evidence with a high degree of clinical certainty. Such evidence as to whether or not malingering is present is almost always essential in court cases involving financial settlements. It is difficult for the most experienced malingerer to fool an experienced neuropsychologist. Such differential knowledge is essential when a treatment team is preparing a plan for independent living, vocational assistance, educational pursuits, family networking, and financial settlements.

NEUROPSYCHOLOGISTS DEFINED

A clinical neuropsychologist is an individual with a degree in clinical psychology who has had advanced training in the field of neuropsychology. According to the

American Psychological Association's Division 40 (1989), a clinical neuropsychologist "is a professional psychologist who applies principles of assessment and intervention based upon the scientific study of human behavior as it relates to normal and abnormal functioning of the central nervous system." A neuropsychologist specializes in evaluating brain/behavior relationships, plans training programs to help the survivor of a brain injury return to the best level of functioning possible, and recommends alternative cognitive and behavioral strategies to minimize the effects of brain injury. The neuropsychologist often works closely with schools and employers as well as with family members, the injured person's physicians, and other health and rehabilitation professionals.

MINIMUM QUALIFICATIONS

Referring professionals need to know that there is a great variability in the training of individuals providing neuropsychological consultations. In addition to being licensed, a neuropsychologist should have, at minimum, a doctoral degree (Ph.D. or Psy.D.) in clinical psychology from an accredited institution, preferably one that has been approved by the American Psychological Association. According to Division 40 (Clinical Neuropsychology) of the American Psychological Association (1989), a neuropsychologist should have:

1. Successful completion of systematic didactic and experiential training in neuropsychology and neuroscience at a regionally accredited university
2. Two or more years of appropriate supervised training applying neuropsychological services in a clinical setting
3. Licensing and certification to provide psychological services to the public by laws of the state or province in which he or she practices
4. Review by one's peers as a test of these competencies

Typical courses that a neuropsychologist will have taken would include at least three courses in neuropsychological assessment of children, adolescents, adults, and seniors, as well as a minimum of three courses in intervention with the above population groups. Courses in neuroanatomy, rehabilitation, case consultation, and report writing round out this vigorous curriculum.

When referring to a neuropsychologist, you may want to investigate if he or she has had field experience in a variety of settings where brain-injured individuals have been diagnosed and treated. Neuropsychologists can be further certified by the American Board of Professional Psychology in either Clinical Neuropsychology (ABCN) or Rehabilitation Psychology (ABRP).

USE OF TECHNICIANS IN TESTING

In some cases, neuropsychological tests are administered by a technician, often called a psychometrist, for later interpretation by the neuropsychologist. A well-trained technician can free-up time for the neuropsychologist, but many are not well enough trained and may be less likely to identify spurious data, or to modify procedures to optimize information regarding the patient's abilities. As a referring professional, it is important to know to what extent technicians are used, and how they are supervised. It is advised that the neuropsychologist perform his or her own mental status examination, and participate in the administration of at least several of the measures, to acquire a "real-world" picture of the patient's performance levels.

TREATMENT SETTINGS FOR A NEUROPSYCHOLOGIST

What does a neuropsychologist do, and in what settings do you find a neuropsychologist? Neuropsychologists can be found in an acute care setting when an individual is first diagnosed with a brain injury or other neurological disorder, such as multiple sclerosis. In the acute care hospital setting, a neuropsychologist is consulted to assess the extent of brain injury and what aspects of behavior and cognition may be affected. In the hospital setting, a neuropsychologist may do preliminary screening of cognition, and then present findings to the rest of the treatment team for integrated team services. The treatment team usually consists of a physiatrist (a physician specializing in rehabilitation), a physical therapist, an occupational therapist, speech therapist, social worker or case manager, and often a recreation therapist. The neuropsychologist will recommend to the treatment team whether or not the patient can understand and comprehend instructions, and whether or not the patient can be cooperative at this time to interventions.

In an outpatient setting, a patient is usually functioning better neurologically and cognitively, therefore a neuropsychologist will usually be consulted to assess the patient's improved level of cognitive processes. Outpatient settings may either be an outpatient office, where an individual comes once or more per week for treatment and ongoing assessment, or it may be in a day-treatment setting. In a day-treatment setting, a neuropsychologist may see patients individually or in groups. These groups may vary, but usually there are "thinking skills" groups, "social skills" groups, and "coping" skills groups. In a day-treatment setting, the neuropsychologist continues to be involved in treatment team decisions based on findings from testing and treatment. As the patient progresses, he or she may be referred to a vocational skills group and be further assessed for the skills needed to return to work.

Some neuropsychologists work in a residential setting, treating individuals with more severe brain injuries who cannot benefit from outpatient treatment and need a more comprehensive range of services. These individuals cannot return home due to their level and type of deficits.

Listings of neuropsychologists can be found in directories such as those compiled by the National Academy of Neuropsychologists or the International Neuropsychological Society, the two major associations of neuropsychologists.

PROCESS OF NEUROPSYCHOLOGICAL ASSESSMENT

What is involved in a neuropsychological assessment? In the past, the purpose of a neuropsychological assessment was to establish the presence of brain injury. In today's settings, neuropsychological assessment is used as well to establish levels of functioning.

According to a 1996 report by the Therapeutics and Technology Assessment Subcommittee of the American Academy of Neurology, "Neurologic examination and neuroimaging are intended to provide localizing information and are usually superior to neuropsychological testing for localizing focal brain lesions; the purpose of neuropsychological assessment is to provide information on cognitive deficits and capacities." It should be emphasized here that neuropsychological tests do not provide information regarding *causality* of deficits, but the *extent* of deficit.

BATTERY APPROACH VS. PROCESS APPROACH

Some neuropsychologists prefer to use a "battery" approach to testing, giving each patient the same group of tests. This contrasts with professionals who use a "process" approach, based on the original works of Arthur Benton, a neuropsychologist in Iowa. This approach is gaining fast recognition as the preferred testing procedure. With the process approach, a clinician probes basic cognitive skill areas, and then chooses tests based on results of the preliminary screen. As deficits are uncovered, further testing in those areas is performed. With the process approach, the clinician highlights the *qualitative* aspects of a patient's performance, and relies less on the *quantitative* aspects. The clinician will write a report based more on how the patient arrived at their answers rather than relying on actual test scores. This approach is usually more cost-effective. There continues to be a debate, however, over whether to use complete test batteries, or test to the deficits. Jarvis and Barth (1994) state, "Because of a lack of research evidence supporting the use of a flexible battery or pure process approach, the use of a fixed battery and a more empirical approach is indicated."

Results of a neuropsychological evaluation must provide insight into brain functions for a particular individual at a particular time. Results must be reviewed within the context of the patient's medical records, age, education, family dynamics, socioeconomic status, cultural background, and previous work history. The evaluation attempts to record the functional strengths and weaknesses in the patient's cognition and emotions so that the clinician can develop a realistic rehabilitation plan and set both short-term and long-term treatment goals. Simply stated, an evaluation should conclude with recommendations on how therapists will assist the patient to "get where the patient wants to be" functionally.

FUNCTIONAL AREAS OF THE BRAIN EVALUATED

The areas investigated include, but are not limited to, an assessment of attention, concentration, memory, visual-motor coordination, visual-spatial processing, comprehension of speech and the production of speech, and a person's ability to plan, organize, generalize, use abstract thought, and benefit from external feedback. The speed with which an individual processes information is recorded, as well as the level of verbal and visual processing. The report should conclude with a clinical diagnosis and treatment recommendations. Treatment recommendations should include all aspects of functioning, and should mention how the patient's level of functioning is going to impact their return to home and previous occupation. Recommendations for job retraining may be indicated in some cases. Referrals, as appropriate, to other professionals should also be included. A patient, for example, may need to be referred to an audiologist, ophthalmologist, or vocational rehabilitation counselor. An outline of a typical neuropsychological evaluation is provided in the following table:

TABLE 15.1
Format for Neuropsychological Evaluation

1. Client Data
2. Evaluation Procedures
   - List of tests
   - Clinical interviews, collateral interviews
   - Review of relevant medical, academic, and vocational records
3. Reason for Referral
4. Presenting Problems
5. Behavioral Observations during Testing and Interview
6. Test Results
   - Level of alertness/orientation/attention/concentration
   - Psychomotor status
   - Memory and learning
   - Speech and language
   - Visuospatial/perceptual processing
   - Intellectual functioning/achievement
   - Executive functioning
   - Emotional and personality characteristics
7. Interpretation
8. Treatment Recommendations
   - Cognitive therapy
   - Speech therapy
   - OT (occupational therapist), TR (recreation therapist), PT (physical therapist)
   - Individual therapy
   - Group therapy
   - Head injury education classes
   - Referrals to other professionals
   - Vocational implications and recommendations
9. DSM-IV Diagnosis
10. Signature and Credentials Block

TESTS COMMONLY USED

What tests are commonly used during a neuropsychological evaluation? The development and use of standardized neuropsychological test batteries began around the 1940s. The two most popular test batteries have been the Halstead-Reitan Test Battery, and the Luria-Nebraska Test Battery. The use of modified test versions of the Halstead-Reitan are not uncommon, as some professionals use a process-approach method and test only those areas they believe are deficient. The Luria-Nebraska Test Battery is always given in its entirety, based on the ability of the patient. Both test batteries have the ability to assess children as well as adults. The Halstead-Reitan Test Battery tests children from age 9 and up. The Luria-Nebraska-Children Battery tests children beginning at age 8. As stated earlier, not all tests are used with each patient. A selection of tests is made to best characterize the patient's strengths and weaknesses and answer the referring question or questions.

When a patient's attention span and concentration levels are being evaluated, a clinician may choose to administer some form of a digit span test. In a "digit span" test, the clinician asks the patient to repeat a string of numbers, which increasingly becomes longer. Once the patient misses two number-strings of the same length (such as seven digits in a row), the technique changes in that the clinician will ask the patient to recite the number-strings that he or she hears, in the reverse sequence. This is referred to as "digits backward" and is designed to assess a person's "working memory" in addition to attention span. Working memory is the area in the brain that can take in information, manipulate it in some fashion, and then release it in another format. It is a much more complicated task than recalling digits in a forward sequence.

Another test for attention and concentration would be the "letter cancellation" exercise. On this test, a patient is presented with a page of numbers, letters, or both, and asked to mark out, for example, the letter "F" every time he or she sees it. Another test, called "Trail Making Test A," asks a patient to simply connect the dots in numerical order on a page that has numbers out of sequence and arranged at random. The patient is told it is a timed test and is timed to completion. Age-appropriate norms are used to indicate level of attention.

The most widely used tests to measure memory are Wechsler Memory Scale III, Rey Auditory Verbal Learning Test, and the California Verbal Learning Test.

Various tests of expressive and receptive language would include the Boston Naming Test, the Multilingual Aphasia Examination, and the Halstead-Reitan Aphasia Screening Test.

To assess visuospatial skills, the Rey-Osterrieth Complex Figure, the Block Design subtest of the Wechsler Adult Intelligence Scale-III (WAIS-III), and the Benton Visual Retention Test can be used.

Executive functioning would include the Wisconsin Card Sorting Test, the Halstead-Reitan Category Test, the Stroop Test, and Part B of the Trail Making Test.

Motor speed is measured with the Finger Tapping Test, the hand dynamometer, and the Grooved Pegboard Test.

Adult intelligence is measured by the Wechsler Adult Intelligence Scale-III, and the Wechsler Intelligence Scale for Children-III (WISC-III) is used for children under age 16. The Wide Range Achievement Test-III (WRAT-III), the Wechsler Achievement Test (WIAT), and the Woodcock-Johnson Tests of Achievement are the three most widely used tests to measure educational achievement. While most neuropsychologists utilize relatively well-known tests, many neuropsychologists also utilize instruments that have been very well validated by virtue of years of their own experience with that instrument. For instance, while there are no neuropsychological norms as such, valuable information can be obtained from instruments such as the

Proverbs Test, the Sentence Completion Test, the Cornell Index – form N-1, Picture Completion Tests, Kinetic Family Drawing Tests, Figure Drawing Tests, and numerous other psychological instruments. The Yacorzynski-Cox Concept Formation Test has been well validated on children and adults and, with a minimum of administration time, yields highly beneficial neuropsychological information. Not all helpful neuropsychological aids have been validated in the research laboratory; some are validated by clinical experience.

We recognize the valuable role of the psychometrician or neuropsychological assistant, but it is particularly important for a doctoral-level neuropsychologist to personally perform the clinical interview with a brain-injured patient. The neuropsychologist him/herself must be personally involved in the clinical interview. The subtleties of thought process, word-finding, word-association, memory sequencing, and other aspects of brain behavior are often noticed only by the experienced clinician. Frequently, many of the most valuable clinical findings are not evident in paper and pencil tests but are obvious to the neuropsychologically astute interviewer.

EFFECTS OF AGE, EDUCATION, GENDER, PSYCHIATRIC DISORDERS, AND SUBSTANCE ABUSE ON TEST PERFORMANCE

Age

As a person ages, there are some common changes in cognitive processing. The affects of aging can reduce psychomotor speed, reduce some aspects of memory, reduce the ability to access words, reduce visuospatial skills, and reduce complex attentional processes.

Education

Educational levels affect test performance. Some neuropsychological tests have norms for individuals based on educational level, but all do not. When education-specific normative data is not available, the clinician must use professional judgment in the analysis. In general, the higher the educational level, the better an individual is expected to do in cognitive domains.

Cultural background/ethnicity

A patient's cultural background and ethnicity must be figured into the interpretive report. Few tests provide normative data on minorities. Minority patients are at a particular disadvantage on tests of verbal skills, especially if English is a second language.

Gender

Gender issues do not provide as much of a change in test performance as do age, education, and ethnicity. In general, women do better on tests of verbal memory than men, and men do better on tests of visuospatial skills.

Psychiatric disorders

Depression, anxiety, apathy, and irritability directly impact a person's cognitive processes, as well as levels of motivation and cooperation with the examiner. Individuals with MTBI often demonstrate slowed cognitive processing, resulting in delay in response time. Patients with slowed cognition do less well on timed tests than untimed tests. Reduced attention, concentration, and memory recall are common manifestations of depression and anxiety, the two most common emotional reactions to mild brain injury.

Substance abuse

Chronic alcoholism and substance abuse is associated with deterioration in abstraction, visuospatial skills, and problem-solving abilities. Evaluations with head trauma patients must include a thorough history-taking of substance abuse issues, as a large proportion of head injuries are associated with substance use and abuse.

USE OF COLLATERAL INTERVIEWS

Collateral interviewing is relied upon heavily in neuropsychological evaluations, as compared to a typical psychological evaluation. When a patient has experienced neurological damage, he or she is not always aware of the kinds of deficits, or the extent that the deficit presents itself to others. Often, not only cognitive skills but also social skills and "graces" are impaired.

Family members are often the first individuals who notice the changes, even subtle changes, in their loved one. For example, a patient may have difficulty modulating their emotions, and may have more anger outbursts. Many patients become depressed, even though they never experienced depression pretrauma. Patients' frustration thresholds are often lowered as increased awareness of their deficits begin to come to light and have significant impacts on returning home or to work. Family members provide another form of assessment of a patient's functioning that can prove to be valuable. It is always best to assess more than one significant other in the family grouping, as there can always be distortion or exaggeration based on the potential for secondary gains in a family member.

SPECIAL GUIDANCE FOR WORKING WITH PERSONS WITH MTBI

Improvement in emergency medical services, more aggressive emergency room procedures, and greater sophistication in managing brain injuries have resulted in a greater number of individuals surviving head trauma. In the past, many of these individuals died due to injuries. In the last 20 years, most of these individuals lived, although mild to severe disabilities often result. Much research initially ensued regarding the cognitive and emotional effects of moderate-to-severe brain injury, but more recently, the effects of "mild" brain trauma have been studied. What has been very common is that many individuals seemed fine at discharge, but when they attempted to resume their normal routines at school, work, or at home, many complained of difficulty performing simple tasks. These tasks were simple and routine before the injury. Many MTBI persons had difficulty concentrating, remembering, organizing their daily routines, were slow to get their work done, and had decreased ability to interact properly with loved ones, peers, and bosses. When direct causes could not be found, many of these individuals were thought to be having purely psychiatric problems, or they were accused of malingering. A surge in research in MTBI began to address the issues surrounding these individuals who appeared to be mending well physically but not necessarily cognitively, emotionally, or socially.

THE DEFINITION OF MINOR HEAD INJURY

Mild Traumatic Brain Injury (MTBI) has been officially defined by the Mild Traumatic Brain Injury Committee of the Head Injury Interdisciplinary Special Interest Group of the American Congress of Rehabilitation Medicine (1993). The definition is as follows: "A patient with mild traumatic brain injury is a person who has had a traumatically-induced physiological disruption of brain function as manifested by at least one of the following:

1. Any period of loss of consciousness
2. Any loss of memory for events immediately before or after the accident
3. Any alteration in mental state at the time of the accident (e.g., feeling dazed, disoriented, or confused)
4. Focal neurological deficit(s) that may or may not be transient but where the severity of the injury does not exceed the following:
   a. loss of consciousness of approximately 30 minutes or less
   b. after 30 minutes, an initial Glasgow Coma Scale (GCS) of 13–15
   c. posttraumatic amnesia (PTA) not greater than 24 hours

No one specific symptom is necessary to diagnose MTBI. MTBI can be caused by anything that can result in injury to the brain itself. For example, individuals can experience a brain injury resulting from automobile accidents, falls, direct blows to the head, being exposed to toxic substances, excessively high fever, and surgical and postanesthetic complications, to name a few. An individual may experience a CVA (cerebrovascular accident), otherwise known as a stroke, which will cause injury to the brain. Other conditions such as seizures or multiple sclerosis can impair brain functioning. Some individuals are diagnosed MTBI by the score they received on their Glasgow Coma Scale (GCS). The GCS is used by hospital personnel upon admittance into the emergency room. An individual receives a score between 3 and 15, with "mild" brain injury being diagnosed with scores from 13–15. A loss of consciousness does not have to occur, however, to accurately merit a diagnosis of MTBI.

THE NATURE OF "MILD" HEAD INJURY

Permanent brain injury can occur without significant loss of consciousness. The neurological exam may be unremarkable, with all imaging studies, such as MRI and CT scans, being negative. This is because the disruptions of nerve processes can only be seen microscopically. Subtle deficits in functioning, in such areas as attention span, memory functioning, and ability to learn new tasks, may be detected, indicating impairment of cortical functioning. Often, these subtle deficits are not noticed in the first month or so of recovery, but appear as the individual tries to return to a normal home and work routine.

The reason for the subtle deficits that go undetected under neurological examination and through numerous scans is easily explained. The brain is made up of many different layers of matter. Each layer has a different weight, or density. Many neuronal axons cross these layers. The axons are long and thin, and when the brain is subjected to an external force, a subsequent internal injury can occur. The axons become "sheared," that is, torn and stretched, as the different layers of brain matter move at different rates due to acceleration/deceleration forces from the external impact to the head. A very common external object of impact to the head is the windshield — as patients frequently come into contact with it or the side window — upon impact in a car accident. Since the role of the axon is to transfer information from one neuron to another, damage to it causes disruption in information flow. Problems in transferring information, then, can occur within the damaged axon, thereby rendering the initial axon incapable of fully "delivering the message" to the subsequent neurons. There is also "insulation" covering the axons, called the myelin sheath. As this protective coating is damaged, the speed and efficiency of information processing is thwarted.

Other impact damage can occur from the soft brain tissue being torn inside the skull, as the brain shifts in response to a blow to the head, for example. Inside the skull are bony protuberances that normally hold the brain in place. Upon impact, the brain shifts back and forth and is torn on these bony structures. The original site of impact is called the "coup" area, with the subsequent shifting of the brain to the opposite side of impact being designated the "contre-coup" area. Damage can occur at both locations. Since shear damage occurs at a cellular level and is microscopic, it cannot be picked up with conventional imaging techniques as can damage resulting in bleeding or edema.

COMMON SYMPTOM PATTERNS

Mild injuries can result in subtle effects that are not easy to measure except by careful neuropsychological evaluation and interview. Many clients perform in "average" ranges on an array of tests, but what they report in everyday living isn't average at all.

One common symptom pattern is that of mild head injury which is diffuse in nature, more so than specific. That is, persons with minor head injury have difficulty with overall speed of processing, capacity to process information, and efficiency, execution, and integration of their mental processes. Most injuries that are considered to be mild involve the prefrontal cortex, an area of the brain that serves as a "master controller" of behaviors.

A patient may find it difficult to maintain focus of attention, or to shift the focus of attention from one thing to another. An individual may find difficulties in the categorization of facts and ideas, and difficulty with abstract thinking and generalization of ideas from one situation to another. Often, there is a difficulty in a person's ability to plan and organize their daily activities. The speed at which thoughts are processed is often slowed, and there is difficulty in finding the right words to put into speech. Patients with MTBI often demonstrate "cognitive rigidity," a term which reflects an inability to shift thinking style. A patient, for example, may experience difficulty being flexible in their thinking style and consequently "lock on" to ideas or facts, not being able to immediately "shift gears" and generate new ideas easily. After a brain injury, even a mild one, there are alterations in the way the brain processes information. For example, the brain may not be able to perform as many operations at one time as it did before. Thought processes are therefore labored and slow. Difficulty paying attention and staying on task can be due to increased problems with distractibility. As a patient tries to attend to one idea or situation, they can no longer "process out" distracting and competing sounds and activities. Subsequently, as attentional processes break down, patients have difficulty learning new information. This is because the brain cannot "encode" the information on a timely basis, and the patient may not have the ability to "rehearse" the information so that it can be stored for later recall. Difficulties in sequential processing and simultaneous processing of information are often a result of MTBI.

Abstract thinking is often impaired or altered by brain trauma. It is harder to compare and contrast ideas, to integrate one idea into another one. Individuals become more "concrete" thinkers, and may have difficulty generalizing from one situation to another.

Language skills are often affected. A person may experience difficulty expressing their thoughts and ideas. They may have trouble searching for the right word to use. For example, a person may try to say the word "clock" but will rather "talk around" the item and explain that "it is something you tell time with." This process of making up for the lost word is called circumlocution. The word is not lost forever, but for the time being the word cannot be accessed properly.

Many of the problems described above occur more frequently when the person is under stress, is fatigued, or is anxious. Problems exacerbate under conditions of drugs or alcohol usage.

A second common symptom pattern in mild brain injury is one of focal injuries. These usually occur when the soft brain tissue is torn by the rough, bony surface inside the skull during trauma. This results in lesions in the frontal and temporal lobes, and in coup/contre-coup injuries. These brain regions are involved in the processes of planning, organizing, attention, concentration, memory for new learning, and emotional control. Focal injuries can co-exist with diffuse injuries, causing a wide array of possible deficits.

PERSONALITY AND TEMPERAMENT CHANGES

Changes in personality and basic temperament style can occur after an MTBI and affect an individual's performance at work and at home, causing those around him to question his or her competency on the job, and limiting social interactions. Some of the changes which occur in personality and mood are caused as a direct physical consequence of the injury itself, and other changes occur as the patient tries to cope with cognitive and personality changes.

Depression and anxiety secondary to the original injury are very common and should be treated as soon as possible with counseling provided by a rehabilitation psychologist. Psychoeducation should be implemented to teach the patient about the causes of their deficits, and to assist the patient and family in adjusting to the sequelae. A rehabilitation psychologist can assist the patient in finding compensatory strategies to assist reduced attention, concentration, and memory processes, or enroll the patient in a course of cognitive remediation. Cognitive remediation is cognitive exercises which help strengthen weak connections between neurons, and help reestablish brain connections.

FAMILY ISSUES

Every person with a head injury represents numerous family issues. Each person presents a unique package of issues emanating from the patient's age, family status, family relationships, and peculiar family dynamics. Even the most psychologically sound families are traumatized by a patient with a head injury. Those families that are already dysfunctional present particularly difficult challenges for the diagnostician and rehabilitation professional.

Since many persons suffering brain damage are in the 15–25 age range, many of them are dependents still living in the parental home, not as yet vocationally settled, and unable to financially take care of themselves. These persons offer particular challenges in that the siblings, parents, and family network are required to deal with any kind of collateral diagnostic knowledge, and most certainly in any kind of rehabilitation. Adolescents offer demanding challenges in normal maturation. When coupled with brain injury, the adaptations and support systems of the family are stretched sometimes to the breaking point, occasionally resulting in divorce and family dissolution.

In all ages, neurologically impaired persons have difficulty with life skills that can push even the most supportive family to, and sometimes beyond, its limits. Such complex issues include sexuality, economics and finances, rapid mood swings, disturbances of sleep/wake cycles, bowel/bladder dysfunction, speech problems, and many more "new and different" behaviors. Frequently, the family of a brain-injured patient will report that "he/she now has a completely different personality." Since many brain injuries result from deviant behavior, the diagnosis and treatment must also include dealing with the family dynamics, relationship abnormalities, and individual psychological dynamics that were part of the premorbid behavioral abnormalities. Families are frequently not able to adapt to the massive changes in relationships and cannot provide the support systems needed in such cases (Kostan and Van Couvering, 1972).

Each age presents its own unique set of circumstances, the discussion of which is beyond the scope of this chapter. However, it is important to note that while the neuropsychologist may well team–up with or refer to a family therapist, he/she must have at least minimal education and training in the diagnosis and treatment of marriage and family dynamics. Patients attempt to utilize every mechanism of defense known, and are usually quite capable of creating their own. Triangulation, i.e., pitting persons against each other, is a particularly common practice for patients with head injury, and, not infrequently, professionals are pitted against each other, family members against each other, and sometimes the patient him/herself against the physician, psychologist, social worker, and other professionals attempting to provide services.

The geriatric brain-injured patient presents a unique set of challenges. Sleep disturbances, fecal and urinary incontinence, mobility difficulties, irresponsible behavior, dangerous risk taking, anxiety/depression, social life restrictions, unwillingness to learn new skills, and severe mood swings are among the difficulties a caring family must face with an aging brain-damaged person. The normal degenerative aspects of aging often severely exacerbate these problems.

The neuropsychologist must be able to differentiate between family dynamics and patient cooperation and resistance. Secondary gain must be considered along with the value to an adolescent when placing blame on parents, or vice versa. The nearly emancipated adolescent may be thrust back into parental dependence, thus producing every emotion from pleasure to rage. While most neuropsychologists pay less attention to the personality and family dynamics than other psychological specialties, it important for the neuropsychologist to have available and, when appropriate, utilize personality and family dynamic measurement tests.

The vast majority of studies done on families with a neuropsychologically impaired individual are clinical and anecdotal in nature. A review of textbooks in medicine and neuropsychology revealed that the word "family" appeared with significantly greater frequency in neuropsychological texts than in the medical ones. This probably indicates that neuropsychologists are more acquainted with family studies, family dynamics, and family systems than are most physicians, with the possible exception of specialized psychiatrists. Neuropsychologists must first train as general clinical psychologists, therefore it would follow that they would have been more literate in family studies than physicians.

The well-trained neuropsychologist often serves as the liaison between physician, rehabilitation team members, and the patient and family for treatment planning and rehabilitation supervision. This is due to the broad education and training neuropsychologists receive in the normal and abnormal functioning of individuals, families, and systems during their graduate studies prior to specializing in neuropsychology. Because of this broad education and training, inpatient rehabilitation programs frequently rely upon the neuropsychologist for team leadership, case conferencing, direction of case management, and life-skills planning in preparation for discharge from an inpatient facility.

RETURN-TO-WORK ISSUES

Many individuals with MTBI find it difficult to return to work soon after discharge. The family and patient should be counseled regarding their cognitive and social/emotional deficits so that a planned return to work schedule can be implemented. Often, return to work should be graduated from part-time to full-time, and should be supervised initially by a vocational rehabilitation counselor or work supervisor. This allows the patient's work to be supervised until all concerned are satisfied that the employee is working up to expected potential. With a return to work too soon, and without assistance, many persons with MTBI fail at their jobs, when perhaps with a little planning and with minor job or workplace modifications, an employee may have had a more successful return to work experience.

There are many potential effects of brain injury on employability. The most rapidly growing area of employment is in the jobs requiring "information highway" skills, that is, in the areas of accessing, storing, and implementing information. We are barraged daily with all kinds of information to sift through and evaluate. The high demand for "white collar" jobs exceeds the "pink-collar" and "blue-collar" trades.

Mild brain impairment affects all jobs to some degree, but particularly those positions that support and interface with the information economy. Brain impairment, which may seem relatively minor, can cause extraordinary loss of income. For example, if an engineer loses the ability to analyze spatial relationships, he or she is out of a job. If a store owner can no longer plan ahead and project outcomes, he or she will have to sell the business or hire a manager to take his or her place.

Deficits in attention and memory, common sequelae of mild head injuries, affect workers in a variety of positions. Many jobs require the ability to understand, remember, and execute written or oral instructions. Someone on an assembly line being trained for a new product line is unemployable if they cannot learn new procedures in the proper order. As one can see, many individuals with MTBI can be literally *vocationally* disabled from just one accident or neurological insult to the brain. As stated by Lees-Haley (1987), "A 10-percent loss of memory is rated as a mild loss by neurologists and neuropsychologists, but employees who forget 10 percent of what they hear in an 8-hour day may be in 100-percent trouble."

It is not uncommon for a worker's interpersonal skills to be affected by mild brain injuries. Vocationally, this can be devastating for the individual who sells for a living, or who is a public relations consultant for a company. It can be equally devastating to a corporate culture, where "team" players must learn to get along with each other and be able to understand each others' viewpoints. Some injuries increase a person's irritability, render them less able to read social cues, increase their aggressive tendencies, and rate them "difficult to get along with" by others. Many MTBI individuals find they can no longer handle the pressure of stressful occupations. When these lowered social skills and reduced ability to tolerate emotional stress are a change from the worker's previous level of functioning, chances for promotion are greatly reduced for these individuals. Individuals with MTBI are much more likely to be in danger of losing their jobs, and often are the first to be let go when "downsizing."

SPECIAL ASPECTS TO LOOK FOR IN TESTING MBTI

Neuropsychological deficits can appear immediately following a minor head injury, or it can take months to realize that cognitive and emotional changes have occurred as a result of that injury. A thorough neuropsychological evaluation a few months after an injury can pick up the more subtle deficits and make rehabilitative efforts and return-to-work efforts more successful. Without proper identification of deficits, individuals may blame other circumstances in order to explain their changes in concentration, memory, personality, and/or resilience to stressors.

A study by Leininger et al. (1990) looked at individuals who had minor head injury, both with and without loss of consciousness. These individuals reported cognitive difficulties at one month post injury. Of those subjects tested, the research concluded that those tested displayed significantly poorer performance than uninjured controls on several neuropsychological tests. Deficits were most evident on tests of reasoning, information processing, and verbal learning. When patients were asked to reproduce a complex geometric design, inefficient organization, poor attention to detail, and faulty error recognition contributed to reduced scores more so than gross visuospatial or motor integration deficits. The authors concluded, "As far as minor head injuries are concerned, the occurrence or nonoccurrence of a traumatic loss of consciousness does not seem to distinguish persons at greater or reduced risk for neuropsychological consequences."

REFERENCES

1. American Academy of Neurology, Assessment: Neuropsychological testing of adults, *Neurology*, 47, 592–599, 1996.
2. Division 40-Clinical Neuropsychology, Definition of a clinical neuropsychologist, *The Clinical Neuropsychologist*, 3(1), p. 22, 1989.
3. Horton, AM, Wedding, D, Webster, J, *The Neuropsychology Handbook*, Springer Publishing Co., New York, 1997.
4. Jarvis, Paul E, Barth, Jeffrey T, *The Halstead-Reitan Neuropsychological Battery: A guide to interpretation and clinical applications*, Psychological Assessment Resources, Inc., Odessa, FL, 1994.
5. Karkut, RT, *Concept formation in normal versus alcoholic individuals: A cross validation study of the Yacorzynski-Cox Concept Formation Test and short form of the Halstead-Reitan Category Test*. Unpublished doctoral dissertation, Forest Institute of Professional Psychology, Springfield, MO, 1988.
6. Kostlan, A, Van Couvering, N, *Clinical indications of organic brain dysfunction*. Proceedings of the 80th Annual Convention of the American Psychological Association, 7, (summary), 1972.
7. Lees-Haley, P, Mild brain injury. *Trial*, November 1987, 83–86.
8. Lezak, Muriel, *Neuropsychological Assessment*, 3rd ed., Oxford University Press, New York, 1995.
9. Leininger, B, Kreutzer, J, Hill, M, Comparison of minor and severe head injury emotional sequelae using the MMPI, *Brain Injury*, 5(2), 199, 1991.
10. Leininger, B, Gramling, S, Farrell, A, Kreutzer, J, Peck, E., Neuropsychological deficits in symptomatic minor head injury patients after concussion and mild concussion, *Journal of Neurology, Neurosurgery, and Psychiatry*, 53, 293, 1990.
11. Miller, LJ, Mittenberg, W, Brief cognitive behavioral interventions in mild traumatic brain injury, *Applied Neuropsychology*, 5(4), 172, 1998.
12. Minor, AC, *A normative study of concept formation in middle-aged men and women as measured by the Yacorzynski-Cox Concept Formation Test*, Unpublished doctoral dissertation, Forest Institute of Professional Psychology, Springfield, MO, 1992.
13. Segalowitz, SJ, Lawson, S, *Journal of Learning Disabilities*, 28(5), 309, 1995.
14. Yacorzynski, GK, Perceptual principles involved in the disintegration of a configuration formed in predicting the occurrence of patterns selected by chance, *Journal of Experimental Psychology*, 29, 401, 1941.

15. Yacorzynski, GK, *Concept formation as a function of personality structure*, Paper presented at the American Psychological Association meetings, 1949.
16. Yacorzynski, GK, Brain dynamism as reflected in illusions, *Genetic Psychology Monographs*, 68, 3, 1963.
17. Yacorzynski, GK, *Frontiers of Psychology*, Philosophical Library, New York, 1963.
18. Yacorzynski, GK, Cox, RH, Cox, Dr, *Yacorzynski-Cox concept formation test*, Forest Institute of Professional Psychology, Springfield, MO, 1988.

16 Auditory/Vestibular Symptoms, Evaluation, and Medico-Legal Considerations

Edward J. Jacobson, Ph.D., DABFE, DABFM

The exact number of individuals in the United States injured each year with a documented brain injury is not known precisely. This is because of statistical variations that result from factors such as: (1) the definition of brain injury[1]; (2) classification as to if it is mild, moderate, or severe[2]; (3) the populations upon which information has been collected[3]; (4) whether the injuries known to result in symptoms generally associated with it are always reported; or (5) if medical assistance is even sought for every injury incurred. Despite this uncertainty recent information indicates that each year approximately 2,000,000, or about 175–200 per 100,000 individuals, sustain a brain injury. Other data note that 51% of these result from automobile accidents, 21% from falling, 12% from violence, and the remaining from sport, recreation, and other causes. Although the reportable incidence of brain injury may vary, the literature does indicate a relatively consistent list of symptoms generally associated with this type of injury. These encompass a wide range of physical and behavioral symptoms attributable to a multiplicity of pathophysiologies. These include symptoms often thought to be associated with the auditory and vestibular systems and might be present with complaints of photosensitivity and other visual difficulties such as diplopia, headache, cognitive dysfunction, emotional aberrations with unpredictable anger outbursts, mood change or depression, or neck, back, and other physical complaints. Any of these may be constantly present — or may be transient in their clinical presentation — but those most frequently reported with MTBI are "...headaches, dizziness, and memory problems."[1] There appears to be nothing in the literature that would indicate what percentage of these individuals had injuries that specifically resulted in auditory or vestibular symptoms. Empirically, however, logic would dictate the incidence to be significant given the frequency with which these symptoms are reported and the large number of MTBI patients believed to present clinically.

A Mild Traumatic Brain Injury (MTBI) is defined as a "disruption of brain function"[6] meeting one or more criteria as defined by the American Congress of Rehabilitation Medicine. These criteria include deficits that result in significant physical and/or behavioral limitations that can temporarily or permanently restrict a patient's ability to function. The MTBI does not necessitate a loss of consciousness and can result from a direct trauma to the head, from the head striking an object, or from acceleration/deceleration injuries.

Because the auditory and vestibular systems contain delicate structures, they are not immune to pathophysiologic change(s) from a direct insult to the head or from the interaction of the ear and its functions with other sensory systems. The symptoms related to the dysfunction of any such abnormality that is present with MTBI require clinical documentation to avoid errors in diagnosis and whatever treatment might be necessary.

GENERAL CONSIDERATIONS

Injury deficits secondary to MTBI are not always easily documented. If behavioral symptoms are present, some believe those that last longer than one year posttrauma indicate the existence of a functional component.[7] If physical complaints are present along with a behavioral abnormality the physical component is also often viewed as psychological and, therefore, nonexistent or suspicious. This may be especially true for neurologically-based symptoms believed to result from MTBI, a category into which auditory/vestibular symptoms can be grouped. There are certainly situations where this is a valid concern, and, indeed, questions should be initiated when any symptom exists beyond a reasonable time period, which in some situations may be in excess of a year or longer. However, if a diagnosis is disputed, considered nonexistent despite the patient's stated persistence of a symptom(s), or if symptoms appear inconsistent with a given diagnosis, there should also perhaps be concern about whether the evaluation was accurate and led to an inappropriate diagnosis. Such inconsistencies may on occasion also be a product of a clinician's inexperience rather than deception on the part of the patient. To simply conclude that a patient's symptom presentation is somehow atypical, or even impossible, or that if symptom resolution or modification does not occur within a specified time is always an indication of malingering or represents another motivation, could be dangerous and perhaps generate a serious error in clinical judgment. Seemingly confusing diagnostic conclusions are at times difficult to confirm not only because of these factors, but because many symptom-producing abnormalities do not readily reveal themselves on imaging studies, including MRI or a CT Scan.[6,8,9,16] Clinicians also at times tend to prematurely offer an opinion of symptom causation that is biased or inaccurate, and may reflect an absence of awareness for certain diagnostic conditions that perhaps were not made apparent during their educational or training programs.

Patients frequently present with symptoms that are quite similar but vastly different in etiology. Establishing an exact causation in these situations is often very challenging, even in routine clinical presentations, since the pathogenesis of many symptoms can be multifactorial. This is quite often true for symptoms traditionally considered referable to the auditory and vestibular mechanisms, either separately or in combination with one another, and may be especially difficult when trauma is the precipitating factor to their onset.

A diagnosis may be additionally complicated when there are medico-legal issues. Relative to auditory and vestibular, or vestibular-like symptoms, a diagnosis may require an especially definitive clarification to reduce potential complications for becoming involved in a lengthy litigation process. This is always in the best interest of all parties involved, not the least of whom is the patient. An unnecessarily lengthy evaluation process can potentially erode a treatment outcome. That definitely applies to dizziness secondary to trauma from a Motor Vehicle Accident (MVA), or if there is a Workers Compensation (WC) injury. This entire process may be even further complicated under current managed care systems because of restrictions imposed relative to obtaining referrals to specialists when there is need for specific testing, or if a complicated examination is necessary to establish a diagnosis and an ultimate treatment. On other occasions this may be brought about by a failure to understand the diagnostic process necessary for a credible differential diagnosis when the traumatically-induced injury and any resultant sequelae has the potential for litigation.

Despite these difficulties, few would disagree that achieving a favorable clinical outcome, designated as Maximum Therapeutic Benefit (MTB) for injuries incurred in an MVA, or Maximum Medical Improvement (MMI) as with a Workers Compensation injury, is best accomplished if the treatment is consistent with a valid diagnosis. It should be obvious that if the diagnosis and treatment are inappropriate, symptoms that are not self-limiting will persist. Patients caught in this dilemma are the ones usually labeled as having symptoms that are functional. If there have been multiple accidents it will usually be necessary to apportion, differentiate, or separate any preexisting injury and conditions, if applicable, and determine to what extent each may have contributed to the last overall clinical presentation. This is sometimes possible only if other existing clinical records are available for review. Unfortunately, this is not always possible. There also are times when symptoms are not the direct result of an accident-related trauma, even though they appear as such, and care must be taken in separating those that are related from those that are not. For example, it is not impossible for an individual to have an onset of dizziness or any other symptom, including hearing loss, at or about the time of an accident and, because of their proximity to the accident, believe they are related.

To this might be added a cautionary note that the more individuals who are at times involved with an evaluation and treatment regimen, the more difficult it can occasionally become for future providers to be effective and objective. This needs to be understood not only by clinicians, but by others who might become involved, such as case managers, insurance agents, and representatives of the legal profession. For those patients with dishonest motives resulting in symptom invention or magnification, overutilization of providers, tests, and clinic visits may add to a patient's sophistication to intentionally deceive.

Another concern is that too many providers over a lengthy series of clinic visits may actually add to the handicapping effects of an injury, or perhaps, as believed by some, create a handicap that otherwise might not have resulted. For example, patients seen by multiple providers receive a lot of attention and are frequently excused from various responsibilities that were required of them prior to the injury; this may result in a dependence on others that would not have occurred otherwise. This is not to suggest that a patient should be abandoned in those situations where ongoing care and treatment is necessary for injuries and any sequelae that are validly documented, only that the clinical evaluation and treatment process should strive to be efficient.

VALIDITY AND RELIABILITY

Because a diagnosis must be consistent with the symptom(s), and, ultimately, any treatment, every clinical test must, whenever possible, be both valid and reliable. This is best accomplished through an understanding of obtaining objective test information and documentation of this data. If clinical studies demonstrate repeatable test results, they might be considered reliable when, unfortunately, it is possible to have reliability without validity. This occurs when a patient is less than honorable in their ability to produce consistent test results. In other words, some individuals are very proficient and capable at presenting clinically in a way that, on behavioral tests, a category into which certain auditory tests belong, can consistently duplicate their responses on multiple occasions. Conversely, if what is being tested or evaluated is valid, that is measuring or assessing what is intended, then that test or examination is also reliable. Therefore, it is possible to have reliability without validity, but if a given test is valid it is also reliable.

ANATOMY

The ear is responsible for the dual sensory functions of hearing and the body's ability to orient itself in space. This ability to orient occurs in conjunction with vision and proprioception.

Auditory function is a marvelous process of energy transition that results from the conversion of acoustic energy events into mechanical energy, then to hydraulic energy, and finally electrical energy. The three divisions of the ear referred to as the outer, middle, and inner ear, respectively, allow for this process to take place, and it occurs without any appreciable loss of energy and is accomplished by what is essentially a step-down transformer. This is created, in part, by the surface area of the eardrum and the footplate of the stapes that have a relative surface area ratio of about 20:1. Upon entering the external canal of the outer ear, acoustic energy is converted to mechanical energy, striking and placing the eardrum into vibration. This energy is then converted to hydraulic energy within the fluid-filled inner ear where it is transformed into electrical energy resulting from stimulation of the sensory receptors located in the inner ear. This process enables the ear, along with its neural projection areas of the brain, to detect approximately 340,000 Just Noticeable Differences (JNDs) for the psychophysical experiences of pitch (frequency) and loudness (intensity).[10]

The sensory system of the ear responsible for orientation commences with the peripheral vestibular portion of the inner ear. It enables detection of linear and angular acceleration. Although delicate, the various structures that comprise this system are generally well protected by their location within the dense petrous pyramid portion of the temporal bone, except for the auricle and cartilagenous lateral third of the ear canal. Despite their relatively protective anatomical location, the various segments and their respective structural contents can still become damaged or physiologically disrupted from traumatic insult. As stated by the definition of MTBI, this can occur with or without loss of consciousness. The damage can be direct or indirect and, at times, from trauma quite distal to the ear, but cause symptoms that are usually referable to the ear.

The following subsections are intended as a general orientation and not as a treatise for each division of the ear and its respective anatomy. However, they should provide a general orientation and, hopefully, an appreciation for the fragile and delicate nature of these structures and their susceptibility to injury.

EXTERNAL EAR

The outer ear consists of the visibly apparent auricle and the external ear canal. Laterally, the auricle has a series of eminences and depressions to which names have been assigned. This elliptically-shaped appendage has a deep depression called the concha that is partially divided by the crus of the helix, which is the thickened outermost margin of the auricle, and extends nearly to the opening of the canal. The divisions are the cymba concha superiorly and the cavum concha inferiorly, which provide the opening into the canal or external auditory meatus. Anterior to the concha is a small projection, the tragus, which extends posteriorly in a somewhat overlapping fashion to the entrance of the external meatus. The latter extends from the cavum concha to the eardrum and has a somewhat S-shaped configuration as it courses its way in a medial, anterior, and inferior direction. It is narrower at the junction of the osseocartilagenous portion, and then widens again as it courses toward the eardrum. The length of the canal is approximately 25 mm along the superoposterior wall and 31 mm along the anteroinferior wall, and it has a width of approximately 6–7 mm.

MIDDLE EAR

Terminating the medial aspect of the external canal is the somewhat translucent tympanic membrane (TM). The position of the TM follows neither an exact horizontal and vertical axis nor a 90° angle relative to the canal. It sets obliquely with its long axis extending from the posterosuperior to the anteroinferior wall of the canal, and slopes at an angle of about 140° to the superior wall of the canal. Measuring along its long axis, it is approximately 9–10 millimeters (mm) in height and 8–9 mm in width. The TM is not flat if viewed directly from the side, but is concave as a result of traction exerted by the manubrium of the malleous of the middle ear. The membrane is thin, having a thickness of about 0.1 mm, yet consists of three separate tissue layers. The lateral layer is contiguous with the epidermal layer of skin of the ear canal. The medial layer has spoke-like fibers radiating toward the periphery to the fibrocartilagenous ring surrounding the TM, and also circular fibers that are denser towards the center, close to the umbo of the malleous and again toward the periphery. The medial layer is continuous with the mucosa lining the tympanum, or middle ear cavity.

The middle ear cavity is an irregular and oblique-shaped space situated along an anteroposterior plane having an approximate vertical dimension of 15 mm, and a width at its narrowest dimension of 2 mm, 6 mm at its widest, and 4 mm inferiorly. It has a volume of about 2.0 milliliters (ml). The cavity is bordered superiorly by the tegmental wall (roof), inferiorly by the jugular wall (floor), anteriorly by the carotid wall, posteriorly by the mastoid wall, the tympanic membrane laterally, and the labyrinthine wall at the medial aspect. Extending from the carotid wall to the nasal pharynx is the eustachian tube. It exits from the middle ear cavity downward in an inferoanterior direction to communicate with the nasopharynx. Its length is approximately 2.5 cm. The function of this structure is to equate the pressure inside the middle ear with the atmospheric pressure surrounding the head.

The middle ear cavity is traversed by three small bones that form the ossicular chain. They are the malleus, incus, and stapes. Laterally, the malleus connects to the TM, and medially to the footplate of the smallest bone in the body, the stapes, where it attaches and covers the oval window of the inner ear. Three ligamentous attachments allow the conduction of sound via a physical system of leverage despite the bones being suspended through the cavity, and does this without any significant impedance of acoustic energy. This is achieved in addition to the lateral and medial wall attachments by the malleus' three ligamentous attachments, the incus' two ligaments, and the annular ligament, which attaches to the periphery of the stapes footplate. There are two muscles, the tensor tympany and the stapedius.

Inner Ear (Cochlea)

The nerves for hearing are contained within the cochlea. This structure is encased in the temporal bone and has a coiled construction resembling a snail's shell, and thus its name. Laid horizontally, it would approximate the appearance of a cone if its apex were pointed along a superior axis, and would measure about 9 mm across the base and 5 mm along the vertical axis. If uncoiled it would have the approximate length of 30–35 mm. The basal turn of the cochlea would lie inferior to the posterior semicircular canal and the apex of the coil or cupula anterior, lateral and slightly superior. It consists of an outer osseous capsule that contains perilymph and fits glove-like to encapsulate a membranous inner portion of similar shape. Within the membranous portion of this tube-like structure is the cochlear duct which contains the most important structure for hearing, the organ of Corti, and is positioned on the basilar membrane. The entire membranous portion contains endolymph. The organ of Corti contains an outer and inner row of hair cells over which is positioned the tectorial membrane. When movement occurs along the basilar membrane, a shearing action is created between the hair cells and the tectorial membrane, resulting in the neuroelectric impulses responsible for sensory input to the brain where auditory stimuli are ultimately interpreted. The hair cells number approximately 12,000 to 16,000–18,000 and must be magnified up to 250,000 times to appreciate their arrangement along the basilar membrane. The organ of Corti is bordered superiorly by the scala vestibuli and inferiorly by the scala tympani.

Inner Ear (Vestibular)

The osseous labyrinth contains the vestibular end that is situated posterior to the anteriorly positioned cochlea. Like the cochlear portion, it also has a membranous insert containing endolymph, and has perilymph between the membranous and osseous segments. Lying between the membranous division of the cochlear and the vestibular semicircular canal segments are two structures: the saccule, which communicates by the ductus reunions with the cochlea, and the utricle with its maculae, which contain otoconia. These are "small calcium carbonate crystals, ranging from 0.5 to 30 microns in diameter"[11] and are responsible for the detection of linear acceleration. Angular acceleration is made possible by the cristae contained within the ampulla of the horizontal, posterior, and superior (anterior) semicircular canals, with the latter two lying in a somewhat orthogonal relationship to one another. The cristae have hair cells numbering about 23,000, and the two maculae about 4,000.[12] The horizontal canal is 30° off the horizontal plain and is taken into consideration during vestibular testing.

Cranial Nerve (CN) VIII is the auditory-vestibular nerve and has three branches: a cochlear branch, and the superior and inferior vestibular branches "The superior division innervates the cristae of the anterior and horizontal canals, the maculae of the utriculus, and the anteriosuperior part of the saccular macula" while the inferior division provides innervation to the "...crista of the posterior canal and the main portion of the macula of the sacculus..."[11] The axons of the primary vestibular neurons divide into ascending and descending branches to form the vestibular tract, and these fibers enter the vestibular nuclei situated near the floor of the fourth ventricle of the brain. These are four in number and are named the superior, inferior, lateral, and medial. The superior nucleus has afferent input from the cristae of the end-organ canals and other anatomic structures. The inferior nucleus receives afferent neural signals from the cristae and maculae and, to a lesser extent, spinal afferents and efferents to the cerebellum and reticular formation. The lateral nucleus is involved with both afferent spinal commissural fibers and efferent fibers to the cervicothoracic and the lumbosacral cord, and these are believed to control vestibulospinal reflexes. Again referring to Baloh and Honrubia,[11] the medial nucleus is an afferent target with "... fibers from the cristae of the semicircular canals...saccular and utricular..." structures. These structures also associate with the Medial Longitudinal Fassiculus (MLF). The medial nucleus has efferent connections "... in the descending MLF to the cervical and thoracic levels by way of the vestibulospinal tract..." and "...efferent fibers pass to the ascending MLF bilaterally to reach...the oculomotor nerves' nuclei." These authors continue that, "Because of its projection in the MLF to the extraocular muscles of the eye and the spinal cord, the medial vestibular nucleus appears to be an important center for coordinating eye, head, and neck movements."[11] These neural pathways and their interactions with other sensory systems would help to explain why MTBI patients with neck injuries frequently have auditory/vestibular symptoms. The interested reader is referred to an excellent text, *Clinical Neurophysiology of the Vestibular System,* for a more detailed anatomical and physiological description of this highly complex and not entirely understood system.

HISTORY

Obtaining a history on an accident patient with auditory and/or vestibular symptoms will generally differ from that of a patient with the same or similar symptom(s) that are not accident related. This type of initial interview is also more time consuming.

As with any evaluation, questioning the patient will help determine not only if an abnormality exists but where, and what tests, examinations, treatment, or referrals might be appropriate or possibly contraindicated. It is also advisable at this time to obtain specifics from the patient about the accident and request pertinent medical records that might be available for review. The first clinician to have contact with the patient will not, of course, have this advantage, but may have access to accident reports. Often, an attorney is already involved and is an excellent resource for acquiring needed records since the patient has probably already signed a release of information. What is alleged and what might have been recorded elsewhere in documents may differ, but there should be little difference in the date, time, and location of the accident. Any differences that are identified need to be clarified. The accident description should help determine the type of injury. Information regarding the use of safety equipment and restraints, number of vehicles, vectors on impact, speed on closure, and position of occupants at time of impact can also be helpful if the incident involves one or more motor vehicles. Similar information is also pertinent for a WC injury, even though a vehicle is usually not involved unless it was used in accordance with job-related responsibilities. A claim number, names of other professionals involved, name of attorney, and the insurance companies implicated also may be needed to facilitate the quality of documentation necessary to generate a thorough evaluation report. All information in the report should be verifiable — that is, valid and reliable — to be credible.

As already noted, various symptoms may appear the same but result from different sources or causes. The following symptoms are an example, although not exhaustive, of what should be considered during the initial interview when the MTBI patient presents with what are thought to be auditory or vestibular complaints, although both are usually present. Included is a section regarding the cervical spine since it can produce or influence auditory and vestibular symptoms, and, probably more than realized, contributes to the auditory and vestibular symptoms present with many MTBI victims.

TINNITUS

This is, at one time or another, present in essentially one-third of the population.[12] It is important to document whether the perceived ear sound is unilateral and to which ear the sound is localized or to determine if it is bilateral; thought to be inside the head; has a pulsatile character; is high-pitched; low in pitch; intermittent or constant; changes with or in the absence of other auditory, vestibular, or bodily symptoms; or causes sleep disturbance. A high-pitched tinnitus may also occur in the absence of documented outer, middle, or inner ear abnormality, and may be myofascial in origin as with Temporal Mandibular Joint (TMJ) Syndrome. This is often present unilaterally, can be intermittent, and usually involves the affected side. Tinnitus may also originate from other trauma sites such as the cervical spine.[13-16] Other causes include aminoglycosides, cis-platinum,[17] or large amounts of aspirin ingestion and various prescription medications.

EAR FULLNESS AND PRESSURE

This, too, can result from various causes. Although clinically reported by trauma patients, it can occur as well with otitis media, external otitis, barometric changes, sensorineural hearing loss, allergy with eustachian tube dysfunction, and with situations as simple as impacted cerumen.

HEARING LOSS AND HEARING FLUCTUATIONS

Many clinical patients complain of difficulty hearing following a traumatic event — or that hearing fluctuates — and this can involve either one or both ears. This may or may not be due to a physiological change in the auditory mechanism. Individuals who state that they can hear but not always understand, especially if attempting to communicate in the presence of background noise or when several individuals are talking, usually have high frequency hearing loss rather than an actual fluctuation of their auditory thresholds. It can also involve a change in auditory discrimination (understanding) ability. Such individuals are at times scheduled for a neuropsychological evaluation assuming the problem is an auditory processing problem associated with a cognitive disorder, rather than considering the fact that a hearing loss may exist. A perilymphatic fistula or fistula tract injury can also cause hearing fluctuations. A Temporary Threshold Shift (TTS) can cause fluctuations in hearing as a result of excessive noise-level exposures.

NOISE EXPOSURE

A question of hearing loss is not only suspect but frequently reported when there has been exposure to a loud blast — referred to as Acoustic Trauma (AT) — or if frequent loud exposures have occurred across time as with Noise-Induced Hearing Loss (NIHL). Tinnitus is generally present in the history, and test findings are usually different from that occurring from trauma associated with MTBI. Any exposure to noise can be work-related, a product of recreational exposures, or both. Because the exposures are cumulative in their affect on the ear, not having been around noise for a long period of time does not mean that the ear has "healed," and the patient needs to be questioned carefully in this regard so as not to confuse causation. These losses are not associated with pain and many patients are unaware that they have a loss, especially if the loss is relatively mild.

OTALGIA

This is generally not reported unless there has been direct trauma to the ear, and is more likely present with outer and/or middle ear disease. An exception would be discomfort occurring with odonoiatric disorders.[14] A periodically present sharp pain, generally brief in duration, is more an otodynia, such as that occurring with TMJ syndrome.

OTORRHEA

This should not be present except in conjunction with an otitis media or external otitis. There are situations, however, where a basal skull fracture results in the accumulation of other types of fluid in the middle ear cavity. This can be a hemo-tympanum or cerebral spinal fluid (CSF), depending on the type of fracture. A longitudinal fracture involving the temporal bone is more apt to involve the middle ear or the external canal and present with a hemotympanum, whereas a transverse fracture involving the petrous pyramid may result in a sensorineural loss of auditory sensitivity, and the middle ear or tympanum could contain CSF. If such fluid is present, this usually does not result in tympanic rupture nor is it considered clinically prudent to initiate a myringotomy to evacuate the fluid. Fluid of this type should be otoscopically observable since the tympanic membrane will appear somewhat bluish in color if CSF, and reddened if a hemotympanum. In either case, the TM will not have its usual translucent character.

AUDITORY DISCRIMINATION

The clinical presentation of auditory and vestibular symptoms secondary to traumatic head injury often result in complaints of difficulty understanding others during conversations, when watching television, or in some other listening situation. As already noted, this raises the question of whether the difficulty is a result of hearing loss or a cognitive disorder involving auditory processing caused by an MTBI. If there is no hearing loss a neuropsychological evaluation can be helpful.

VESTIBULAR

The clinical presentations of dizziness vary. It may result in a description consistent with a pseudo-sensation of motion described as a whirling or spinning as with vertigo, or some other characterization. It may be described as a lightheadedness where the individual at times feels like he/she is going to experience a loss of consciousness, or does lose consciousness as with syncope, or simply feels woozy. At times the symptom is orthostatic in nature and occurs only when getting up quickly. Dysequilibrium or imbalance may be present in isolation, or in conjunction with other described symp-toms. At times it may be more noticeable at night when the immediate environment is dark because of being unable to visually compensate for a vestibular deficit. There are those who describe it as being present in a near constant manner, or it can be episodically present. Still others describe it as infrequently present, that it varies in intensity, gradually improving or worsening since the traumatic event, had an onset immediately post accident, occurred for a brief time or that it had an onset with a significant latency after the trauma, that it was accompanied by nausea with or without emesis, or any combination of these. Some patients describe a sensation of tumbling forward when squatting down or looking downward, while others fall backward when looking upward. It may also be present in only certain body positions, but may or may not meet the criteria for true Benign Paroxysmal Positional Vertigo (BPPV). The dizziness may be especially present or intensified with straining or lifting because of a perilymphatic fistula. There are also descriptions that cause even the careful clinician to suspect Meniere's disease or cochlear hydrops. As noted by Baloh and Honrubia, "Several diseases are known to produce Meniere's syndrome but in the majority of cases the cause is unknown."[11] Relative to etiology, if the only symptom is dizziness and not the classic presentation of coexisting ear fullness or pressure, fluctuating hearing loss, and a buzzing or roaring tinnitus, all of which occur in close proximity with one another, that raises the question of whether Meniere's disease is present. It is dubiously acknowledged by some as to whether it can be traumatically induced. As stated by Ruth and Lambert, "… a hallmark of Meniere's disease is its variable expression from one patient to the next or even in the same patient over time. The array of terms applied to this disorder such as *Meniere's-like*, *vestibular hydrops*, and *cochlear hydrops* reflect this diagnostic uncertainty."[18] Symptom inquiry may also be especially difficult at times since vestibular-like symptoms can result from causal dysfunction indirectly related to the ear. This can involve the cervical spine but may, for example, result from vascular disease,[17,19,20] demylinating disease,[21] autoimmune disease,[18,22] migraine,[23] and metabolic causes.[22,24]

CERVICAL SPINE

There are multiple symptoms that can occur because of traumatically-induced physiological changes involving the neck and the neural projections and interactions that its structures have with various other sensory systems. Discomfort involving the cervical spine is frequently reported as pain, stiffness, decreased range of motion, or occurring when tilting the head in one direction or the other. The symptoms can be constant, intermittent, involve one side only, or be bilaterally present. There may be times when dizziness occurs while tilting the head backward. These symptoms do not always appear immediately following an injury-producing situation, and at times commence latent to the injury-causing incident, perhaps even by years. This requires, therefore, that a history include whether there have been prior accidents, and should note even those that have resulted from sport and recreational injuries to the neck. They tend to be more common with acceleration/deceleration injuries resulting from automobile accidents, and have been noted to be more prevalent with seatbelt use.[9] Although MTBIs are reportedly more common in males,[5] clinical experience suggests that individuals with this diagnosis that have auditory and vestibular symptoms are more often female. This may reflect their generally slighter musculature in this area of the body.

Careful questioning will produce testimony that the neck symptoms can occur in conjunction with tinnitus, vertigo, headache, ocular anomalies,[15] dysphasia, dynophasia, numbness or tingling of the upper extremities, or a myriad of other physical symptoms presenting in various combinations. Postural changes are common and have developed to compensate or avoid certain body positions that the patient has learned may result in noxious symptoms. There is often an accompanying Vestibular Ocular Reflex (VOR) abnormality, diplopia, and metamorphopsia or a suspect change in vision post injury. When headache is reported it often originates suboccipitally, and may migrate or radiate forward to include the temporal and other areas of the head. These may also be present with cognitive problems, an emotional problem, hearing loss, auditory processing difficulties, and memory deficits.

Several theories have evolved to account for the various symptoms associated with cervical spine injuries. These include vertebral artery occlusion, dysfunction within the cervical sympathetic system, proprioceptive changes, and altering of muscle reflexes specific to this region of the body. The literature has referred to the various complexes of symptoms resulting from injury to the neck as a Barre-Lieou syndrome,[15] which first appeared in the literature in 1926. It has also been called a "posterior sympathetic syndrome." The symptoms occurring with this disorder are consistent with those associated with MTBI. It is in fact recognized that acceleration/deceleration injuries involving the neck are "...a true head trauma even if there is no contact of the head with an object."[14]

EVALUATION

Diagnostic audiological tests are invaluable and necessary when attempting to establish the derivation of auditory or vestibular symptoms. The test results become a part of the patient's permanent record. Although often referred to as "hearing tests," diagnostic tests are administered for purposes different than those done at work, school, or in a physician's office to screen hearing. Rather than testing just for hearing, they are designed relative to the known physiology of the ear and psychophysical and psychoacoustic principles to either assist in determining whether a loss of hearing or ear symptoms are of outer, middle, or inner ear origin, retrocochlear, or some combination of these. All testing is conducted in a controlled environment, but that portion specifically used to establish auditory thresholds must be accomplished in a sound booth. Both the diagnostic audiometer used to establish these thresholds and the sound booth must adhere to specific standards. The instrumentation must be routinely calibrated and inspected for proper performance. Because air and bone conduction studies are considered "behavioral" tests, it is essential that both the instrumentation and test technique adhere to rigid criteria that have been established to help assure validity and reliability. This objective is essential if the obtained test data are to provide any meaningful diagnostic information or have medico-legal credibility. A complete assessment includes not only air and bone conduction, but middle ear studies, nonbehavioral tests such as Auditory Brainstem Evoked Potentials (ABR) and Electronystagmography (ENG), and possibly other tests depending on need. Such additional tests may include techniques specifically designed to detect functional losses.

Prior to any of the various tests that comprise a complete diagnostic evaluation, an otoscopic examination is necessary. If there is any obstruction in the external meatii from cerumen or foreign bodies such as cotton or broken-off Q-Tips®, these obviously should be removed, and only then should the various tests be administered.

AUDIOLOGICAL

The initial portion of the test battery uses air-conducted auditory stimuli introduced into the ear through earphones to determine auditory thresholds. All test data or thresholds are obtained on each ear and recorded on a graph called an audiogram.

The audiometer is operated manually using one of three psychophysical techniques to establish thresholds, generally, The Method of Limits.[25]

A Speech Reception Threshold (SRT) is then acquired using spondaic words. These are bisyllabic words with equal stress on each syllable, e.g., "baseball," "airplane," "cowboy," etc. The words are presented in an ascending-descending manner, crossing threshold several times. "Threshold" is considered the point at which 50% of the words can be identified and repeated by the individual being tested. As a quick check on validity, the decibel (dB) level at which this occurs should be within 5 dB of the puretone average established for auditory thresholds at three of the frequencies tested. These are 500, 1000, and 2000 Hertz (Hz), or cycles per second, although a complete audiogram requires testing at the frequencies of 250, 500, 1000, 2000, 4000, and 8000 Hz. In many instances it should also include 3000 Hz and 6000 Hz.

After the SRT is established, a list of Phonetically Balanced (PB) words are presented at a Supra-Threshold Level (SL) to determine auditory discrimination (understanding) ability, usually at 30 dB relative to the SRT. Normal discrimination is 100%. This, too, is accomplished separately in each ear.

Bone conduction testing is then initiated using an oscillator placed behind the ear on the mastoid process, but not touching the auricle. Touching the auricle with the oscillator sets up air-conducted stimuli in the canal much the same as with earphones. This portion of the test is used to assess or measure inner ear nerve or cochlear function. The thresholds are also recorded on the same audiogram with the air conduction thresholds. The frequencies tested are 250, 500, 1000, 2000, and 4000 Hertz (Hz) and employ the same test technique as that used to establish air conduction thresholds.

If there is a significant interaural asymmetry, masking noise is introduced into the better (non-test) ear while puretone or speech thresholds are being obtained in the contralateral (in this case, poorer) ear. This is necessary to avoid unwanted responses from the better ear when the poorer ear is being tested.

TYPES OF HEARING LOSS

There are three types of hearing loss: sensorineural, conductive, and mixed. These can occur at levels considered mild through severe, and at times profound, with the latter sometimes being referred to as a "dead ear." The classification for these is determined according to the relative thresholds for air and bone conduction.

If the bone conduction thresholds are something other than normal, generally considered to be 0-25 dB HL on the audiogram, and are at the same level as the air-conduction levels on the audiogram, this represents what is referred to as a sensorineural or nerve loss. This category of loss can involve the cochlea of the inner ear and, at times, retrocochlear structures, such as with an acoustic tumor on the eighth cranial nerve (CN VIII), or both.

If the bone conduction threshold is at a better level than air conduction, the test will show an air-bone gap. This results in what is referred to as a conductive loss if the thresholds by bone conduction are normal and the air-conduction thresholds abnormal. A conductive loss is indicative of a problem lying within the outer and/or middle ear. These can often be eliminated or improved with medication or surgery, depending on the cause.

A third type of loss is a mixed loss and is simply a combination of the other two. These can occur at levels considered mild through severe. The conductive portion of the loss can also often be improved with medication or surgery.

MIDDLE EAR FUNCTION

Electroacoustic impedance or immittance measurements are used to assess middle ear function and integrity. This is done with a small amount of air for the compliance and tympanogram portions of the testing, and acoustic stimuli introduced at suprathreshold levels for stapedius reflex responses. All measurements are accomplished using a soft, pliable probe tube placed into the external meatus of each ear. These tests are also recordable. They are helpful in determining the presence of a tympanic membrane perforation, ossicular chain continuity, middle ear fluid, and other conditions involving the middle ear. This does not duplicate what was identified on the audiogram establishing a conductive loss or the conductive component of the mixed loss, but helps clarify the cause for the conductive element.

ELECTROCOCHLEOGRAPHY (ECOG)

This test is based on the presence of short-latency auditory-evoked potentials and consists of three components. These are the Cochlear Microphonic (CM), the Action Potential (AP), and Summating Potential (SP). The CM and SP are generated by the hair cells in the cochlea, while the AP is a product of the auditory nerve nearest the cochlea. The test can be administered from electrodes positioned in the canal, or by needle electrodes introduced into the middle ear transtympanically. It is helpful in establishing a diagnosis of Meniere's disease and for identifying the presence of a perilymphatic fistula.

AUDITORY BRAINSTEM-EVOKED POTENTIALS (ABR)

This test is used to evaluate the neural integrity of the cochlea and auditory pathway of the brainstem. It uses electrodes variously placed in the ear canals and on the forehead to record evoked electrical potentials resulting from the introduction of auditory stimuli into the ear. The electrical potentials evoked represent responses generated at various levels along the ascending auditory neural pathway within the first 10 ms following stimulation. These neuroelectric events consist of five to seven wave responses occurring at latencies relative to their anatomical origin(s). The first five waves tend to be most useful clinically, and are labeled as Roman numeral I, II, III, IV, and V. In the human adult, latencies can differ relative to age, the specific instrumentation used to record the responses,[26] and, obviously, from various disruptions in the continuity of the neural pathway. The test can be used to help establish auditory thresholds, but its greatest clinical application is in its ability to determine if the auditory symptoms have a retrocochlear component, and the probable level within the brainstem that such dysfunction might be occurring. It is, for example, especially sensitive for space-occupying lesions such as an acoustic neuroma, and for auditory symptoms that appear neurologically-based when, for example, an MTBI is suspect. The neural generator believed responsible for Waves I and II is believed to result from the auditory nerve.[27] Wave III is considered by van der Honert to result from the ventral cochlear nucleus "...or their axonal projections in the trapezoid body..." and from "...activity within the medial nucleus of the contralateral superior olivary complex, with possible contribution from the fiber tract of the trapezoid body."[28] That Wave III is generated by the cochlear nucleus is supported by Moller.[27] Wave IV generation is believed to result from the medial aspect of the brainstem, and may result from more than one source and possibly involve the superior olivary complex.[27] It is stated by van der Honert[28] that Wave IV is a product of a "bilateral discharge of neurons of the lateral lemnisci." Wave V results from "...the central nucleus of the contralateral inferior colliculus..." or possibly further along the ascending pathway, and this is generally agreed upon by others.[27]

As with all tests considered technically sophisticated, special instrumentation is necessary for recording these electrically minute responses. It is a test that requires experience to administer and interpret.

VESTIBULAR

Electronystagmography (ENG) is by far the most time-consuming and technically difficult test to administer in a complete test battery. Its purpose is to document whether vestibular symptoms are attributable to the vestibular portion of the inner ear, are of CNS origin, are a combination of these, or are perhaps unrelated to the vestibular system.

The vestibular system does not function only as a product of its inner ear structures but interacts in conjunction with other neurologic structures and systems. These include the vestibulo-ocular and vestibulospinal reflexes. These consist of three known neural pathways, two of which are the lateral and medial segments of the vestibulospinal tract and arise from the vestibular nuclei, and the third is the reticulospinal from the reticular formation. These interact with the cervico-ocular and vestibulo-ocular reflexes. The latter, along with the negative potential of the retina of the eye and positive potential of the cornea, result in the corneal-retinal potential to create an electric dipole. This provides the basis for the ENG test. Changes in this potential can be recorded when active electrodes are positioned close to, above, and below the eye relative to a ground electrode. The electrical field in this situation will intensify or become more positive when the eye moves towards it, and lessens or becomes more negative when the eye moves away. This change in electric potential can be amplified and recorded. Instrumentation used for ENG includes a recorder that is preferably dual-channeled, and a differential amplifier capable of recording minimal eye movements. The patient is coupled to the system using electrodes. These can be gold cup electrodes used with alternating current recordings, or silver/silver chloride electrodes that can be used with alternating or direct current recordings. Eye movements and calibration for visual stimuli are obtained using a light bar with automated light-moving capability for the various visual tests. An open loop irrigation system provides the capability of introducing water directly into the external auditory canal while controlling water temperatures necessary for bithermal ("hot" and "cold") caloric irrigation. Testing is accomplished using either a chair or table that is appropriate for the test demands of proper patient positioning. Variations exist regarding the type of equipment and components and should be selected relative to the intended use and capability of the person(s) responsible for patient testing. The test protocol will always commence with calibration, and may be complicated if conjugate eye movement is absent. The difficulty can usually be remedied by placing electrodes on the outer and inner canthi of the eye best able to track a moving object. The protocol will include testing for spontaneous nystagmus, which should be accomplished immediately following calibration since the information derived will be needed for other measurements. The Dix-Hallpike maneuver should be completed early in the test and before the positional testing is completed because of the potential for fatiguing the response once the patient lies down, which is one of the criteria that allows for distinguishing between a Classical Hallpike and an Atypical Hallpike. A Classical Hallpike would be consistent with a BPPV, whereas an Atypical Hallpike is a CNS finding. The test also includes oculomotor tests that are necessary for assessing gaze nystagmus, saccades, pendular tracking, and Optokinetic (OPK) nystagmus. Positional testing is a part of the overall test sequence and includes having the patient assume sitting, sitting with head turned right, sitting with head turned left, supine, supine with head turned right, supine with head turned left, whole body right, and whole body left positions. The caloric test provides best results when specifics relative to this portion of testing such as water temperature, duration of irrigation, sequence of irrigation, patient preparation and control, and other variables are controlled.[29]

ADDITIONAL REASONS FOR TESTS

The audiological test battery answers several questions relative to auditory and vestibular functions. There are several reasons why they should be administered when an MTBI patient presents clinically since there are usually medico-legal questions that will arise if symptoms are secondary to an accident. These tests, when properly administered, are:

1. Considered objective
2. Necessary to establish a diagnosis
3. Needed if proper treatment and therapy is to be initiated
4. An acceptable entry to permanent records
5. Noninvasive and, therefore, do not pose risk to the patient
6. Able to be used to establish permanency or disability ratings if necessary, and in certain situations may void any permanency
7. Repeatable, and can thus serially monitor change in function
8. As with ENG, able to test certain aspects of vestibulo-ocular function with eyes closed
9. Able to correlate CNS findings on ENG with those that may be identified on ABR

10. Often the only tests that are instrumental in establishing a differential diagnosis
11. Provide information frequently not amenable to verification on imaging studies

THERAPIES AND TREATMENT

The treatment of auditory vestibular symptoms may range from medication to surgery or require no treatment whatsoever. Any treatment will depend on a diagnosis. If symptoms are originating from a structural change in the middle ear from significant head trauma, resulting in, for example, an ossicular discontinuity, perilymphatic fistula, or a TM perforation, surgery can restore the system to a safe status and generally improve any hearing loss or vestibular symptoms that resulted from the anomaly. If there are vestibular symptoms, medication may be recommended. However, there appears to be a growing population of clinicians who feel medication such as meclazine is contraindicated since it may disallow central compensation in situations where there is a peripheral vestibular deficit identified on objective studies. Antivertiginous medications do not consistently result in clinically gratifying symptom relief for large populations of patients having CNS-mediated symptoms, especially those falling into the MTBI group. There are also those individuals who cannot safely use medications to suppress vestibular function. Additionally, there are patients who have experienced an acute episode of dizziness from a labyrinthitis, and who, in a reasonably short time, achieve symptom resolution without any assistance.

The management of dizziness or balance dysfunction is often accomplished through exercise programs. The clinical objective is to facilitate CNS compensation through repetition and habituation of the dizziness. The therapy is often administered by various clinicians including physical or occupational therapists, and involves an attempt to extinguish the noxious symptom by instructing patients in various exercises or placing them in certain positions to extinguish the problematic symptoms. This category of treatment also includes body positioning strategies for Benign Paroxysmal Positional Vertigo (BPPV) in which otoliths become "dislodged," especially within the posterior semicircular canal. This is referred to as "cupulolithiasis," and therapy is directed towards repositioning these free-floating particles. An example of the latter would be those situations where the ENG demonstrates a Classical Hallpike, a peripheral test finding. An Atypical Hallpike is not a peripheral finding, and patients who have this finding on the test do not usually appear to respond favorably to therapy. Therapy does not appear to be entirely effective for symptoms that are CNS or cervicogenic in origin, even though patients whose symptoms fall into this category are frequently referred for therapy. However, the nonsuccess of therapy may, and probably does at times, reflect poor selection of patients for therapy since its application success will depend on whether the symptoms are an imbalance; dizziness, as with vertigo; or a sensory integration failure. This can be determined only by appropriate testing and patient assessment prior to therapy. All too often, patients are simply described as being "dizzy" without regard to its characterization or origin, and the therapy may not be appropriate. Another variable additional to patient selection relative to type of vestibular-like dysfunction is that patients who are motivated tend to be more successful since therapy includes the active participation of the patient at home or elsewhere to maximize therapeutic goals. It does assist some patients with compensating visually or proprioceptively for their peripheral vestibular deficits, and perhaps helps some patients avoid an otherwise unnecessary fall.[30]

Optometrists provide another approach to treatment. Therapy may be initiated in situations where there is, for example, a vestibulo-ocular abnormality. Results vary and, again, the success appears related to an appropriate diagnosis and selection of patients for therapy.

Chiropractic treatment is common with symptoms associated with MTBI resulting from accidents. These can be as adjustments, heat, or other therapy modalities.

The final treatment category of significance involves the surgical or chemical destruction of the inner ear nerves. This can involve the auditory or vestibular segments. Obviously, the selection of patients who will benefit from this approach is specific to the diagnosis.

As with any clinical entity, all treatment approaches have claimed their share of success. Perhaps the success rate would be even greater, as indicated, if patients were selected based on a more exacting diagnosis relative to the treatment being considered.

CASE REPORTS

The following is intended to help exemplify patient presentations having similar symptoms but a significantly different diagnoses. Each presented clinically subsequent to an accident upon referral from their primary care physician, a medical specialist, or their insurance carrier for a second opinion or Independent Medical Evaluation (IME). The cases depict how a diagnosis might affect treatment. There is one example of a faulty cause-effect relationship, one representing a workers compensation injury, and the other examples are somewhat typical of automobile accidents. At least one example represents test findings that are considered unusual and unexpected to what is generally identified on test.

CASE #1

TR was a 51-year-old seat-belt-restrained driver involved in a low impact accident while backing out of parking space, striking another car. He had been involved in two previous minor accidents without injury. Subsequent to the most recent accident he experienced neck discomfort and, three days post event, scheduled an appointment with a chiropractor for treatment that involved high-velocity manipulation of the cervical spine. Following the third treatment he presented to a local hospital with numbness involving the left upper and lower extremities, diplopia, and concerns of a possible metamorphopsia involving the left eye, probable Vestibular Ocular Reflex (VOR) abnormality, imbalance, continued neck symptoms with decreased range of motion when turning the head to the left, cognitive dysfunction, near constant tinnitus perceived as a "roaring" sound in the left ear, and headache greater over the left mastoid area. He was admitted to the hospital with a diagnosed "blow-out stroke," and an MRI of the brain noted abnormalities compatible with "...ischemia or infarction involving the left posterior circulation in the left cerebellar hemisphere, left thalamus, left posterior occipital lobe, and in the midbrain and pons." He was released from the hospital six days later but his auditory and vestibular-like symptoms persisted and prompted his neurologist to refer him for complete auditory/vestibular studies. The patient shortly afterward was performing poorly with job-related responsibilities and lost his job because the employer believed there was a significant psychiatric or functional component to his symptoms. The insurer also was hesitant to approve a referral for testing, and there was considerable delay before tests were administered, unfortunately, post stroke.

On audiological tests he demonstrated a mild, nearly symmetrical high frequency loss of hearing. Middle ear function was normal, bilaterally. The ENG demonstrated peripheral vestibular physiology to be within normal limits with only a 6% decrease on the right and a 10% DP to the right. There was low-intensity upbeating nystagmus with eyes open and also closed, abnormal sinusoidal tracking to the right and vertically, equivocal vertical OKN, right-beating positional nystagmus with an upbeating component, and equivocal saccades to the left that showed multiplestep activity on a significant portion of the tracing. The abnormal results were interpreted as being CNS in origin, with the upbeating nystagmus considered consistent with dysfunction involving the dorsal central medulla in the region of the medial vestibular nucleus, resulting from probable infarction.[1]

Comment

This patient initiated a malpractice claim against the chiropractor, who settled at considerable cost to the carrier. The accident symptoms were less than those occurring from treatment in this situation, with the former resulting in symptoms consistent with MTBI by definition, but the latter becoming another diagnosis. A psychiatric component was not present and documented as such on neuropsychological testing, with the report stating that the "...stroke and subsequent deterioration of functioning, to the point at which he has become unemployable, has shattered his sense of importance and value to his family and has significantly diminished his self-esteem and sense of self-worth." Prior to the unfortunate treatment, he had been a committed and hard-working employee. When this work pattern changed, a hasty opinion was initiated by others at his former place of employment as being a product of a functional disorder. Another concern was the delay in attempting to document the validity of his auditory/vestibular symptoms, which added to his frustration and were not considered until his neurologist felt such testing to be necessary in trying to facilitate treatment.

CASE #2

MO was a 71-year-old female when first seen for evaluation September 24, 1998. She noted a bilateral hearing loss of unknown duration that had been gradually progressive. About eight years earlier, at her then stated age of 63 years, the vehicle she was driving was broadsided. The accident caused her to strike her head, and she eventually had an audiological evaluation because of then reported hearing loss which noted a bilateral sensorineural loss, but not an ENG, despite her reporting occasional vestibular-like symptoms. While living in another state, she had a neurological evaluation that reportedly revealed nothing in terms of a neurologic basis for her symptoms, but that evaluation did not include imaging studies or complete audiological testing. At the time of her last evaluation she was experiencing periodic episodes of dizziness characterized as a sensation of movement, as with vertigo, that was present near daily; imbalance; and, at times, lightheadedness and several syncopal events that were preceded by nausea and an occasional emesis. Tinnitus was present as a high-pitched sound in either ear. She denied otalgia, otorrhea, or otodynia. Familial history of hearing loss and known ototoxic drug usage was unremarkable. She was having difficulty understanding others during conversations, but more with competing background noise. There was no apparent fluctuation in hearing, but she questioned this because of her difficulty at times understanding speech. Fullness or pressure in the ears was further denied, as was any use of medication, and general health was stated as essentially normal.

Her referring physicians questioned whether the cause for her symptoms were accident-related or represented another etiology. A complete audiological evaluation noted an interaurally symmetrical, high-frequency sensorineural loss of hearing; auditory discrimination was within normal limits and symmetrical; middle ear function studies were normal and stapedius reflexes present without abnormal adaptation; but ENG showed a minimal 10% left peripheral deficit with 0% directional preponderance (DP); and right warm calorics showed a Failure of Fixation Suppression (FFS) and a direction-changing positional nystagmus. An ABR study demonstrated an interaural asymmetry with Wave III on both sides delayed in latency, and Wave V on the left delayed to produce an abnormally prolonged Wave I-V Interpeak Interval.

The audiological report stated that there was "…nothing by test that would be highly suspicious for an acoustic tumor, although there are other space-occupying lesions that can present with symptoms of this type…" and that it was doubtful that her complaints were related to the accident. This prompted avoiding conservative treatment with Antivert and on October 21, 1998, an MRI of the brain with and without IV contrast identified a "…7x6x8 mm meningioma …located in the left temporal fossa."

Comment

This woman had another accident November 27, 1998, followed by worsening of her symptoms. A complete audiological evaluation corroborated this when results were compared to her first full work-up. Again, nothing was felt to be accident related, but that she then was experiencing a coexisting vascular reason for the increased symptoms consistent with her age. The second accident did not result in litigation for auditory/vestibular symptoms. It is unclear why an earlier complete evaluation was never ordered since there appeared to be a correlation between her symptoms and the initial accident, and also because of persistent ongoing auditory/vestibular symptoms.

Case #3

DL was a 34-year-old male when initially seen for testing June 6, 1988. He questioned progressive loss of hearing occurring secondary to noise exposure from a punch press at work. The job description noted his left ear as being closest to the noise because of the position of his body when operating the press. He also had occasion to lift heavy objects, but claimed no ear symptoms with lifting or straining. He did use ear protection in compliance with OSHA which was required at his place of employment because of the noise. Tinnitus was present in the left ear as a high-pitched noise. He experienced occasional lightheadedness and imbalance which was occasionally accompanied by nausea and ear fullness, experienced no fluctuation in hearing after noise exposures, and used the ear protection that his employer provided. He denied otalgia, otorrhea, known ototoxic drug use, familial history of hearing loss, medications, accidents, prior ear problems during childhood, or any other history often associated with ear symptoms. The company physician and nurse felt the loss was probably NIHL and they were opposed to him seeing an outside provider. A CT scan was negative for tumor when evaluated by an otolaryngologist (ENT) who thought the man was suspect for "a leak," a perilymphatic fistula. He wanted another opinion and prior records were not available.

Testing demonstrated a high-frequency sensorineural loss for the right ear, having a characteristic notch often noted with NIHL. The left ear showed an audiometric configuration involving all frequencies but greater for the high frequencies, consistent with a mixed loss having an air-bone gap ranging from 20-45 dB. The SRT was commensurate with the auditory thresholds in each ear, and auditory discrimination within the range of normal at 96% on the right and 92% on the left ear. Middle ear function tests were essentially normal except for the absence of the stapedius reflex on the left. The ENG revealed a minimal 10% decrease in left vestibular physiology, 18% DP to the left, and nonlocalizing CNS findings. Because of the interaural asymmetry and absence of tumor, middle ear fluid, or familial history of hearing loss, a fistula was again suspect, and the second ENT physician who examined him clinically also felt he was suspect for a fistula. The patient still felt the loss was due to noise, despite the conductive component to his loss perhaps contraindicating this diagnosis, and also because of the influence of medical personnel at his place of employment.

He returned on three more occasions for tests, with each showing an additional decrease in hearing on the left that was sensorineural. Auditory discrimination showed deterioration, and the ENG showed unilateral weakness and had dropped to 16%, 20%, and 16% on subsequent tests, respectively. At the time of his third follow-up visit, discrimination had deteriorated to 20%. An ABR and ECOG was abnormal for the left ear. He consented to a surgical exploration of the left ear. A fistula was present and repaired. Subsequent testing postoperatively demonstrated improved hearing on the left, and his dizziness and nausea resolved. His tinnitus was far less severe than it had been and was no longer causing sleep disturbance as it had prior to surgery. Auditory discrimination had improved to 88%. Date of follow-up was May 15, 1989. On December 14, 1990, he again presented with all of the symptoms he had been experiencing prior to surgery, but dizziness was worse and discrimination had dropped to 28%. Even though he was instructed post-operatively to limit lifting heavy objects at work and given written instructions, his employer disallowed the instruction almost immediately upon his returning to work. He was again operated on, and again symptoms improved, as did his test results. He was again instructed on limiting the lifting, but pressure to maintain his job disallowed this and, when symptoms again worsened, his test demonstrated a "dead ear" on the left and 26% decrease in peripheral vestibular function. He was not seen again clinically.

Comment

This was a work-related injury resulting from a job requirement that involved occasionally lifting up to 100 pounds. Because of the employer's refusal to allow postoperative restrictions, a bad situation became worse. Given the patient's testimony and hesitancy of the employer to obtain an evaluation outside of their clinic, there appeared to have been a suspicion by the employer that DL was trying to avoid responsibilities necessary to perform his job. Perhaps there was an initial attempt to avoid a reportable WC injury.

CASE #4

EJ was a 44-year-old woman when initially evaluated on October 2, 1996. She denied tinnitus, fullness/pressure in the ears, fluctuations of her hearing, absence of noise exposure, otalgia, otorrhea, or otodynia. Familial history of hearing loss and known ototoxic drug use were unremarkable. She did believe she had an ear infection in the right ear as a child, and was aware of a TM perforation on the right and, possibly, a mild loss of hearing in that ear. She also had experienced an occasional imbalance, and at times some unexplained nausea, neither of which she had ever conveyed to anyone until asked at the time of the audiological evaluation. She had occasional numbness involving the right hand and leg, and further questioning revealed an automobile accident five to six years previously, for which she saw a chiropractor because of a "pinched nerve in her neck." She further reported severe headache every two to three weeks since that accident that resulted in her taking pain medication. Otoscopically, a small perforation was present in the posteroinferior portion of the right TM.

On testing, EJ showed a mild conductive loss of hearing for the right ear that involved all frequencies, and it had an air-bone gap ranging to 20 dB. The left ear had entirely normal auditory thresholds. Middle ear function studies demonstrated a large compliance for the right ear consistent with the perforation, and normal middle ear function on the left. Stapedius reflexes were absent on the right, again consistent with the perforation, and the reflexes on the left were normal without evidence of auditory recruitment or abnormal reflex adaptation. These results did not explain her imbalance, so an ENG was completed and showed a left-beating spontaneous nystagmus, equivocal vertical sinusoidal tracking, and a direction-changing positional nystagmus that showed an upbeating component in nearly all test positions. The test used air calorics instead of water because of the TM perforation. Test responses using air are generally greater on the side with a perforation. This was apparent, but the response on the left was weaker than expected, and when the responses for the two sides were compared, a very large interaural difference was identified and suggested a unilateral weakness on the left side. She was scheduled for a TM repair but question remained as to whether her vestibular-like symptoms were a product of the previous accident or some other CNS abnormality.

Because this was felt to be CNS in origin, an MRI was scheduled on October 10, 1996, and revealed a small acoustic neuroma measuring 2-4 mm in diameter "...located in the deep portion of the internal auditory canal." Interestingly, this was on the side with the normal auditory thresholds, but the location of the tumor still did not explain the headaches. She was then seen by a neurosurgeon and the decision was made to do nothing with the acoustic tumor since there was no facial nerve involvement, but that she should be followed at periodic intervals and reevaluated, both with MRI and audiologically.

On April 15, 1999, EJ again presented clinically for audiological testing because of auditory/vestibular symptoms reportedly resulting from a fall several months earlier. In November 1998 she had slipped on ice and struck her head while carrying boxes to the trash at a business she was managing. There was no apparent loss of consciousness, but she did feel she had been "dazed" briefly before an employee assisted her back into their place of employment. She has experiencing vertigo and lightheadedness since the fall, and there was a change in the pitch of her previously present tinnitus. She also reported headache, neck stiffness, and decreased range of motion when turning the head to the left or the right since the slip-and-fall accident.

Numbness was present involving the right arm and leg, there where TMJ symptoms with ear discomfort, cognitive abnormalities, and she reported often feeling "angry for no apparent reason." She was examined by various providers who felt that her symptoms were a result of the previously diagnosed acoustic tumor and not the WC incident. This added to her frustration since she was in disagreement with this opinion, the symptoms she was experiencing were different post accident from those present before her fall. Since the fall, she had been referred for therapies which included those specifically for dizziness/balance, vision therapy, and medication, but none resulted in any symptom resolution.

She is being scheduled for follow-up ENG and also ABR studies, but this is being delayed because of insurance reasons. She will be seen either under her WC or individual insurance.

Comment

There appears to be three separate situations. The acoustic tumor is not likely causing her cognitive or psychological difficulties, nor does it account for her neck symptoms or numbness of the right arm and leg. The second issue pertains to the previous surgery in the right ear and it has remained normal, as has the left ear. A third question exists as to whether the initial accident several years previous was still causing headache and neck symptoms, if there has been an exacerbation of a preexisting neck injury since there had been an acceleration/deceleration neck injury when her car was struck from behind, or if the slip-and-fall accident is responsible for all of her recent symptoms. These questions will need to be answered upon completion of her scheduled ENG and ABR, and her evaluation will probably also result in further evaluation by a physician familiar with Barre-Lieou syndrome.

CASE #5

LW is a 41-year-old female seen for an IME who, on June 15, 1997, at about 0900 hours, sustained a job-related accident when she fell from a ladder while hanging pictures above eye level. She was employed as a domestic. She subsequently noted tinnitus perceived as a "seashell-sounding" noise, greater for the left ear, that at times became high-pitched. Vestibular-like symptoms are reported as "very rarely spinning" but occur as more of an imbalance, and at times she feels near syncopal. The symptoms seem to worsen if she has just gotten up after sleeping. There was reported fullness/pressure in both ears, and she related this to her allergies. Head-aches were initially present for a couple months post event, but further questioning indicated that these were also present prior to the accident. She believed these to be associated with the allergies and probable sinus problems. Her headaches post event were specific to the left parietal and temporal regions that at times originated in the lower occipital area, and there was a coexisting discomfort extending down the left neck into the shoulder. She felt that her hearing fluctuated at times. Narcolepsy was also diagnosed subsequent to her fall. Further questioning indicated that she had neck symptoms while in the fourth grade and had been "dizzy" at about that time.

LW was seen by a large number of providers and was no longer driving or working because of her symptoms. On a report generated shortly post accident, she was diagnosed as having struck her head and that there was a loss of consciousness. At the time of the IME, however, she stated that she had been on the bottom rung of the ladder when she slipped, and that she reflexively extended her left arm to break her fall which resulted in a wrist fracture, but that she never struck her head nor was there a loss of consciousness. Her daughter, who was working with her at the time, observed her mother getting up from the floor almost immediately after falling and noted no loss of consciousness. She was seen medically almost imme-diately after her fall to reduce the wrist fracture, and at that time there were no lacerations, areas of edema, or contusions noted anywhere, including the head. A review of available records revealed several inconsistencies regarding not only the head-injury questions, but also with respect to her auditory and vestibular symptoms.

Her persistent vestibular-like symptoms resulted in a referral to an otolaryngol-ogist (ENT) for evaluation. She was then referred by the ENT physician to a neuro-otologist who felt that she had a probable Meniere's disease, even though his report stated that it was "...not classical Meniere's disease..." On a follow-up visit he counseled the patient relative to a surgical procedure to resolve her symptoms. This was based on the history, primarily because of aural pressure and test-retest differ-ences on the auditory threshold tests that were thought to be related to fluctuations in hearing. A review of the audiological tests did appear to change on multiple testing, and the ENG was interpreted as having"... some central signs..."

Comment

When seen for the IME, the audiological tests demonstrated auditory thresholds to be normal, bilaterally. At the beginning of testing, she did, on the SRT portion, offer half-word responses, and these are at times noted with individuals attempting to provide results different than what is actually present. She was reinstructed. A review of the fluctuating thresholds obtained elsewhere was suggestive of threshold variations that may have reflected differences in test techniques or some other variable resulting in those differences. The ENG and ABR results at the time of the IME were not consistent with Meniere's, but did show findings that were CNS in origin and were most consistent with what is generally obtained on patients having neck-generated auditory and vestibular symptoms. A clarification of her reported symptoms for hearing fluctuations, fullness in the ears, and description of her dizziness also helped to provide insight into the probable diagnosis that the neck was instrumental in her symptoms. She is being referred for further evaluation of the neck — since this is less aggressive than irreversible ear surgery — to see if her symptoms can be modified and resolved.

SUMMARY

The incidence of auditory and vestibular symptoms are common with MTBI. With an incidence of about 2,000,000 cases reported annually, it is relatively easy to extrapolate that the number of patients in this group who have auditory and vestibular symptoms is very large. Logic for the latter is derived from data indicating that the three most often indicated symptoms are headache, dizziness, and memory disorders. To what extent they are appropriately identified and evaluated is questionable given the case reports used as examples. This perhaps accounts for why at least some patients report poor symptom resolution and clinical outcomes from therapy, and suggests that the diagnosis leading to therapy may at times be inappropriate. This exists, at least in part, by the lack of awareness some exhibit for recognizing the role that the neck plays in MTBI complications. When auditory and/or vestibular symptoms are reported, there is no question that the vestibular component is the most difficult for establishing a diagnosis and, ultimately, any therapy. As stated by Norre[31] dizziness can be complex in its presentation, and a "Simplistic interpretation…" without regard for "… total context, is a very dangerous strategy and is to be condemned." Because headache is so common with MTBI, an additional comment by Edmeads[32] is equally appropriate since neck surgery is at times considered to resolve the symptom. He states that, "…any surgical adventures in these patients are most ill-advised, at least until all litigation has been concluded." Obviously, he is reflecting on the fact that errors in judgment do occur, and that a conservative approach to treatment is advised when there are medico-legal issues.

Further clinical investigation is needed to better distinguish between various types of dizziness occurring secondary to trauma, especially if there is a coexisting neck injury. Why this has not received more research attention is somewhat curious since dizziness associated with the neck is mentioned in publications from many countries and in the professional literature of otolaryngology, neuro-otology, neurology, orthopedics, and audiology. This may reflect an excessive clinical reliance on imaging studies that frequently do not reveal abnormalities of the type present with MTBI. Hesitation to further research this area may also result from the complex nature of symptom presentation and the amount of clinic time needed for these patients. Additionally, there are opinions that a large number of these patients have psychological disorders, but evidence on postmortem investigation has "…showed focal contusions in frontal and temporal cortex, corpus callosum, subcortical structures, diencephalon, and subdural and subarachnoidal microbleeding as consequences of sudden angular accelerations."

Germane to every evaluation is an appropriate history. This assists in establishing a diagnosis and successful treatment protocol that, in conjunction with valid and reliable tests, lessens the potential for unnecessary or delayed treatment and perhaps avoidable litigation. To this end, a complete audiological test battery and description is presented and suggested as a means to clarify whether the symptoms are peripheral, CNS in origin, some combination of these, or caused by insult to structures distal to the ear, such as with cervical spine trauma. This is not to imply that these tests are the only ones that may be necessary. This is a complicated and challenging area of clinical inquiry because of the complexities associated with MTBI, and, therefore, a multidisciplinary approach is generally needed for appropriate diagnosis and treatment. Equally important is the fact that this requires experience that can sometimes be achieved only by many years of patient encounters.

It was noted that the tests provide a record that may be required with litigation inquiry often associated with MTBI since various disputable accidents are frequently cited as causative. For records to be credible they must be valid, and considerations were presented to help facilitate this objective.

This chapter was intended for the wide variety of individuals most often involved with this type of patient, not all of whom are expected to have a medical background or similar training and experience. Therefore, the information contained is considered an overview. Although certain specialties were mentioned in the case reports included for purposes of illustration, any difficulties occurring during patient care by members of a specialty is not intended as a criticism for that specialty, but to demonstrate a probable discrepancy between diagnosis and treatment. There is no question that most providers of care are reputable representatives of their respective professions.

There is extensive information in the literature specific to the topic of MTBI and various symptoms that frequently accompany this diagnosis. A more in-depth discussion of testing, instrumentation, anatomy, and the complicated neurophysiology related to this topic can be readily acquired through topic-specific, computerized library searches, and from many of the references presented in the bibliography.

BIBLIOGRAPY

1. Rosenthal, M, Mild traumatic brain injury syndrome, *Annals of Emergency Medicine*, 22, 115, 1993.
2. Esselman, PC, Uomoto, JM, Classification of the spectrum of mild traumatic brain injury, *Brain Injury*, 9, 417, 1995.

3. Sosin, DM, Sniezek, JE, Thurman, DJ, Incidence of mild and moderate brain injury in the United States, 1991, *Brain Injury*, 10, 47, 1996.

4. Kraus, JF, McGarther, DL, Epidemiological aspects of brain injury, *Neurol. Clin.*, 14(2), 435, 1996.

5. Brain Injury Statistics, Shepherd Center: A Specialty Hospital, *http://www.biausa.org/costand.htm*, April 7, 1999.

6. Kay, T, Harrington, DE, et al., Definition of mild traumatic brain injury, *J. of Head Trauma Rehabilitation*, 8, 86, 1993.

7. Goodyear, B, Neuropsychological Evaluation of Mild Traumatic Brain Injury: Detection and Other Functional Disorders. *The Forensic Examiner*, Nov/Dec., 32, 1998.

8. Jay, GW, Goka, RS, Arakaki, AH, Minor traumatic brain injury: review of clinical data and appropriate evaluation and treatment, *J. Insurance Medicine*, 27, 262, 1996.

9. Jonsson, H, Jr, Cesarini, KB, Sahlstedt, Rauschning, W, Findings and outcomes in whiplash-type neck injuries, *Spine*, 19, 2733, 1994.

10. Oyer, HJ, *Auditory Communication for the Hard of Hearing*, Prentice-Hall, Inc., Englewood Cliffs, NJ, 1966.

11. Baloh, RW, Honrubia, V, *Clinical Neurophysiology of the Vestibular System*, F. A. Davis and Co., Philadelphia, 1990.

12. Schulman, A, Aran, J, Tonndorf, J, et al., *Tinnitus: Diagnosis/Treatment*, Lea and Febriger, Philadelphia, 1991.

13. Jongkees, LB, Cervical Vertigo. Presented at the Seventy-Second Annual Meeting of the American Laryngological, Rhinological and Otological Society, Inc., New Orleans, La., March 25, 1969.

14. Cesarini, A, Alpini, D, Bovniver, R, et al., *Whiplash Injuries, Diagnosis and Treatment*, Springer-Verlag Italia, Milano, 1996.

15. Bland, JH, *Disorders of the Cervical Spine, Diagnosis and Medical Management*, Second Edition, W. B. Saunders Co., Philadelphia, 1987.

16. Tamura, T, Cranial symptoms after cervical injury: aetiology and treatment of Barre-Lieou syndrome, *J. Bone Joint Surg.*, 71-B(2), March 1989.

17. Dennis, MJ, Neely, J, Otoneurologic Diseases and Associated Audiologic Profiles, *Diagnostic Audiology*, Jacobson, JJ, Northern, JL, Eds., Austin, Texas, 77-79, 88, 1991.

18. Ruth, RA, Lambert, PR, Evaluation and Diagnosis of Cochlear Disorders, *Diagnostic Audiology*. Jacobson, JJ, Northern, JL, Eds., Austin Texas, 1991.

19. Baloh, RW, Vestibular insufficiency and stroke, *Otolaryngology-Head and Neck Surgery*, 112, 114, 1995.

20. Hotson, JR, Baloh, RW, Acute vestibular syndrome, *New Eng. J. Med.*, 680, 1998.

21. Rubin, W, Brookler, KH, *Dizziness: Etiologic Approach to Management*, Thieme Neducak Publishers, Inc., NewYork, 1991.

22. Hurley, RM, Sells, JP, Autoimmune inner ear disease (AIED): a tutorial, *Amer. J. of Audiology*, 6, 22, 1997.

23. Curtrer, MF, Baloh, RW, Migraine-associated dizziness, *Headache*, 300, June 1992.

24. Rybak, L, Metabolic disorders of the vestibular system, *Otolaryngology-Head and Neck Surgery*, 112, 128, 1995.

25. Hirsh, IJ, *The Measurement of Hearing*, The McGraw-Hill, New York, 1952.

26. *The Short Latency Auditory Evoked Potentials*, ASHA Audiologic Evaluation Working Group on Auditory Evoked Potential Measurements, Amer. Speech-Language-Hearing Association, Rockville, MD, Dec. 1988.

27. Moller, AR., Jannetta, PJ, Neural Generators of the Auditory Brainstem Response, *The Auditory Brainstem Response*, Jacobson, J, Ed., College-Hill Press, San Diego, 1985.
28. van den Honert, C, Sensory and Neurologic Aspects of Evoked Potentials, Proceedings of a Symposium in Audiology, Mayo Clinic-Mayo Foundation, Dept. of Otolaryngology Section of Audiology, Rochester Methodist Hosp., Rochester, MN, April 24-25, 1987.
29. Evans, KM, Melancon, B, Back to Basics: A Discussion of Techniques and Equipment, *Seminars in Hearing*, 10, 123, 1989.
30. Shumway-Cook, A, Horak, FB, Vestibular Rehabilitation: An Exercise Approach to Managing Symptoms of Vestibular Dysfunction, *Seminars in Hearing*, 10, 196-208, 1989.
31. Nörre, ME, Neurophysiology of vertigo with special reference to cervical vertigo, *Medical Physica*, 9, 183, 1986.
32. Edmeads, J, Headaches and head pains associated with diseases of the cervical spine, *Med. Clinics of North Amer.*, 62, 533, 1978.

17 Vision Function, Examination, and Rehabilitation in Patients Suffering from Traumatic Brain Injury

Thomas Politzer, O.D., FCOVD, FAAO

INTRODUCTION

Vision is our dominant sense. More than just sight measured in terms of visual acuity, vision is the process of deriving meaning from what is seen. It is a complex, learned, and developed set of functions that involve a multitude of skills. Research estimates that 80% to 85% of our perception, learning, cognition, and activities are mediated through vision.

The purpose of this chapter is to review visual dysfunctions that commonly occur following TBI (Traumatic Brain Injury), and discuss functional, nonsurgical rehabilitative strategies for remediating those dysfunctions. There is a glossary included at the end of the chapter.

PREVALENCE OF VISUAL DYSFUNCTION IN PATIENTS WITH TBI

A recent United States National Health Interview Study states that approximately 2,000,000 head injuries occur yearly in the United States.[1] Mild traumatic brain injury (MTBI), defined as a "traumatically-induced physiologic disruption of brain function" accounts for 80% of patients hospitalized for TBI.[1]

Visual dysfunction is one of the most common devastating residual impairments of head injury. Gianutsos[2] reports an extremely high incidence (greater than 50%) of visual and visual-cognitive disorders in neurologically-impaired patients (traumatic brain injury, cerebral vascular accidents, multiple sclerosis, etc). According to Padula,[3] "The majority of individuals that recover from a traumatic brain injury will have binocular function difficulties in the form of strabismus, phoria, oculomotor dysfunction, convergence, and accommodative abnormalities."

OVERVIEW OF THE PATHOPHYSIOLOGY OF VISION PROBLEMS FOLLOWING BRAIN INJURY

Vision is frequently disrupted following head injury, stroke, and other neurologically-compromising conditions (e.g., multiple sclerosis, cerebral vasculitis, aneurysm, hypoxia, etc.). The anatomy and physiology of the visual system, the vascular network of the brain, and the dynamics of head trauma all contribute to the incidence of ocular trauma and visual dysfunction.

Injury to the visual system can be diffuse and/or focal, and can localize to any, or a combination of, the ocular structures, cortical areas, the mid-brain, or cranial nerve nuclei. Brain injuries affecting vision typically occur via axonal shearing, hemorrhage, infarct, inflammation, and/or compression.

The third cranial nerve and third nerve nuclei are vulnerable to injury following trauma, aneurysm, and stroke. The third nerve innervates 8 of the 12 extra-ocular muscles (the medial, inferior, and superior recti, and inferior oblique muscles), the ciliary muscle, the levator muscle, and the pupillary sphincter muscle. Consequently, injury to this area causes some classic signs and symptoms that will manifest as:

Exotropia/Exophoria
Convergence Insufficiency/Convergence Infacility
Accommodative Insufficiency/Accommodative Infacility
Ptosis
Fixed and Dilated Pupils
Limited Motility (Adduction, Sursumduction, Infraduction) of the affected eye

The sixth cranial nerve and nuclei are prone to injury in TBI and stroke. These control 2 of the 12 extra-ocular muscles (the lateral recti muscles) which are responsible for abduction of the eye. Injury to the communication pathways between the sixth nerve nuclei and their paired third nerve nuclei (medial longitudinal fasciculus (MLF) can occur and is termed an "internuclear ophthalmoplegia" (INO). Sixth nerve problems will manifest as:

Esotropia/Esophoria
Divergence Insufficiency/Divergence Infacility
Limited Abduction of the Affected Eye

Internuclear Ophthalmoplegia will manifest as:

Exotropia
Limited Adduction of the Affected Eye
Paralysis of Gaze to the Affected Side

The fourth cranial nerve is very frequently injured in TBI and stroke. It is more frequently injured by direct trauma. The fourth nerve and nucleus control 2 of the 12 extra-ocular muscles, the superior obliques. These muscles are responsible for inferior gaze of the eye when it is adducted. Damage to this area will manifest as:

Hypertropia
Limited Down Gaze of the Affected Eye when Adducted

The optic nerve, radiations, and pathway back to the occipital and associated corticies can be injured in TBI and stroke. The location of the injury will determine the nature of the deficit. Visual field loss is the manifestation of these injuries.

If the optic nerve is damaged between the eye and the optic chiasm, there will be a monocular loss of sight and an afferent pupillary defect (positive Marcus-Gunn). This is seen in direct trauma and multiple sclerosis.

When the damage is at the optic chiasm there will be a classic bitemporal visual field loss. This is found frequently in pituitary disorders.

If the injury occurs in the optic radiations coursing back from the chiasm to the lateral geniculate nucleus (LGN), there will be an incongruous bilateral visual field loss. This can manifest as an hemianopsia, or quadrantanopsia.

When the injury is posterior to the LGN and ranging back to the occipital cortex there will occur a homonymous bilateral visual field loss. The visual field loss will show more frequently as a hemianopsia, but can also be a quadrantanopsia. Posterior cerebral occipital lobe lesions may spare the anterior geniculo-calcarine radiations, and thus leave some preserved temporal crescent peripheral field on the side of the hemianopsia.

Visual fibers feed forward to other areas of the brain. One area in particular, the parietal cortex, is frequently referred to as the "association cortex." It is called this because it integrates information from the various senses in an attempt to derive meaning from the "whole picture." When there is damage to the parietal area (particularly the right side) there will frequently be a visual neglect to the left.

Visual neglect is a perceptual loss of vision. The person is unaware of their sight, or lack of sight, to the affected side. If the nerve pathways and occipital cortex are spared and only the parietal cortex is affected there will be a sparing of vision (to a good degree), but the person will "ignore" and not attend to vision on the affected side. If the pathways and/or occipital cortex are injured as well as the parietal cortex, then there will be an actual visual field loss in addition to the person having a neglect, and/or denial of loss of vision.

The occipital lobes are the primary visual sensory areas of the brain. Occipital lobe injuries cause visual field losses. Lesions in these areas will cause hemianopic visual field losses, with or without macular sparring, as well as other significant visual field losses. Because of the association between the occipital cortex and the parietal and temporal corticies, damage to this area can manifest as deficits in the formulation of complex visual stimuli and comprehension of visual stimuli into meaningful information.

DIZZINESS AND BALANCE PROBLEMS RELATED TO VISION

Vision plays a significant role in balance. Approximately 20% of the nerve fibers from the eyes interact with the vestibular system. There are a variety of visual dysfunctions that can cause or associate with dizziness and balance problems. Some-times these are purely visual problems, and sometimes they are caused by other disorders such as stroke, head injury, vestibular dysfunction, deconditioning, and decompensation.

In vestibular dysfunction, it is felt that visual dysfunction occurs in the following manner. Initially, with vestibular dysfunction that causes dizziness and balance problems, the person will commonly adapt by relying more on their visual system for input. In doing so, they typically become more visually focused, rely more on visual anchoring techniques, and attempt to block out peripheral visual stimulation. While initially helpful, if the vestibular dysfunction continues, this type of visual adaptation will eventually break down.

In actuality, it is the peripheral and ambient portion of vision that is most important for vision contributing to balance and spatial orientation. By deempha-sizing this part of vision to use focal visual anchoring, the dizziness and balance problem will eventually become worse. Treatment is aimed at reinforcing the periph-eral ambient vision (with prism and partial selective occlusion) while vestibular therapy is conducted.

There are several visual dysfunctions that can cause, or contribute to dizziness and balance problems.

ANEISOKONIA

When magnification difference becomes excessive, generally more than about 4%, the effect can cause disorientation, eyestrain, headache, dizziness, and balance dis-orders. Treatment is with contact lenses, or magnification size-matched lenses — isokonic lenses.

VERTICAL IMBALANCE

Vertical imbalance is fairly common following TBI. It can also be triggered by fever, stroke, deconditioning, or sometimes for no apparent reason. In an effort to adjust to the vertical misalignment of the eyes, the patient will frequently tip their head to mechanically help align them. This, in turn, can cause disorders in the fluid of the inner ear and resultant dizziness and balance disorders. Treatment is with therapy to correct the muscle imbalance and prisms.

BINOCULAR VISION DYSFUNCTION

Binocular vision disorders can occur following TBI. Higher amounts of exophoria or esophoria, and certainly exotropia and esotropia, will cause eyestrain, double vision, muscle spasm, and perception of excessive peripheral visual stimulation, which, in turn, can trigger dizziness and balance problems. Treatment is with lenses, prisms, and therapy.

Double Vision (Diplopia)

Double vision is among the most disorienting and devastating vision disorders. Patients suffering diplopia will oftentimes go to great lengths to eliminate it. Many will patch, or cover, an eye. Disorientation from double vision will frequently trigger dizziness and balance problems. Treatment is with lenses, prisms, therapy, partial selective occlusion, and, rarely, surgery.

Ambient Visual Disorder

Disorders of the ambient visual system (the peripheral spatial visual system addressed later) can cause an individual to misperceive spatial relationships. Dizziness and balance problems arise when the attempts to orient to the misperceived environment by showing a tendency to lean to the side, forward, or backward occurs. Treatment is with specially-designed prisms and partial selective occlusion. These techniques work effectively in conjunction with physical and occupational therapy attempting to rehabilitate weight bearing for ambulation.

Eye Movement Disorders

Eye movement disorders may present as nystagmus, ataxia, apraxia, and/or limitation of gaze. Eye movement disorders may be congenital or acquired. With acute adult onset of nystagmus, the brain does not register that the eyes are shaking, but that the world and objects in it are moving. This is termed "oscillopsia" and will frequently cause dizziness and balance problems. Treatment is aimed at correcting (if possible) the underlying cause for the nystagmus, and concurrently the use of lenses, prisms, visual therapy, and partial selective occlusion are often helpful.

ASSESSMENT OF VISUAL FUNCTION

Given the high incidence of visual dysfunction in the TBI population along with the importance of vision in daily functioning, a comprehensive eye and vision examination is indicated for patients suffering a TBI. Examination should include tests for acuity, refraction, eye movements, reflexes, binocular vision, accommodation, stereopsis, visual field, eye health, and, as indicated, visual perceptual skills, electrodiagnostics, and low vision.

VISUAL ACUITY AND DISORDERS OF REFRACTION

Myopia, hyperopia, astigmatism, and presbyopia will all cause blurred visual acuity. Changes in refraction, as well as decompensation of preexisting refractive errors, can occur following TBI. Gianutsos found that nearly all of the patients in her study who were referred for vision evaluation had inadequately corrected visual acuity.[2]

EYE MOVEMENTS

FIXATION

Ocular fixation refers to the ability to hold eye gaze steady while viewing an object. There are different types of disorders of fixation, which are referred to as eccentric fixation, unsteady fixation, and nystagmus. Eccentric fixation is most typically found in congenital or early age acquired strabismic deviations with amblyopia. In these cases, the individual uses a nonfoveal portion of the eye for aligning. On observation, the eye is generally stable in fixation. Unsteady fixation is seen in cases of TBI and manifests as an intermittent loss of fixation. It is generally felt to be more of an attention or binocular problem than a true oculo-motor dysfunction. Nystagmus can occur as a result of TBI. It will manifest as an uncontrolled shaking of the eyes. As opposed to vestibular nystagmus with fast and slow phases, it will typically show random pendular movements, fast or slow, horizontal or vertical. Disorders of fixation can associate with blurred vision, dizziness and balance problems, and oscillopsia.

PURSUIT

Pursuit movements refer to the ability of the eyes to smoothly and accurately track a moving object. They are limited in speed to about 30 degrees per second. When attempting to track faster than this, they will exhibit correctional saccadic movements, or "cogwheeling." The two most common disorders of pursuit following TBI are limitation of gaze and ataxia. With ophthalmoplegia, muscle entrapment, or muscle damage, there will be a limited range of motion of pursuit to the involved muscle's field of action. More commonly, the quality of smooth and accurate pursuit will degrade, manifesting as jerky movements. Disorders of pursuit can associate with using head movements for tracking and poor eye-hand coordination.

SACCADES

Saccades are fast-scanning eye movements used to change fixation from one object to another. They can be voluntary (e.g., reading) or involuntary (e.g., looking at an object that suddenly appears in the peripheral vision). Saccadic disorders following TBI include limitation of gaze (as with pursuit), ataxia (saccadic movements that overshoot or undershoot the target), and hypometropia (slowness in initiation and execution of saccade). Saccadic dysfunctions will tend to associate with reading problems such as losing place, slowness, and inaccuracy, and with problems in scanning the environment.

OCULAR REFLEXES

VESTIBULO-OCULAR REFLEX (VOR)

The VOR, while not a true eye movement, works in conjunction with the vestibular system to stabilize fixation during head and body movements, VOR disorders include loss of fixation during head/body movement with and without regaining fixation.

Symptoms that tend to associate with VOR dysfunction include decreased visual acuity, oscillopsia, dizziness, and balance problems.

PUPILLARY REFLEXES

Pupillary abnormalities are not uncommon following TBI. Pupillary reflexes should be evaluated for direct and consensual response to light, accommodation, roundness, and size. A dilated and fixed pupil is associated with third cranial nerve involvement. A Tonic, or Adie's pupil, can result from general trauma. Anisocoria needs to be investigated, but physiological anisocoria of less than 1mm is not uncommon in the general population.

STARTLE RESPONSE

A startle, or guarding, response is an expected finding when an object is suddenly and abruptly introduced near the eye in the field of view. It is generally not found in patients with very low-level function following TBI, who do not exhibit a startle response.

CORNEAL SENSITIVITY

Using a fine wisp of cotton from a swab, the cornea is lightly stroked in the inferior portion while the patient looks up. This is done to both eyes and the patient is asked to judge if the feeling is equivalent between the eyes. This tests for patency of the corneal branch of the fifth nerve. In lower-level patients, a light puff of air can be blown at the cornea and the patient observed for a blink response.

LIGHT SENSITIVITY

Patients who have suffered a traumatic brain injury will often suffer from photophobia (sensitivity to and intolerance of light). Photophobia, which is a subjective symptom, is not completely understood. There are some direct causes, including eye disease, corneal abrasion, and albinism, but many times an etiology is unclear. While evaluation may include glare recovery testing, most of the time diagnosis is made on observation and history.

BINOCULAR VISION

Binocular vision refers to using both eyes together. It is comprised of convergence and divergence. Convergence is the ability of the eyes to work together tracking an object as it approaches the individual, and divergence is the ability to track an object as it moves away. There are a variety of objective and subjective standardized methods of measuring binocular vision.

Strabismic deviations occur when the eyes do not align together. When acquired, as with TBI, and as opposed to congenital or infant onset, strabismus will frequently result in double vision. Double vision is one of the most disorienting of visual dysfunctions and people will go to great lengths to alleviate it, including covering or closing an eye and adopting aberrant head positions.

Binocular dysfunctions are disorders of "eye-teaming" ability that do not result in an actual strabismic misalignment. There can be convergence or divergence insufficiency, convergence or divergence infacility (poor flexibility), or convergence or divergence excess. The most common problems in patients with TBI are convergence insufficiency and infacility. These dysfunctions can cause eyestrain, headache with use of the eyes, intermittent diplopia, and blurred vision.

ACCOMMODATION

Accommodation is the ability to focus the eyes. The age-related loss of accommodation is referred to as "presbyopia" and onsets in the early to mid 40 years of age due to size, and decreased elasticity of the intra-ocular lens. Acquired dysfunctions following TBI are typically accommodative insufficiency or infacility, but there can also be spasm. Symptoms include blurred vision, eyestrain, and headache with use of the eyes.

STEREOPSIS

Stereopsis is a form of depth perception and is true "3-D" vision resulting from the eyes working together properly. (There are many forms of depth perception, and even a monocular person will have depth perception.) Even subtle binocular dysfunctions will frequently disrupt stereopsis and result in complaints of problems judging distances, a tendency to bump into objects, and problems with eye-hand coordination.

VISUAL FIELD

Visual field losses are frequently found in TBI patients, especially in the more severe injuries. Assessment of visual field relies on both compliance and understanding by the patient, and can be difficult in lower-level functioning patients. Measurement can range from confrontation visual field testing to automated computer perimetry. Among the most common visual field losses are hemianopsia, constriction, and quadrant losses.

EYE HEALTH

It is important to thoroughly assess ocular health, as numerous injuries are possible following TBI. A careful external exam and dilated fundus exam are indicated. Lacerations of the lid and adnexal regions are possible. Eyelid abnormalities such as ptosis or lagophthalmos are fairly common. Corneal desiccation and exposure keratitis leading to scarring from lagophthalmos can occur. Traumatic iris ruptures, angle abnormalities, and cataracts may be present. Retinal tears, hemorrhage, and papilledema may also occur. Increased intra-ocular pressure can occur secondary to traumatic angle changes, iritis, uveitis, and intra-ocular hemorrhage.

VISUAL PERCEPTUAL SKILLS

Visual perceptual dysfunction is a common residual impairment following TBI. According to Zoltan,[4] recovery from visual perceptual deficits takes longer than physical recovery, and research has shown a correlation between resolution of perceptual deficits and functional outcome. Problems with visual memory, spatial relationships, visual cognition, pattern recognition, and visual attention can occur.

Visual memory is the ability to visually process stimuli and information, memorize, and then recall upon command.[5] Furthermore, the individual must be able to match visual information with previous memory.

Spatial relationships refer to the ability to know "where I am" in relation to objects and space around me, and to simultaneously know where objects are in relation to one another.

Visual cognition refers to the ability to mentally manipulate visual information and integrate it with other sensory information. Included in this is the ability to analyze visual information; compare to present, previous, and future stimuli; and reason about the nature of the stimuli.

Pattern recognition is the ability to recognize the salient (e.g., shape and contour) and specific features (e.g., color, shading, and texture) of an object. This is important in achieving perceptual constancy: the ability to recognize objects when viewed from different angles and positions.

Visual attention refers to the ability to sustain attention on, and shift attention between, visually presented stimuli and information. This relates to focal and ambient, central and peripheral visual processes as described under Post Trauma Vision Syndrome and Visual Midline Shift Syndrome. The focal process relates to detailed discrimination, attention, and concentration. The ambient visual process relates to spatial orientation, motion detection, and balance.

LOW VISION

Visual impairment resulting from a loss of visual acuity can occur following TBI. This can result from direct trauma to the eye causing conditions such as cataracts, retinal tears, and macular hemorrhage; or from damage to the optic nerve, pathways, or cortex. Many patients with visual loss cannot achieve their full potential with ordinary eyeglasses. In low vision, telescopes, microscopic lenses, magnifiers, electro-optical systems, and other sophisticated optical devices are used to enhance sight by magnifying the image on the retina of patients with partial sight. The right device can help people improve their vision.

POSTTRAUMA VISION SYNDROME AND VISUAL MIDLINE SHIFT SYNDROME

There are two integrated visual systems responsible for the ability to organize the individual in space for balance and movement (ambient), as well as to focalize on detail such as looking at a traffic light (focal). Following a neurological event such as a TBI or stroke, patients have been noted to complain of a variety of visual symptoms. Some include seeing objects appearing to move that are known to be stationary; there is also the perception of the floor or walls appearing tilted, and significant difficulties with balance and spatial orientation when in crowded, moving environments. Recent research utilizing Visual Evoked Potentials (VEP) has documented that the ambient visual process may become dysfunctional after a neurological event such as a TBI or CVA.[6] Dysfunction in or between the ambient and focal process can cause the types of symptoms noted above.

Visual Midline Shift Syndrome (VMSS) results from dysfunction of the ambient visual process. It is caused by distortions of the spatial system causing the individual to misperceive his or her position in the spatial environment. There results a shift in the concept of perceived visual midline so that it does not correspond with the actual physical neuro-motor midline.

It has been found that Visual Midline Shift Syndrome tends to occur and associate with certain characteristics and symptoms. These include hemiplegia, hemiparesis, and side neglect. Associated symptoms include the floor appearing slanted or tilted; walls and/or the floor appearing to shift and move; and the affected person tending to lean forward, backward, or to one side, and there will likely be associated neuromotor difficulties with balance, coordination, and posture. There are associated visual and ocular findings with VMSS. They include aneisokonia, hemianopsia, visual neglect, and high phoria or strabismus.

VMSS can affect balance, posture, orientation, and mobility. The visual spatial perception of the environment appear compressed in one portion and expanded in another. As a result, perception of the world appears slanted, or tipped, and walls may appear bowed and distorted. Balance is disrupted when attempts are made to orient to that perception of the visual world. For example, imagine a patient who has suffered a TBI with right hemiparesis and right hemianopsia. This patient will be observed to weight bear left, and a shift of their visual perception of their midline to the nonaffected side will often be found. Since vision is the dominant sense, attempts are made to orient to the distorted visual-spatial perception reinforcing the weight bearing and leaning to the left. To this person, the world will likely appear slanted up to their right and down to their left, reinforcing problems with balance, orientation, and mobility.

Post Trauma Vision Syndrome (PTVS) is a constellation of signs and symptoms felt to represent another dysfunction between the ambient and focal process. In PTVS, patients tend to be overwhelmed by details and movement around them. It is as though their peripheral (ambient) visual system has become hypervigilant rather than operating on a more subconscious and automatic level. Peripheral visual stimulation becomes disorienting as attention is continually drawn to any motion or stimulus.

Characteristics common to PTVS include exotropia or high exophoria, accommodative dysfunction, convergence insufficiency, low blink rate, spatial disorientation, and balance problems. Symptoms common in PTVS include diplopia, perception of stationary objects moving, visual memory problems, staring behavior, and asthenopia.

TABLE 17.1
Signs and Symptoms of Visual Problems Associated with Brain Injuries and Their Suspected Correlates

Behavior Observe	Suspected Deficit
Focusing problems	Accommodative problem
	Possible third nerve injury
Covering or closing an eye	Strabismus
	Third, fourth, sixth nerve injury
Blurred or fluctuating vision	Accommodative spasm
	Binocular disorder
	Refractive error
Headaches with use of eyes	Accommodative insufficiency
	Convergence insufficiency
	Binocular disorder
Diplopia (Double vision)	Strabismus
	Third, fourth, sixth nerve injury
Loss of place when reading	Oculomotor dysfunction in saccades
	Visual attention deficit
	Spatial relations deficit
Visual field loss and/or neglect	Occipital cortex injury
	Parietal cortex injury
Tendency to reread and/or reversals	Oculo-motor dysfunction in saccades
	Visual attention deficit
	Spatial relations deficit
Head tilt	Hyper- or hypotropia
	Fourth nerve injury
Asthenopia (Eye strain)	Binocular disorder, accommodative or convergence problem
Poor attention for visual tasks	Visual perception deficit
An eye turns in, out, up, or down	Strabismus
	Third, fourth, sixth nerve injury
Visual confusion	Visual perception deficit
Poor eye-hand coordination	Ataxia of smooth ocular pursuits
	Visual-motor integration deficit
Poor localization	Spatial relations deficit
	Depth perception deficit
	Visual Midline Shift
Orientation and Mobility	Strabismus
	Visual Midline Shift
	Ataxia of ocular fixations, nystagmus
Balance and Posture	Strabismus
	Visual Midline Shift
Dizziness	Strabismus
	Nystagmus
	Visual Midline Shift

TREATMENT OF VISUAL DYSFUNCTIONS

VISION THERAPY

Vision therapy (also referred to as vision training, orthoptics, and eye exercises) is a clinical approach to treat eye movement disorders, binocular dysfunctions, strabismus, accommodative disorders, amblyopia, and certain visual perceptual disorders. The practice of vision therapy uses a variety of nonsurgical procedures to modify visual function. The goal of vision therapy is to help the patient achieve stable, single, comfortable binocular vision.

Vision therapy will typically involve a series of treatments. During therapy sessions, individually planned activities are conducted under professional supervision. The specific procedures and necessary instrumentation are determined by the individual patient's needs, and the nature and severity of the diagnosed problems. Vision therapy techniques employ the use of lenses, prisms, computers, biofeedback, stereoscopic devices, and a variety of other instrumentation to address visual function.

The visual skills which can be treated and improved with vision therapy include ocular fixation, pursuits and saccades, convergence, divergence, accommodation, binocularity, stereopsis, certain forms of amblyopia, certain strabismic dysfunctions, stereopsis, and certain visual perceptual disorders. Symptoms associating with these disorders that can be expected to improve include double vision, eye strain, focusing problems, headache with use of the eyes, certain reading problems, depth perception, suppression of binocular vision, visual memory, visual attention, eye-hand coordination, and peripheral vision awareness.

LENSES

Lenses are ophthalmic tools that bend light simultaneously in multiple directions. They are best known for their use in prescriptions for nearsightedness, farsightedness, and astigmatism. Minus lenses are used for myopia, plus lenses are used for hyperopia, and astigmatic lenses are used for astigmatism. Single-vision lenses are used for general needs, and bifocal lenses are used for both general and near-vision focusing.

Since lenses simultaneously bend light in multiple directions, they can also be used therapeutically. Lenses can be used to affect peripheral vision, binocular vision (how the eyes work together), and visual aspects of balance.

Lenses affect peripheral vision through their size, shape, and power. A larger lens would seem to be better for enhancing peripheral vision, but as a lens is made larger it exponentially increases in its amount of aberrations (distortions) which cause instability of peripheral vision. A round lens, as opposed to an aviator shape, is best for enhancing peripheral vision because the shape is similar to the visual field and produces the fewest aberrations.

Minus lenses constrict space and encourage focal visual attention with less attention to peripheral vision. They can be used in therapy to focus central vision. Plus lenses expand space. They can be used in therapy to blur central vision and encourage attention to peripheral vision. Too much lens power will cause peripheral vision distortion and perception of motion.

Binocular vision is the coordination of convergence and divergence (eye teaming skills) with accommodation (focusing) for single, comfortable, clear vision. Good binocular vision allows for stereoscopic depth perception, and ease in using the eyes for tasks such as reading and computer work. Convergence, divergence, and accommodation are neurologically connected, so change in any one of these areas will affect the others.

Minus lenses directly stimulate accommodation and, secondarily, convergence. Plus lenses relax accommodation and, secondarily, convergence. Plus lenses aid accommodation when deficient and reduce effort when excessive. Minus lenses are generally not used to stimulate accommodation as this will frequently cause muscle spasm, fatigue, and eye strain.

When lenses are too strong or weak, off-angle on astigmatism, too large, distorted, or made of unequal curves, they can cause visual distortions and the perception of movement in space. This occurs because the improper lens distorts the focus and causes movement of the images on the retina of the eye. The brain then interprets this as distortion and movement in space, which in turn can cause dizziness, vertigo, and balance problems.

Since the stability and coordination of central and peripheral vision can be impaired following a neurologic disease or injury, patients may perceive distortions and movement in space as though they are wearing improper lens prescriptions. Appropriate intervention with lenses for general wear, as well as in therapy activities, can help to stabilize vision and improve balance and disorientation.

PRISMS

Prisms, like lenses, are ophthalmic tools that bend light, but do so in a single direction. Prisms are used clinically in a therapeutic manner to help remediate a visual dysfunction, or in a compensatory manner to offset the effects of a visual problem.

Therapeutically, prisms are used to build what are called "fusional ranges." These are the amounts of convergence, divergence, or vertical or rotational range of motion while maintaining single binocular vision. Prisms exercise these components of binocular vision by stimulating or relaxing the corresponding ocular muscle groups and causing the individual to make compensatory adjustments to maintain single vision. This use of prisms is administered as part of vision therapy and is effective in treating binocular vision disorders.

Another therapeutic use of prisms is to prescribe them (manufactured in the lenses of eyeglasses) for intermittent or temporary wear. The theory is that a smaller than full compensatory amount worn by the patient on a part-time and temporary basis will help stimulate appropriate adaptation and can be tapered off in the future. Applications for this type of use are Post Trauma Vision Syndrome, Visual Midline Shift Syndrome, certain binocular vision disorders, and certain types of strabismus.

For Post Trauma Vision Syndrome, it has been found that the use of prisms can effectively demonstrate functional improvement. The application of relatively small amounts of base-in prism has been demonstrated on VEP studies to statistically significantly increase brain wave amplitude. Clinically, it is observed in these patients to improve binocular function and ambient (peripheral) vision awareness.

In Visual Midline Shift Syndrome, it has been found that specially designed yoked prisms can be prescribed to shift visual perception. Yoked prisms are applications where prisms are placed before each eye with the base of the prisms oriented in the same direction. By doing so, the individual's perception of their midline can be shifted to a more centered position, thus matching the physical midline. Oftentimes this enables individuals to begin weight-bearing on their affected side, and reduces or eliminates their perceived spatial distortions.

In binocular and strabismic dysfunctions, use of prisms can reduce symptoms, improve function, and hasten recovery while doing vision therapy. In these situations, prescription of therapeutic prism (an amount, type, and orientation of prism to reduce or neutralize the binocular/vision dysfunction, or to stimulate visual function and fusion) can help reduce or eliminate symptoms and aid treatment. A thorough review of this type of prism application is beyond the scope of this chapter, and the interested reader is referred to any number of good binocular vision texts on the subject.

Use of prisms for visual neglect is a relatively new application and one with great promise. Visual neglect is a perceptual loss of vision. The person is unaware of their sight, or lack of sight, to the affected side. If the nerve pathways and occipital cortex are spared and only the parietal cortex is affected, there will a sparing of vision (to a good degree), but the person will "ignore" and not attend to vision on the affected side. If the pathways and/or occipital cortex are injured as well as the parietal cortex, there will be an actual visual field loss in addition to the person having a neglect and/or denial of loss of vision. It has been found clinically that utilization of yoked prisms stimulates awareness of the visual neglect side with or without the presence of an actual visual field loss. The prisms are oriented to shift visual perception to the side of the loss, thereby increasing visual stimulation to that side and away from the other. Frequently, after using prisms in this fashion on a nearly full time basis, breakthroughs in the neglect can be achieved in one to two weeks.

The application of a prism to enhance visual field has existed for many decades. However, the development of the Gottlieb Visual Field Awareness System (Dr. Daniel Gottlieb, O.D., FCOVD, FAAO)[7] has greatly improved the success in aiding patients after hemianoptic visual field loss. This novel approach places a small wafer of base-out prism in a round shape on the side of the visual field loss. In this manner, as the patient looks to the side of their visual field loss, the image is shifted into their still functional field as they make natural scanning movements. The Visual Field Awareness System has been helpful for patients with hemianoptic field loss. The lens is mounted in one lens on the side of the loss. It shifts the image about twenty degrees nasally, allowing it to be detected within the remaining functional field as the patients make mild scanning movements. Along with the prism system, therapy is prescribed to assist adaptation and improve scanning. In addition to the Gottlieb Visual Field Awareness System, systems have been manufactured by individual ophthalmic labs using Fresnel prisms (temporary film prisms), and by InWave, a lab that uses a molded lens with less prism power.

Compensatory Use of Prisms

There are times, patients, and situations when remediation of a visual problem is not possible or feasible. In these situations, prescription of a compensatory prism (an amount, type, and orientation of prism to reduce or neutralize the binocular/vision dysfunction) can help reduce or eliminate symptoms. A thorough review of this type of prism application is beyond the scope of this chapter and the interested reader is referred to any number of good binocular vision texts on the subject.

OCCLUSION

Double vision (diplopia) is a serious and intolerable condition that can be caused by strabismus, ophthalmoplegia, gaze palsy, and decompensated binocular skills in patients with brain injury, stroke, and other neurologically compromising conditions. Prisms, lenses, and/or vision therapy can often help the patient achieve fusion (alignment of the eyes) and alleviate the diplopia. If and when these means are not employed, the patient may adapt by suppressing the vision of one eye to eliminate the diplopia. If lenses, prisms, and/or therapy are not successful and the patient does not suppress, intractable diplopia ensues.

In this population of patients, patching (occlusion) has frequently been used to eliminate the diplopia. Although patching is effective in eliminating diplopia, it causes the patient to become monocular. Monocular as opposed to binocular vision will affect the individual primarily in two ways: absence of stereopsis and reduction of the peripheral field of vision. These limitations will directly cause problems in eye-hand coordination, depth judgments, orientation, balance, mobility, and activities of daily living such as playing sports, driving, climbing stairs, crossing the street, threading a needle, etc.

A new method of treating diplopia that does not have these limitations has been successfully evaluated. It is called the "spot patch" (invented and named by this author) and is a method to eliminate intractable diplopia without compromising peripheral vision. It is a small, usually round or oval, patch made of dermacil tape, 3-M blurring film (or another such translucent tape). It is placed on the inside of the lenses of glasses and directly in the line of sight contributing to the diplopia. The diameter is generally about one centimeter, but will vary on the individual angular subtense required for the particular strabismus or gaze palsy.[8]

LOW VISION

TELESCOPES

Telescopes are used to help distance vision. They may be mounted to a spectacle prescription so the patient can alternate vision from the telescope to the carrier (regular portion) of the lens. Telescopes provide magnification for improved detailed vision, but reduce the peripheral field of vision. They are used as spotting devices and are not intended for full-time continuous vision.

MICROSCOPES

Microscopes are used to help near vision. They provide good magnification and a relatively large field of view. They are worn like glasses and so do not rely on hand/arm strength or dexterity. They require a very close working distance to the object of regard, sometimes just a couple of inches.

MAGNIFIERS

Magnifiers are used to help mid-range and near vision. They may be stand-mounted, handheld, or a combination. They come in a variety of sizes, shapes, and weights. Some are available with lighting built in. They give less magnification and have a smaller field of view than microscopes, but have longer (near normal) working distance.

ELECTRO-OPTICAL SYSTEMS

Electro-optical systems are used to help reading. They are stand or tabletop mounted. Reading material is placed on a slide, which goes under a scanner that magnifies the image onto a monitor. The systems provide excellent magnification, contrast, and working distance, but are fixed (nonmobile) and have a relatively small field of image view.

SUMMARY

Visual problems are common following traumatic brain injury. Visual dysfunction can be caused from injury to any lobe of the brain, midbrain, or ocular structure. Deficits can manifest as impairment of visual acuity, oculomotor dysfunction, strabismus, binocular vision disorder, accommodative dysfunction, visual field loss, visual neglect, photophobia, and visual perceptual disorders.

While visual problems are common after TBI and will affect normal activities of daily living, they are unfortunately frequently overlooked. There is, however, an increasing awareness of the importance of vision in the rehabilitation of patients with TBI. Given its importance and prevalence, vision examination and intervention should be addressed once TBI patients are medically stable.

There is a wide variety in subspecialties of vision care providers. Vision care specialists who specialize in work with TBI, low vision, neuro-optometric rehabilitation, and vision therapy are appropriate for consultation and treatment. Resources can be found through the Neuro-Optometric Rehabilitation Association (www.noravc.com), American Optometric Association (314-991-4100), College of Optometrists in Vision Development (314-991-4007), or the Optometric Extension Program (714-250-8070).

REFERENCES

1. Reinhardt, DL, Neuromedical aspects of mild traumatic brain injury, Weintraub, A, van der Ark, Eds., *CNI Review*, 8, 19, 1997.
2. Gianutsos, R, Ramsey, G, Perlin, RR, Rehabilitative optometric services for survivors of acquired brain injury, *Arch. Phys. Med. Rehabil.*, 69, 573, 1988.
3. Padula, WV, Neuro-optometric rehabilitation for persons with a TBI or CVA, *Journal of Optometric Vision Development*, 23, 4, 1992.
4. Zoltan, B, *Rehabilitation of the Adult and Child with Traumatic Brain Injury, 2nd ed., Remediation of Visual-Perceptual and Perceptual-Motor Deficits*, FA Davis Company, Philadelphia, 1990.
5. Raymond, MJ, Bennett, TL, Malia, KB, Bewick, KC, Rehabilitation of visual processing deficits following brain injury, *Neurorehabilitation*, 6, 229, 1996.
6. Padula, WV, Argyris, S, Ray, J, Visual evoked potentials (VEP) evaluating treatment for post-trauma vision syndrome (PTVS) in patients with traumatic brain injuries (TBI), *Brain Injury*, 8(2), 125, 1994.
7. Gottlieb, DD, Freeman, P, Williams, M, Clinical research and statistical analysis of a visual field awareness system, *Journal of the American Optometric Association*, 63(8), 581, 1992.
8. Politzer, TA, Case studies of a new approach using partial and selective occlusion for the clinical treatment of diplopia, *NeuroRehabilitation*, 6, 213, 1996.

GLOSSARY OF TERMS

Accommodation – The ability to accurately focus on an object of regard, sustain that focusing of the eyes, and to change focusing when looking at different distances

Agnosia – Difficulty in object recognition

Attitudinal Loss – Loss of the upper or lower portion of the visual field

Anisocoria – Unequal pupil sizes

Apraxia – Difficulty in manipulation of objects

Ataxia – Impaired muscle coordination causing jerky movements

Binocular Vision – The integration of accommodation, convergence, and alignment so the eyes work together as a team

Convergence – The ability to accurately aim the eyes at an object of regard and to track an object as it moves toward and away from the person

Diplopia – Double vision

Esotropia – An eye turns in relative to alignment with the fellow eye

Exotropia – An eye turns out relative to alignment with the fellow eye

Figure-Ground Discrimination – The ability to discern form and object from background

Fixation – The ability to steadily and accurately look at an object

Hemianopsia – Loss of half of the field of view right or left

Hypertropia – An eye turns up or down relative to alignment with the fellow eye

Lagophthalmos – Incomplete blink

Nystagmus – Uncontrolled shaking of the eyes

Ocular Alignment – Determination of eye posture, or aiming

Ophthalmoplegia – Paresis of nerves controlling eye muscles and function)

Photophobia – Sensitivity to light

Pursuits – The ability to smoothly and accurately track, or follow, a moving object

Quadranopsia – Loss of about one-quarter sector of the visual field

Saccades – The ability to quickly and accurately look (scan) from one object to another

Spatial Relationships – The ability to know "where I am" in relation to objects and space around me, and to know where objects are in relation to one another

Stereopsis – Binocular depth perception

Visual Acuity – This refers to clarity of sight; it is commonly measured using the Snellen chart and noted, for example, as 20/20

Visual-Auditory Integration – The ability to relate and associate what is seen and heard

Visual Closure – The ability "to fill in the gaps," or complete a visual picture based on seeing only some of the parts

Visual Neglect – A perceptual loss of vision and visual awareness

Visual Field – The complete central and peripheral range of vision

Visual Memory – The ability to remember and recall information that is seen

Visual-Motor Integration – Eye-hand, eye-foot, eye-body coordination

18 Pertinent Legal Aspects of MTBI

Michael Sawaya

Mumbo jumbo. Why do lawyers talk the way they do? What is in the mind of the lawyer that makes that person so different from the rest of the mortals of the world? Legal matters do differ from ordinary transactions since there is so much history and precedent that is followed in legal issues. Legal matters involve jumping through hoops, fitting into legal precedent, following rules, complying with the rule of law, and other arcane methods of contortion. Truly, the training that good lawyers receive rather quickly changes the way they look at formal human relations. They learn that from the legal standpoint, wrongs cannot be made right without carefully following legal procedures and methods to make sure that the right can be secured. Legal procedure is similar from one type of case to another, and the law has been likened to "a seamless web." This author has distilled his 24 years of legal experience as a trial lawyer working with brain trauma cases to outline the important areas and issues of concern to the brain trauma victim, his family, and his lawyer. This outline is one lawyer's method of conceptualizing the brain trauma case from its beginning to the end, showing methods and procedures for identifying and securing legal rights.

OUTLINE

1. Pretrauma history of the victim (specifically how the person functioned before the trauma).
2. Event of injury: giving specifics and showing as exactly as possible how the injury occurred.
3. Identifying who is responsible for the event of injury. (What person, agency, business, etc. caused the event to occur.)
4. What is the theory of liability? Is someone strictly liable (as in a defective product or dangerous activity), or was injury foreseeable such that negligence law applies?
5. What state or federal laws, agency rules (such as OSHA regulations), or general principles of law apply?
6. What notice needs to be given either that the injury occurred or that there may be liability (such as Uniform Commercial Code notice for breach of warranties in the event of a defective product), what insurance company or companies must receive notice, what governmental entity needs notice to make it liable, etc.?

0-8493-1955-2/00/$0.00+$.50
© 2000 by CRC Press LLC

7. What proof needs to be acquired to prove the event of injury and the causation by some person or entity?

8. What is the injury that has occurred? Is it primarily physical (causing organic damage to the brain and nervous system), or does it also (as it almost always does) involve psychological trauma?

9. Do the treating medical and psychological providers have experience in dealing with brain trauma cases? Are they sympathetic enough, empathetic enough, and open-minded enough to accept the constellation of injuries and the overall effect that the injury has on the victim, family, friends, co-workers, employers, etc.? Will the treating providers be willing and able to testify on behalf of the victim?

10. Does the attorney or law firm reviewing the case have the knowledge, experience, capabilities, and wherewithal to take the case and see it to fruition?

11. What will it cost to enforce the legal rights of the victim and who will pay for them? What will it cost to hire an attorney and when will payment be required?

12. Where will the legal action be filed (what state, or federal court)? What state or federal laws will apply?

13. How will the damages (provable losses to the victim) be proven? What additional experts will be necessary (such as vocational rehabilitation experts, life planners, economists, toxicologists, accident reconstruction experts, engineers, etc.)? What nonexpert testimony will be needed (such as friends, co-workers, teachers, relatives, etc.)? How will physical evidence need to be presented, and how will it best be presented to convince the insurance company, governmental entity, judge, or jury that the damages are extensive and justify the compensation requested?

14. When and if a settlement or an award is made for the injury, *how* will that money be paid, right away, in a structure over time, or in a trust to avoid losing or being ineligible for government benefits such as Medicaid and social security supplemental income?

15. What governmental benefits are available to the victim?

16. Is any particular claim for injuries time-barred under a relevant Statute of Limitation?

PRETRAUMA HISTORY

Do not take it for granted that those responsible for paying for the damages caused the victim will believe that the victim had a life that functioned without problems before the trauma occurred. They will try to prove the opposite. Proof should be found to provide both the level of functioning and the quality of life of the victim before accident. In the case of function, such as high school and college performance, function on the job, etc., actual proof by way of school transcripts, personnel files, etc. should be located as soon as possible to prove the pretrauma level of functioning.

The quality of life issue can be of great importance in proving how the victim lived before the accident. This can be proven with witnesses, but that should not be the only way to prove it unless there is nothing else available. Photos of the victim alone and with friends and family are very useful. If the victim ever produced any craft items, had any hobbies that produced tangible results, received any awards, etc., find proof of it. Find ways to prove that the victim had a life, and a good life, before the trauma.

EVENT OF INJURY

Every brain trauma has an event or events of injury (or injuries) or toxic exposure(s). In many cases the event or events are easy to identify, in many others they are not as clear. This can be especially true in the case of toxic exposure that may involve more than one exposure, and more than one person, agency, or business entity causing the exposure. There may be numerous chemicals over a long period of time.

It is important to identify how the injury could have occurred. More will be discussed with regard to this issue in the section regarding witnesses and identifying evidence, but the starting point is to discover how this event could have caused injury. Some cases are very obvious, with abundant evidence of either loss of consciousness, trauma to the head, or high exposure to known toxic substances. Other cases will be much less obvious, either with no loss of consciousness, little to prove an actual physical impact to the brain, or transient, minor exposure or prolonged exposure to lesser substances less likely to cause immediate harm. Understanding what happened is very important as soon as there is any likelihood of trauma. Unfortunately, in many cases the victim will deny injury, friends and relatives may not realize what has happened until much later, and what has happened will remain mysterious for too long to effectively investigate and gather evidence.

IDENTIFYING WHO IS RESPONSIBLE FOR THE EVENT OF INJURY

It frequently is not obvious who was actually responsible for the act or series of actions that caused the injury or injuries. For example, in many instances a company may have subcontracted a service to another, in which case it may be that both the contractor and subcontractor are responsible. In the case of on-the-job injuries, the presence or absence of a subcontractor may make the difference between a full and a partial recovery of losses. If there is a governmental entity involved, this must be ascertained right away so that the required notices can be given.

As soon as it seems that an injury has occurred, it is essential to identify all parties who have anything to do with the activity that may have caused the injury. Who worked for whom? Who designed the structure or product that was involved? Were there any other companies or groups in the vicinity of the activity that may have been involved? Ask as many questions as come to mind to try to find out who may have been involved in the activity that caused the injury.

WHAT IS THE THEORY OF LIABILITY?

Different theories of liability require different standards and elements of proof. For automobile accidents, in about half the states there are no-fault statutes which allow for payment of medical and rehabilitation expenses up to a certain amount without question as to who was at fault. Also, for certain accidents on real property there may be insurance policies that pay medical expenses up to a certain amount. However, for the balance of injuries caused by the fault of others it is necessary to have a legal justification to require that another pay for the damages caused in the accident. Even if there is legal liability for the damages, it will likely take a legal action to enforce that legal liability.

Negligence is a legal cause of action that allows one whose person or personal property are injured or damaged due to the fault of another to receive a monetary award if certain elements are proven. First, it is necessary to prove that the person causing the damages had a duty to act (affirmative duty) to protect your person or property, or a duty to refrain from acting in a way that would harm your person or property. Second, it is necessary to prove that the person failed to do what a reasonable prudent person would have done in the same or similar circumstances. Third, it is necessary to prove that the acts or omissions of the person were the cause of your damages or injuries. Fourth, it is necessary to prove those damages or injuries.

Strict Liability is a legal theory that makes a person or business entity liable for injuries or damages caused to another under certain limited circumstances. Strict liability for dangerous products is one circumstance. Strict liability for ultrahazardous activities (such as electrical transmission) is another. When strict liability is the theory of liability it is not necessary to prove a duty, nor is it necessary to prove that the person or business entity knew or should have known of the consequences of its actions.

Intentional Torts (a tort is a legal cause of action for damage to person or property and includes negligence, assault and battery, slander and libel, outrageous conduct) differ from negligence and strict liability in that it must be proven that the person or entity causing the injury intended the consequences. In the case of battery (unlawful touching of another) it is simply necessary to prove that the touch was intended, and not necessarily that the detriment resulted from the touch. With respect to assault it is necessary to prove that the person causing the assault (which does not necessarily need to result in someone actually being battered) intended to cause someone else to be in reasonable fear of being unlawfully battered or touched. For intentional torts and for reckless activities it is usually possible to make a claim for punitive damages. (Punitive damages allow one to receive a monetary award that is intended simply to punish the person or business entity that was sued.)

WHAT STATE OR FEDERAL LAWS, AGENCY RULES, OR GENERAL PRINCIPLES OF LAW APPLY?

Many activities are regulated by the states and by the federal government. Those activities include aviation, trucking, public transportation, utilities, food production and distribution, restaurants, public recreation (such as skiing and swimming), amusement parks, and industrial and business facility safety, among others. It is very important that any accident or toxic exposure be reviewed from the standpoint of government regulation. The reason is that if there has been a violation of one of those regulations there may be a cause of action for negligence per se. In other words, in such cases, it is enough to prove negligence by simply proving that the regulation or statute was violated.

NOTICE REQUIREMENTS

In many cases it is a legal requirement that there be notice given of an injury. This is true in automobile crashes. The insurance company for all parties involved should be given notice. The stated reason for this is that the insurance company cannot begin its investigation until it is given notice. Failure to give notice may result in the insurance company avoiding the responsibility it would have under its contract of insurance. Some states require proof of prejudice to the insurance company (that is to say that the insurance company is materially and substantially affected in a detrimental way) by the failure to give notice. Other states do not require proof of such prejudice.[1]

Notice is required under the Uniform Commercial Code to hold the seller and manufacturer of defective products liable under theories of express or implied warranties.[2] Those warranties include warranties of fitness for particular use and warranties for general merchantability (free of those defects that would make them not saleable). Those warranties are very useful theories and come in handy when other legal causes of action or theories are not accessible either due to problems with proof or statute of limitation problems.

One very important type of case in which notice is mandatory is the case of a claim against a governmental entity of a state or the federal government. Under old English principles of law the King could not be sued unless he had given his permission to be sued. The idea was that the King could do no wrong. This same old principle has been codified in the states and the federal government under the principle of governmental immunity. It is still held to be true that the government cannot be sued unless it has given its permission to be sued. It might be surprising to know, for instance, that in some states a teacher cannot be sued for activities carried out in the classroom unless they involve an intentional tort. Not all governmental activities have been exempted from governmental immunity from suit. It is clear, in any event, that when a governmental entity is involved there must be notice given which complies with the notice requirements of the entity involved. Any governmental immunity notice required by statute must be given by the required method of notice as soon as possible. Failure to give such notice may be fatal to the claim.[3]

Whenever a statute is being used it is mandatory that the statute be read and followed to the letter. Even for lawyers it is not advisable to rely upon memory when following the dictates of a statute.

For all types of cases it is advisable that notice be given to all parties and insurers of the event of the injury, the claim of legal responsibility, and the extent of damages known or expected. This avoids any claim of surprise, and may help later to make the person or business entity receiving notice liable should it intentionally or negligently destroy evidence in its control.

WHAT EVIDENCE NEEDS TO BE ACQUIRED TO PROVE THE EVENT OF INJURY AND THE CAUSATION BY SOME PERSON OR ENTITY?

As soon as it appears that there has been an injury or a toxic exposure, it is essential to start gathering information as to what occurred. Witnesses have a way of disappearing very quickly and thus it is necessary to get names and addresses of anyone who saw the event of injury occur. If the injury involved the use of a product, that product (all of it) must be saved. If it cannot be actually gathered because it is in the possession of another, and if you cannot feel comfortable that the product will be kept safe from destruction or degradation, a lawyer should be contacted immediately so that a court order can be obtained if there is time to do so. If the exposure involves poisoning or some tainted product, not only the product should be saved, but body fluids and excretions must also be saved and frozen. This should preferably be done with an expert such as a toxicologist, but your home freezer will do at least for a time if an expert is not available.

Photos of the scene where the injury occurred should be taken quickly. Measurements of any actual physical evidence such as skid marks should be taken. If an expert investigator is not available, get a witness to watch you do it if you are helping another. If it is your own case, do it with a witness watching so that you can later prove what was done.

Photos of the immediate injuries and bruising also are very important and should be taken as soon as possible and developed as soon as possible. In serious cases it is advisable to have a professional photographer take the photos, but that is not legally necessary. If the photos are ever to be used in a court it will be necessary to have testimony that the photos accurately depict what the photographer saw at the time the photos were taken. Therefore, if a friend is available to do it in a pinch, that would be helpful. If you have retained a lawyer, that lawyer should be able to assist in getting the photos that are necessary. In many events a video of the scene or of other evidence will be very helpful. A home video camera will do.

Identifying witnesses and getting their statements and their understanding of the facts is essential whether the case is one of injury or toxic exposure. It is better to get statements of witnesses sooner than later. There may be other unknown witnesses or evidence that can be located and secured. Legal counsel should be engaged for this service as soon as it is determined that there may be a claim for injuries. Never rely on the assertion that "everything will be taken care of," or anything of that nature. For instance, in cases of slip-and-fall injuries, the store personnel will often indicate that there is no worry and that all the bills will be paid. That is frequently said and very seldom done, and if it is, it is usually only to a small amount of available "med pay" insurance. Those statements are made to get the victim and friends or family out of the way so that the only investigation will be by the company or its agents or insurers. In those cases it is often that helpful evidence just never materializes.

If there have been paramedics or ambulance attendants involved, speaking to them may be very important to identify what occurred shortly after the event of injury.

Proving the Injury/Physical and Psychological

In many cases it will not be readily apparent whether the injury is psychological, physical, or a combination of both. What is the injury that has occurred? Was there loss of consciousness? Does the victim deny loss of consciousness when it is nonetheless clear that he or she cannot perfectly recall all that happened before the incident, during, and after? If so, there may well have been a loss of consciousness. When did the victim first start complaining of symptoms that are associated with brain trauma? It is a sad fact that many emergency rooms are staffed with physicians and attendants who are not trained or accustomed to asking questions about brain trauma, and do not give proper advice regarding it to their emergency room patients. The extent of questions may simply be "Did you lose consciousness?," which is a poor question since most victims of traumatic loss of consciousness do not remember losing consciousness unless a good deal of time has passed and locations have changed (such as by riding to a hospital while in a coma).

These sorts of questions are not just academic. In so many cases it is clear that the victim was not a good historian of what occurred, what were its effects, and where the actual injury to the body occurred. Many healthcare providers take skimpy histories, have incorrect histories in their records, and have ignored asking about injuries (such as symptoms of brain trauma). If one healthcare provider asks a question about a specific injury and another does not, an impression may be left that either the victim has been exaggerating, pretending, or that the problem is not very severe. All of this may simply be that histories have either not been thorough or were taken incorrectly.

A thorough and detailed medical history is absolutely critical in each case in which there may be a question of brain trauma. Although many healthcare providers will not have such a history form that is routinely provided to patients, a good injury lawyer should have access to such a history form.

Brain trauma inevitably involves psychological symptomatology.[4] In some cases this can occur to a great extent, and in others it may be somewhat limited. Telling the difference between the two and being able to identify the interrelationship between the two is important in every case. If the psychological symptoms are ignored or scantily treated, the proof of the actual organic (physical) trauma will be made more difficult. Unfortunately, many healthcare providers are not wise to the legal requirements of proof and look at the case only from a narrow vantage point of a specific specialty. This frequently leaves the hapless victim in a bad position to prove whether his problems were really due to the physical injury, or due to psychological disorders not properly addressed. This is made doubly important since there are many insurance company-oriented experts who are very much aware of the confusing relationship between actual physical injury and psychological symptoms. For example, it is a standard insurance company expert line to say "the neuropsychological testing for cognitive deficits will be invalid if there was untreated depression or anxiety."

Although it is obviously a healthcare question as to which type of treatment and diagnosis should be first initiated, psychological or actual physical trauma, it is, from a legal standpoint, essential that the psychological symptoms get treatment as soon as possible. This not only inevitably assists in the victim's and their family's overall recovery, but it eliminates a source of potential problems with respect to proof of the brain injury.

This discussion leads most easily into the next section which discusses why it is so important that *all* the treating healthcare providers are experienced in brain trauma cases.

Do the Treating Medical and Psychological Providers Have Experience in Dealing with Brain Trauma Cases?

Good personal injury attorneys are accused of constructing their cases. Good personal injury attorneys do take a part in making sure that their cases are well constructed. The brain injury case too frequently has inadequate documentation history and diagnosis and care. Too often there is a lack of coordination between healthcare providers. Also, all too frequently the insurance company that should be providing all the care needed will be seeking a limitation of treatment by the use of healthcare providers known to limit care. Ignorance in this event is not bliss. This author has discovered after hundreds of brain trauma cases that brain trauma victims do not progress well in treatment if the brain injury is not well understood and well communicated *in addition to* being well treated. Good treatment requires documentation and coordination of care.

One sometimes hears the complaint that attorneys suggest their clients into a case of brain trauma when proper psychological treatment would be more than sufficient to treat the "trauma." This may in fact be true in some cases. However, it is probably true only in those cases where the actual treating healthcare providers are not well experienced and well trained in treating brain trauma. Well-experienced providers will understand, for instance, the interrelationship between the psychological trauma and the true brain injury symptomatology. The well-experienced provider will not ignore either the psychological or the organic brain trauma symptoms. The experienced provider will have associates capable of providing the proper cognitive retaining, the proper speech therapy, the proper vocational rehabilitation, etc. Furthermore, the well-experienced provider will know that the physical symptoms of pain will need to be well treated so that the cause and effect between pain and depression/anxiety can be minimized or eliminated.

By contrast, the inexperienced provider will allow some or all of the psychological and physical symptoms to be ignored or untreated. The era of managed care, as well as the basic conservative nature of the healthcare field, tends to encourage the ignoring of symptoms until there is a clear and vocal complaint about them (and even after that to save costs for the "system"). When symptoms are ignored, the result will likely be a dilemma for the victim to prove that later "discovered" symptoms are related to an event of trauma or a toxic exposure.

Coordinating treatment between various providers is of great importance to the outcome of both the medical and the legal case. If each of the providers know what the others are doing and saying, it keeps the victim/patient better informed and better treated. With provider coordination, the lawyer will have a much tighter and easier case to present. For instance, if one provider wants an MRI to eliminate the possibility of multiple sclerosis and the MRI is not performed, another treating provider may be on shakier ground finding symptoms due to brain trauma. While this is debatable from a medical standpoint, it is not debatable from a legal standpoint since questions that cause doubt about the causation of the brain trauma never help the trauma victim in court.

How to get coordination when there is no medical coordinator and no diligent primary physician in the case can be difficult. It is a decidedly awkward position for a lawyer to be doing medical coordination. If there is sufficient value to a case, the lawyer might consider hiring a medical coordinator. It is risky to ask the insurance company to provide a coordinator because they will likely find someone sympathetic to insurance company desires to close the case as soon as possible. The best that the lawyer may be able to do in a case of more ordinary value is to be sure that all providers are receiving the reports of the other providers. The providers can be called on the phone and requested to send copies of reports to the other providers. If the providers will take calls from the lawyer, then an occasional call to check in on treatment is a good idea. If the provider will not take calls from either the lawyer or other providers, it may be advisable to recommend different providers in subsequent cases.

How does one find out if the providers are experienced in brain trauma cases? The best way is to ask the provider how many cases he or she routinely has. If the injury lawyer has never heard of the provider or has a negative opinion about the provider, that is a good hint that there may be a problem. Other providers can be asked about the reputation, in brain trauma cases, of the provider in question. The question should *in no event* be ignored.

It is a bad sign if the provider does not appear to be both sympathetic and empathetic to the brain-injured person and the family. If the provider does not like dealing with lawyers, does not like writing reports, or is reluctant to testify in court, these are also bad signs. Like it or not, the lawyer is part of the treatment team since what he or she does for the victim will impact all parties involved. If the lawyer does not know the provider involved, and is not certain of his or her willingness to be cooperative with respect to the documentation or legal testimony required, then the provider and the lawyer should meet. If such a meeting is declined or ignored, there is a problem with the case.

Does the Attorney or Law Firm Reviewing the Case Have the Knowledge, Experience, Capabilities, and Wherewithal to Take the Case and See It to Fruition?

The brain trauma case is, as are all personal injury cases, substantially, if not primarily, a medical case. It is usually only secondarily a legal case. That is to say that the majority of the issues and time in the case will be spent in understanding, managing, coordinating, and documenting the medical aspects of the client's case. As has been stated above, the lawyer must understand the legal claims and legal theories of injury cases, know how to preserve evidence, and must know how to present the issues in court. However, if the attorney knows only the legal aspects of the case and does not know or will not become educated in the medical aspects of the case, he or she will not likely succeed with the case.

Working with brain trauma cases is frightening to many. Why they are frightening is perhaps a matter of speculation, but it seems that those who are frightened are unable to accept the profound and detrimental changes that the victim has suffered. Brain injury is not contagious, but some treat it as if it is. The brain trauma lawyer, like the brain trauma healthcare provider, must work with the trauma victim from where he or she is, not where they were before. No one can pretend that the trauma did not occur, and all must realize that, from the point of suffering, and from the new condition, deficits and all, life must begin again. If the lawyer appears reluctant to speak of the brain trauma, and is unable to comfortably confront family and significant others about the issues of living with the brain trauma, he or she is indicating an unwillingness to embrace the brain trauma case. Any person involved with the brain trauma victim who is unwilling to embrace the issues of the case is a risk for the case. Lawyers who want to downplay the brain injury, act as if they do not believe it, tell the victim that a jury won't believe it because he or she does not "look injured," and is unwilling to accept the victim's condition, is a risk to the victim's case. This is a frequent example of brain trauma cases that come out of auto crashes that on the surface do not appear to have been able to cause such extensive brain trauma. Surely those cases are difficult, but to work such a case well, it must be embraced, problems and all. Although it may not be worthwhile in the last analysis to take such a case to a jury, it is either sufficiently worth the lawyer's while to embrace the case for all its issues, or a new lawyer should be retained.

Lawyers who want to make more out of the case than there really is are also a risk for the victim. They can make the victim much worse by creating an artificial condition of disability and debilitation. This type of lawyer can be spotted quickly by the not-so-subtle suggestions that the victim is much worse than he or she may appear, and that the victim should always maximize his or her complaints to the healthcare providers. Furthermore, this type of lawyer will often tell the victim that he or she has a serious brain trauma before it has even been diagnosed.

The victim, or the family, needs to search for a lawyer who has experience with the brain trauma case. Recommendations for an experienced brain trauma lawyer can be solicited from healthcare providers or other attorneys. The lawyer should be interviewed and asked about his or her experience in such cases. The lawyer can be asked if he or she has tried such cases before, how much reading he or she does in the field, and whether he or she belongs to any brain injury associations or groups. The lawyer should be asked what he or she will do to stay in contact with the treating providers, and what he or she will do if there is an apparent conflict between providers in the care needed for the victim. The issue to be determined is how active the lawyer will be in the victim's case, both in terms of understanding it and in terms of being the victim's advocate.

COSTS OF LEGAL ACTION

Without a doubt, a brain trauma case can be very expensive in terms of out-of-pocket costs. From the beginning of the investigation to the presentation at trial, a brain-trauma case can involve major expenses, sometimes into the tens of thousands of dollars. Engineers and accident investigators will charge hourly and expect to be paid monthly. Expenses for ordering files and doctors' reports will likewise be an immediate expense. The healthcare providers working on the case will want to be paid an hourly rate (usually from leaving the office to returning to the office), sometimes into the several hundreds of dollars per hour.

Nearly all personal injury lawyers charge by the hour. It is a rare case in which the victim wants to pay a lawyer by the hour, because the outcome is often less than certain and the victim is often in a compromised position, financially. The percentage fee agreement is known as a "contingent fee" agreement as the fee paid to the lawyer will depend upon whether there is money received in the case. The percentage can vary widely and will depend upon the amount of time and effort that the lawyer can expect to spend in the case. For the very serious case in which the recovery is limited, the victim and his family are urged to inquire whether it can be arranged to have a fee below that commonly charged for the ordinary injury case. Frequently those cases are really easier for the lawyer, and he or she will not be reluctant to lower the percentage below that usually charged in his or her standard fee agreement.

Lawyers are ethically allowed to advance legal costs directly related to the case. Strict legal ethics prohibit attorneys from lending money to clients for expenses not directly related to the case. The fee agreement should spell out what the anticipated level of advanced costs will be.[5] Furthermore, the victim and family should inquire of the attorney what costs they will be expected to advance, and when. Very often, in the serious case, the lawyer will have no reluctance to agree to advance all the costs through trial. That willingness may vary depending upon the apparent risks of the case. If the lawyer is not capable, for financial reasons, of assisting in advancing any costs, it is strongly advised to look for another lawyer. If the lawyer asks for a fee to investigate the case, also look for another lawyer.

WHERE WILL THE LEGAL ACTION BE FILED?

In the United States, each state has separate jurisdiction over its court system. Laws vary from state to state. The extent of recovery may well be different depending on the state involved. For instance, California allows unlimited punitive damages, while Colorado has a strict limit not allowing more than twice the amount of the actual compensatory damages, except that a judge may extend that to three times under special circumstances. Also, so-called "tort reform" in some states has severely limited the amount that can be recovered for the noneconomic parts of the case.[6] This is frequently called the "pain and suffering" award, and it is the amount that is paid to a victim for losing all those things that were part of the joy of life, such as reading, bowling, walking, talking, or anything that does not directly involve earning money. If there is a chance of applying more than one state's laws, it pays to decide which one is most generous.

In the United States there is also a federal judiciary with federal courts in each state. For some claims there may actually be a federal law giving the federal court jurisdiction in the case. In many cases the laws to be applied in the federal court will be same as those applied in the state courts in which the federal court sits, but if there is a choice of state laws involved in the case, the federal court may be more likely to apply a more balanced view than the state court would.

Proving Damages

The word "damages" has the legal meaning of the extent of the injury, but it also means the monetary award to be attached to that injury. For the trauma victim, proving damages involves identifying all those physical and psychological injuries together with economic losses, and all those ways that the injuries have affected the quality of the victim's life.

Identifying all the injuries is the first step. If the victim, for instance, suffers from headaches, it may take months before the source of the headaches can be determined. If, to use the same example, those headaches are causing the victim to lose sleep and, thereby, be more depressed, finding the cause of the headaches may have a very strong bearing on ultimately determining the extent of the victim's cognitive loss from actual brain trauma. Although this is not a legal issue per se, it becomes a legal issue in that it is not possible to know the extent of the legal damages until the true extent of physical and psychological injuries can be determined. This is true in almost every case of brain trauma. The entire team of healthcare providers and legal counsel must be aware of the fact that the extent of injury is a mystery that takes many clues and many good minds to ultimately determine.

Once it is determined that there is actual organic brain trauma, the victim and his or her team of healthcare providers and lawyers must be aware that for a period of up to 2 years there may be recovery of function. Although the recovery over time does diminish, any knowledgeable provider will admit that recovery up to $1\frac{1}{2}$ years is not uncommon, and for up to 2 or more years there can still be recovery. If a case is prematurely put into litigation (to be tried in court) and a trial is held before the reasonable period to expect recovery, the victim may be shortchanged by a jury that believes the insurance expert that substantial recovery can be expected.

For many brain trauma victims returning to former employment at the same level of functioning is not possible. In those cases it is essential to determine what level of employment function remains. This will, in most instances, not be clear from the physicians or the psychologists/neuropsychologists, etc. Vocational rehabilitation counselors with knowledge of brain trauma issues are probably the best source of assistance in determining what is the victim's level of employability. The vocational rehabilitation counselor becomes an essential part of the victim's team. In some instances there will be insurance coverage for this part of the team, but in many instances it will be the victim or his lawyers who will be called upon to pay for this service. In some cases there are state agencies that can be called upon for assistance. More about that is included in the section below discussing government benefits available to the trauma victim.

Economic losses are frequently the largest and most important part of the victim's "damages." The extent of losses is almost never obvious. For instance, how much it will cost to provide essential services to the victim over his or her life will involve getting the opinion of someone knowledgeable in those issues, and an economist, to value that over the person's lifetime. In the serious case, the services of a "life planner" will help to determine what the victim will need by way of services and living expenses. In all but the simplest case the services of an economist will be very important to determine what the present value of the dollar losses are. The economist will need to work with the vocational rehabilitation counselor to determine what differences in pay exist in work that the victim may now be able to do in comparison to what he or she could do before the accident.[7] In years past it was not as common to use economists for this purpose, and lawyers often attempted to do this on their own at trial. That is becoming much less common and is probably not now recommended for the serious case. The lawyer cannot ethically testify in his or her own case except in the rarest of circumstances. Experts are recommended to assist in putting together the complicated information that will be necessary to prove the true extent of the victim's losses.

Proving the "pain and suffering" loss of enjoyment of life and loss of quality of life can be the most challenging, as it requires the greatest skill of the advocate to have the jury identify with and provide compensation for something that is essentially intangible and very personal. Every good lawyer has a different take on how that is best accomplished, and to some extent it depends upon the lawyer's personality and talent. Whatever the skill level of the lawyer, it is essential to show what the victim was like before the trauma or toxic exposure, and what he or she has become since.

Many lawyers urge their clients to start a diary of daily events so that the victim can easily recall the difficulties that he or she encountered during recovery. Although this is indeed a good idea, it can be expected that if it is ever used at trial, the lawyer for the defense will ask the victim who asked him or her to keep a diary, and it may look as if the lawyer is trying to "cook something up." In most injury cases, anyway, the defense tries to make the jury believe that the whole case is a carefully orchestrated attempt on the part of a greedy person and his or her lawyer to get a windfall, like winning the lottery. The more legitimate and credible the case appears, the more likely a jury is to accept the case presented and to award money for the real losses suffered.

The victim and their family will know more than anyone will how to show the quality of the victim's life before the event of trauma or toxic exposure. For example, they will know what awards he or she received. They will have the photos that show happier and fuller times. They will know the friends and co-workers who can testify about the life of the victim before the brain trauma. One photo of happier times will speak volumes to the jury. Several photos may describe an entire life. Enlarging those photos will make this visibly clear to the jury.

Day-in-the-life videos are becoming more popular as a way of showing how the victim lives his or her life after trauma. For such videos, a professional videographer will follow the victim during one or more days to document how the victim and their family live their lives with the burden of the injuries received. It tends to make the victim and family very credible. Such videos are relatively expensive, but if properly done can be very useful as a way of presenting the case both to the insurance company before trial (in hopes of settlement without risk) and to the jury at trial.

METHODS TO AVOID TAXES AND MAXIMIZE AVAILABLE GOVERNMENT BENEFITS

In general, personal injury settlements and awards are not taxable unless the award is for punitive damages. However, when the money is invested, the interest earned will be taxable.[8] A way to avoid paying taxes on the interest generated is to enter into a "structured settlement," which means that the insurance company will purchase an annuity at the time of settlement. Since the annuity is part of the settlement, the interest earned on the annuity as it is paid out will not be taxable. The structured settlement also avoids the pitfalls that come with having too much cash in one's hands at one time. So many trauma victims spend the money received in a foolish fashion, leaving much less available for later years when it may be needed the most. In recent years it has been discovered that some insurance companies have been far less than truthful in terms of describing what the annuity costs for the company to purchase. There have been large kickbacks to certain insurance companies for purchasing annuities. Some companies are purchasing annuities from companies that might not be considered to be the strongest. Furthermore, the insurance company purchasing the annuity will usually try to avoid any responsibility if the annuity company goes bankrupt or goes out of business. Some lawyers will not agree to a structure unless the insurance company making the settlement stands behind the annuity company. A word to the wise: look into the structured settlement since it has many good aspects to it, but be very careful.

The indigent trauma victim will have the right to Medicaid benefits and Social Security Supplemental Income (SSI) support. Such benefits are need-based, and a person with even moderate assets is disqualified from receiving those benefits. Federal law allows for "special needs trusts" to fund expenses not generally paid by SSI. Special needs trusts are very complicated and should be drafted by a knowledgeable lawyer and reviewed by the state Medicaid administrator.

When a settlement is offered, the victim or his family must decide how the money will be paid. Is it appropriate to receive the money all at once? Is a trust needed to avoid losing or being ineligible for government benefits such as Medicaid and Social Security Supplemental Income? Is it appropriate or necessary in the case to have the money paid out over time from an annuity investment? These are difficult questions that need careful study and review by both an expert attorney and advisors familiar with investments and tax consequences.

GOVERNMENTAL BENEFITS AVAILABLE TO THE TRAUMA VICTIM

As discussed above, Medicaid and SSI are very important benefits that the injured person may have a right to receive. If the victim had been employed, paying social security taxes prior to his or her disability, the victim may have a right to social security benefits that are not needs-based, that is pure disability insurance.[9] The Social Security Administration is very accessible to ask questions about availability of social security. Applicants are frequently denied. If denied, absolutely seek a knowledgeable lawyer's opinion.

STATUTES OF LIMITATION

Nearly every legal claim has a time-fuse that is described in what are called "statutes of limitation." Those laws, found in the statutes of each state and, when applicable, in federal statutes, detail how soon a claim needs to be filed in a lawsuit before it expires. If the statute of limitations expires, the victim is not necessarily foreclosed from filing suit, but if the person sued defends by alleging that the statute of limitations has expired, the case will fail unless there is an exception to the expiration of the statute. Some exceptions to statutes of limitation are as follows: (1) the victim was under a disability that kept him or her from knowing that he or she had been injured, (2) the victim did not know that there was a claim, and (3) the victim was a minor child. A minor child is considered to be under a legal disability from suit until he or she reaches majority (between 18 and 21 years depending upon the specific state's laws), or until a guardian or conservator has been legally appointed for him or her. Parents are not considered legal guardians or conservators as far as this concept is concerned.

The best advice to give to any injured person is to seek the advice and counsel of a reputable injury lawyer. Don't sit on your rights.

REFERENCES

1. *Marez v. Dairyland Ins. Co*, 638 P.2d. 286 (Colo. 1982).
2. Colorado Revised Statute 4-2-607(3)(a) (Other states with the Uniform Commercial Code will have different statutory citations).
3. States and federal governmental immunity notice requirements differ. The federal government immunity notice requirement is found at 28 U.S.C. 2675, and state notice requirements can be found in the state statutes.
4. Proving Cognitive and Behavioral Brain Injuries, Trial, September 1996.
5. Rules of Professional Conduct, Rule 1.8 (e).
6. Colorado Revised Statute 13-21-103.
7. The present value of $1.00 in the future is held to be less now than it will be at some time in the future as it must take account of inflation and the fact that a dollar invested will earn interest and thereby compound itself.
8. Section 104, United States Internal Revenue Code.
9. 20 Code of Federal Regulations 404.110.

Index